Urogynecology in Primary Care

Patrick J. Culligan and Roger P. Goldberg (Eds)

Urogynecology in Primary Care

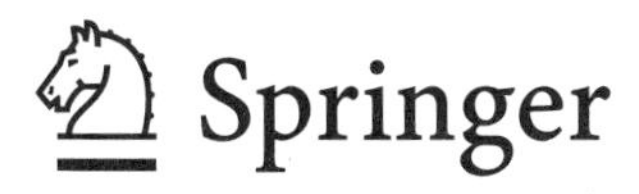

Patrick J. Culligan, MD
Director, Division of Urogynecology and Reconstructive Pelvic Surgery
Atlantic Health System
Morristown, NJ, USA
and
Clinical Associate Professor of Obstetrics and Gynecology
UMDNJ
Newark, NJ, USA

Roger P. Goldberg, MD, MPH
Director of Urogynecology Research
Evanston Continence Center
Evanston, IL, USA
and
Assistant Professor of Obstetrics and Gynecology
Northwestern University Medical School
Evanston, IL, USA

British Library Cataloguing in Publication Data
A catalogue record for this book is available from the British Library

Library of Congress Control Number: 2006926446

ISBN-10: 1-84628-166-0 e-ISBN 1-84628-167-9 Printed on acid-free paper
ISBN-13: 978-1-84628-166-2

9 8 7 6 5 4 3 2

Springer Science+Business Media
springer.com

With love from Pat to Kim, Brian, Clare and Molly—for their support, encouragement and love. And to my mom who I miss every day. (P.C.)

With love from Roger to Elena and Lucia, Carlo and Dante Leo. (R.G.)

And with much appreciation to Dr. Peter Sand, whose passion as a teacher inspires both of us to keep learning and to teach others. (R.G., P.C.)

Preface

The field of urogynecology and reconstructive pelvic surgery encompasses not only urinary incontinence and pelvic organ prolapse, but disorders such as chronic urinary tract infections, sexual dysfunction, defecation dysfunction, and pelvic pain as well. This textbook is designed as a clinical guide for treating women suffering from this wide variety of pelvic floor disorders. Written with busy practitioners in mind, this textbook will be useful as a quick reference guide for anyone with an interest in female pelvic floor disorders.

Patrick J. Culligan

Contents

Contributors

Laura A.C. Berman, PhD, L.CSW
Feinberg School of Medicine
Northwestern Memorial Hospital
Berman Center
Chicago, IL, USA

Patrick J. Culligan, MD
Division of Urogynecology and Reconstructive Pelvic Surgery
Atlantic Health System
Morristown, NJ;
Obstetrics and Gynecology
UMDNJ, Newark, NJ, USA

Eman Elkadry, MD
Department of Obstetrics and Gynecology, and Reproductive Biology
Harvard Medical School
Division of Urology and Reconstructive Pelvic Surgery
Mount Auburn Hospital
Cambridge, MA, USA

Roger P. Goldberg, MD, MPH
Urogynecology
Evanston Continence Center;
Obstetrics and Gynecology
Northwestern University Medical School
Evanston, IL, USA

Neeraj Kohli MD, MBA
Department of Obstetrics, Gynecology and Reproductive Biology
Division of Urogynecology and Reconstructive Pelvic Surgery
Brigham and Women's Hospital
Harvard Medical School
Boston MA, USA

Christine A. LaSala, MD
Urogynecology Division at Hartford Hospital
Obstetrics and Gynecology
University of Connecticut School of Medicine
Hartford, CT, USA

Vincent R. Lucente, MD, MBA
The Institute for Female Pelvic Medicine and Reconstructive Surgery
Temple University College of Medicine
Allentown, PA, USA

Kerrie A. Grow McLean, PsyD, LPC
Berman Center
Chicago, IL, USA

Jay-James R. Miller, MD
Obstetrics and Gynecology
Northwestern University
Feinberg School of Medicine
Evanston Continence Center
Evanston, IL, USA

Miles Murphy, MD, MSPH
Institute for Female Pelvic Medicine and Reconstructive Surgery
St. Luke's Hospital
Allentown, PA, USA

Deborah L. Myers, MD
Division of Urogynecology and Reconstructive Pelvic Surgery
Brown University Medical School
Women and Infants' Hospital of Rhode Island
Providence, RI, USA

Sujatha S. Rajan MD
Department of Obstetrics, Gynecology, and Reproductive Biology
Division of Urogynecology, and Reconstructive Pelvic Surgery
Brigham and Women's Hospital
Harvard Medical School
Boston, MA, USA

Charles R. Rardin, MD
Brown Medical School
Division of Urogynecology and Reconstructive Pelvic Surgery
Women's and Infant's Hospital of Rhode Island
Providence, RI, USA

Robert M. Rogers, Jr., MD
Northwest Women's Healthcare
Department of Gynecology
Kalispell Regional Medical Center
Kalispell, MT, USA

Peter L. Rosenblatt, MD
Department of Obstetrics and Gynecology, and Reproductive Biology
Harvard Medical School
Division of Urogynecology and Reconstructive Pelvic Surgery
Mount Auburn Hospital
Cambridge, MA, USA

Marie C. Shaw, MBA
The Institute for Female Pelvic Medicine and Reconstructive Surgery
Allentown, PA, USA

Peter K. Sand, MD
Division of Urogynecology
Northwestern University
Feinberg School of Medicine;
Evanston Continence Center
Evanston Northwestern Healthcare
Evanston, IL, USA

Paul Tulikangas, MD
Urogynecology Division
Department of Obstetrics and Gynecology
University of Connecticut
Hartford Hospital
Hartford, CT, USA

1 Incontinence and Pelvic Floor Dysfunction in Primary Care: Epidemiology and Risk Factors

Sujatha S. Rajan and Neeraj Kohli

Introduction

Urinary and fecal incontinence, pelvic organ prolapse (POP), and female sexual dysfunction are increasingly common conditions and fall in the realm of pelvic floor dysfunction. It is unclear if the true incidence of these conditions is increasing or if they are being detected more frequently due to increased willingness from physicians, patients and the media to address them.

It is clear that primary care clinicians should expect to encounter these conditions on a regular basis in the years ahead. Based on data from the Bureau of Census, postmenopausal women will comprise 33% of the population in the year 2050 compared to 23% in 1995. Since incontinence and pelvic organ prolapse predominantly affect perimenopausal and postmenopausal women, the demand for evaluation and treatment is projected to steadily increase. In addition, our society continues to enjoy longer life expectancy and there remains a strong focus on improved quality of life, thereby bringing disorders of pelvic floor dysfunction to the forefront of women's health.

Definitions: Pelvic Floor Dysfunction

Urinary Incontinence (UI): Defined by the International Continence Society as the complaint of any involuntary urine loss.

Fecal Incontinence (FI): Either the involuntary passage or the inability to control the discharge of fecal matter through the anus.

Pelvic Organ Prolapse: Protrusion of the pelvic organs into or out of the vaginal canal.

Female Sexual Dysfunction (FSD): Persistent or recurring reduction in sex drive, aversion to sexual activity, difficulty becoming aroused, inability to achieve orgasm, or dyspareunia. Sexual dysfunction is defined by the World Health Organization as the various ways in which an individual is unable to participate in a sexual relationship as he or she would wish.

Urinary Incontinence

Prevalence, Incidence, and Natural History

The prevalence of Urinary Incontinence varies widely due to varying definitions of the condition, different populations studied, and differing research methodologies. Population-based studies estimate that as many as three fourths of women in the United States report at least some urinary leakage, with 20% to 50% reporting current leakage.[1] The NIH sponsored comprehensive study[2] of UI in the United States reported a 38% prevalence of UI among community dwelling women 60 years of age and older. Of greater clinical relevance is the number of women with *severe or more frequent* leakage, estimated fairly uniformly at 7% to 10% by various researchers.[3] This group of women is probably the most socially impacted by this condition and, hence, will tend to seek evaluation. Approximately 50% of nursing home residents have urinary incontinence, making

UI a leading cause of nursing home admission. One in five women with urinary incontinence will also suffer from fecal incontinence or "dual incontinence."

Stress and mixed urinary incontinence are the two most common forms of UI. The prevalence of stress incontinence is reported at 49%, followed by mixed incontinence at 29% and urge incontinence at 22%.[4] Information on the incidence of urinary incontinence is limited and ranges from 3% to 22.4%, increasing with age. Because urinary incontinence is transient in some women, there is a yearly reported remission rate of 12%.

The severity of UI is usually assessed by the number of incontinence episodes per week. Among women with UI, 50% report at least one loss per week. Among women with mixed UI, 40% report four or more incontinent episodes per week.

Risk Factors for Urinary Incontinence

A number of different risk factors have been proposed for UI and have been summarized by Bump in the following model (Figure 1.1).

Age

Many studies have shown an increased prevalence of UI with advancing age. Melville[5] has recently reported that the prevalence of UI was 28% in women of 30 to 39 years of age and 55% in those of 80 to 90 years. The severity of UI also increases with age; this may be explained by the interplay of multiple factors during the aging process, including increasing medical comorbidities, medication use, impaired mobility, menopause, and alteration in volume status and excretion.

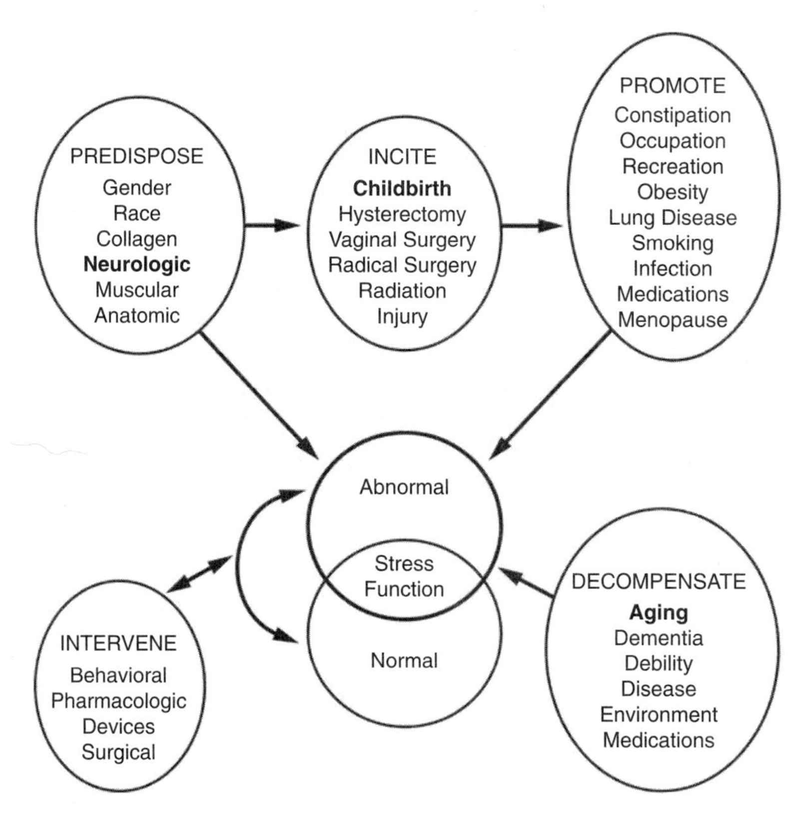

FIGURE 1.1. Factors related to the development of urinary incontinence. (From: Bump RC, Norton PA. Epidemiology and natural history of pelvic floor dysfunction. *Obstet Gynecol Clin North Am.* 1998;25:723. Copyright 1998, with permission from Elsevier.)

Sex

UI is two to three times more common in women than in men, especially among community-dwelling adults younger than the age of 60. Very few young men report UI. The gender gap starts to narrow, especially after the age of 70, as a result of more men reporting bladder problems secondary to an enlarged prostate.

Ethnicity

The relationship between ethnicity and UI is complex. Although it had been believed that African American women have a greater prevalence of urge incontinence compared to white women, Fultz[5a] reported a prevalence of UI of 23% in white women and 16% in African American women. More recently, results from the SWAN study,[6] which included multiethnic women in the age range of 42 to 52 years, indicated that nonwhite women were less likely to report any incontinence and that there was no association between ethnicity and the severity of UI. Social and cultural expectations and access to care, among other factors, may certainly play a role.

Obesity

This is a well-established risk factor for UI, and higher BMI (body mass index) is associated with an increased severity of UI. The SWAN study[6] has shown a 5% increase in the probability of leakage with each unit increase in BMI.

Pregnancy and Childbirth

Most women develop UI during pregnancy, but for the majority of them this is a transient condition. In a study[7] of 305 primiparas, 4% had stress incontinence before pregnancy, 32% during the pregnancy, and 7% in the post partum period. Pregnancy and obesity do place an added burden on the pelvic floor structures and could certainly contribute to their weakening, thereby leading to UI.

Vaginal childbirth is believed to be a strong inciting factor for UI, especially stress urinary incontinence. Vaginal birth can cause direct damage to the pelvic floor soft tissues. This effect is compounded by the long-term pelvic floor muscle dysfunction that results from damage to the pelvic nerves at the time of delivery. Allen et al.[8] have shown that a significant prolongation of nerve conduction was seen among nulliparous women who delivered infants weighting more than 3.4 kg. A large Swedish study[9] has reported that the first birth seems to be the most harmful to the pelvic floor; subsequent deliveries only moderately increase the risk for incontinence. An association between the number of vaginal deliveries and stress incontinence has been reported by multiple other studies.[10,11] A recent analysis of 542 identical twin sisters, with a mean age of 42 years, found birth mode (vaginal or cesarean) to be a major "environmental" determinant of stress urinary incontinence. In that study, vaginal delivery was associated with a 2.3 times higher risk of stress urinary incontinence within the predominantly premenopausal cohort.[12]

The effect of parity on urinary incontinence disappears with increasing age. Results from the Norwegian EPINCONT study[13] have shed light on the roles of vaginal delivery and cesarean birth in the development of UI. The study concluded that the risk of urinary incontinence is higher among women who have had cesarean deliveries than among nulliparous women and is even higher among women who have had vaginal deliveries. When compared to a nulliparous status, cesarean birth was associated with stress incontinence and mixed-type incontinence, whereas vaginal delivery further increased the risk of stress incontinence only. However, the authors of the study stated that these results should not be used to justify an increase in cesarean deliveries.

Studies analyzing the effects of operative vaginal deliveries (forceps and vacuum), episiotomy, length of the second stage of labor, infant head circumference, and birth weight on UI are inconsistent.

Menopause

An abundance of high-affinity estrogen receptors have been identified in the pubococcygeal muscle, urethra, and trigone of the bladder. Low estrogen production after menopause results in atrophy of the superficial and intermediate layers of the urethral epithelium with subsequent atrophic urethritis, diminished urethral mucosal seal, loss of compliance, and irritation—changes that can predispose to the development of both stress and urge urinary incontinence and recurrent bladder infections. Despite these well-founded theoretical concerns, various studies[6,14] have shown conflicting results regarding the role of menopause in the development of UI.

Oral estrogen has been associated with an increased risk of UI in current users. The Women's Health Initiative (WHI) study[15] has shown that menopausal hormone therapy increased the incidence of all types of UI at 1 year among women who were continent at baseline. The risk was highest for stress urinary incontinence (SUI).

Hysterectomy

The role of hysterectomy in the development of UI is controversial. Alteration of anatomical relationships, as well as denervation of the pelvic floor at the time of a hysterectomy, could certainly lead to postoperative UI. Thom and Brown,[14] in a review of the literature, noted that there was no increased risk of incontinence within the first two years after a hysterectomy. But multiple other studies[16,17] have consistently found an increased risk of UI after a hysterectomy.

Melville[5] reported, in an age-stratified postal survey of 6000 women aged between 30 and 90 years, that current major depression, diabetes, and a history of hysterectomy were significantly associated with severe UI.

Fecal Incontinence

Prevalence of Fecal Incontinence

The true prevalence of fecal incontinence is difficult to estimate given that fewer than one third of patients with this condition ever discuss it with their physicians—certainly a reflection of the enormous stigma surrounding this disorder. Prevalence estimates also vary considerably depending upon the definition used and the method of inquiry. The reported prevalence rates[18] vary from 11% to 15%, with markedly higher rates in the elderly. Fecal incontinence is nearly twice as common among women than men,[22] and is observed in up to 47 % of nursing home residents.[19,20] Among patients with urinary incontinence and prolapse, roughly one third report loss of fecal control.[21] Primary care providers encountering urinary incontinence and prolapse should be cognizant of these associations and consider incorporating a few simple screening questions focusing on bowel control.

Risk Factors for Fecal Incontinence

Obstetric Factors

Vaginal delivery is believed to be one of the major risk factors in the development of FI. Weakening of the anal sphincter mechanism after vaginal delivery is attributed to both direct trauma to the muscle and indirect trauma to the pudendal nerves (unilateral or bilateral). Anatomic injury usually occurs in the anterior portion of the anal sphincter complex. In a prospective study[23] of the effect that vaginal deliveries have on the pelvic floor, 80% of primigravidas sustained reversible pudendal nerve damage that in some women persisted for up to five years postpartum.

A majority of these sphincter injuries remain silent and information on their natural history is limited. Anal sphincter tears were detected by anal endosonography in 35 % of primiparous and 44 % of multiparous women, of whom symptoms of anal incontinence or fecal urgency were present in 13% and 23 %, respectively.[24]

Ryhammer et al.[25] found a significant long-term association between the number of vaginal deliveries and several anorectal parameters in perimenopausal women. They noted lower perineal position at rest, increased perineal descent with maximal straining, decreased anal sensibility to electrical stimulus, and prolonged latency in the pudendal nerves, to be associated with increasing parity. Other obstetric risk factors for FI include forceps delivery and midline episiotomies.

Age

Increasing age is a risk factor for developing anal incontinence, even before the postmenopausal years. Pollack et al. reported that a 30-year-old woman has twice as high a risk of developing anal incontinence as does a 20-year-old woman.[26] Physiologic changes in the anal continence mechanism could explain the increased risk of FI with advancing age. Findings from anal manometry studies[27] have shown age-dependent decreases in anal resting and squeeze pressures. These parameters decline even more rapidly after menopause. With aging, anal closing pressure (the difference between maximum resting pressure and rectal pressure) is reduced, and this is an important determinant of anal continence.[27]

Sex

Some studies have shown a higher prevalence of FI in females, and the female-to-male ratio is reported at 1.5:1.[28] Other studies do not support an increased prevalence in women.

Other factors

The patient's ambulatory status is also important when considering the etiology of the disorder. Wheelchair-bound patients and those who are dependent on others for access to bathroom facilities may have episodes of *functional* incontinence yet have totally normal anorectal function.

Quander et al.[29] have reported that subjects who were taking anticonvulsant, antipsychotic, hypnotic, antiparkinsonian, and antidepressant medications were two to three times more likely to have fecal incontinence. These results persisted in a logistic regression analysis after adjustment for age, sex, race, and comorbid illnesses of stroke and diabetes. Whether this increased prevalence of fecal incontinence is due to the medications themselves or to the comorbid illnesses requiring these medications could not be explained in this study.

Pelvic Organ Prolapse (POP)

Prevalence of POP

Accurate estimates of the prevalence of POP were limited earlier because of variations in the definitions of POP, population differences, and variation among examination techniques. Among ambulatory women, the prevalence of POP varies widely in different populations, ranging from 30% to 93%.[30,31,32]

In a large study of 16,616 women[33] who each have a uterus, the rate of uterine prolapse was 14.2%; the rate of cystocele was 34.3%; and the rate of rectocele was 18.6%. For the 10,727 women who had undergone hysterectomy, the prevalence of cystocele was 32.9%; of rectocele, 18.3%. This study did not grade the severity of prolapse. Nygaard et al.[34] reported that among 270 nonhysterectomized women, 25.6% were considered to have prolapse when it was defined as the leading edge of vaginal descensus at or below the hymeneal ring.

The Pelvic Organ Support Study (POSST)[35] reported a 7% prevalence of prolapse to or beyond the level of the hymen among 1004 women. There is little information available on the natural progression of prolapse. In a study of 412 women evaluated over a two-to-eight-year period, new-onset cystocele, rectocele, and uterine prolapse occurred in 9%, 6%, and 2% of women per year, respectively. The general tendency of POP is to worsen with time. Some studies have reported natural regression of POP, and this is more common among the milder (grade 1) forms of POP.

It is also important to specifically address the prevalence of surgery for POP. It has been reported that a woman's lifetime risk for needing surgery for POP was 11% by the age of 80. Approximately one third of women undergoing surgery will need a second operation for recurrent prolapse.

Risk Factors for Pelvic Organ Prolapse

Age

Advancing age has been shown to be an independent risk factor for POP, and the prevalence of POP increases with age. In a Swedish study of women between the ages of 20 and 59, the prevalence of any form of prolapse was 6.6% in women 20 to 29 years old and 55.6% among those 50 to 59 years old.[32] An American study by Swift et al. reported a 12% increased incidence of severe POP with each advancing year of life or a doubling of the incidence for every additional decade.[36]

Obstetric Factors

In the above-mentioned Swedish study,[32] prolapse was noted in 44% of parous women, and the corresponding prevalence among nonparous women was 5.8%. Increasing parity and, maybe more significantly, increasing number of vaginal deliveries are important risk factors for prolapse. It has been postulated that as the fetal vertex passes through the pelvis, there is a stretching and tearing of the soft tissues and fascial supports of the pelvis and compression and stretching of the pudendal nerve. Both of these mechanisms could explain the increased risk of all pelvic floor disorders associated with vaginal delivery. Instrumented vaginal deliveries, especially forceps-assisted, may increase this risk even more.

According to the Oxford Family Planning Association study,[37] the likelihood of a woman developing prolapse increased approximately 8-fold after 2 vaginal deliveries and about 12-fold after 4 or more vaginal births.

The risk of developing future prolapse grows with increasing birthweights. Swift and his colleagues have reported that there is a 24% increase in the incidence of severe POP for every 1 lb increase in the weight of a vaginally delivered infant.[36]

Demographic

POP is more common among women with lower levels of education. It has been postulated that this may be due to some unmeasured risk factor, such as socioeconomic status, nutritional status, or a lifetime of work. In comparison to white women, African American women have the lowest risk of POP, and Hispanic women have the highest risk

Obesity and Occupation

Chronic increased intraabdominal pressure has been proposed as a risk factor for POP, caused by increased strain placed on the suspensory support structures throughout the pelvis. Women with chronic obstructive lung disease or chronic constipation, weight lifters, nursing assistants, marathon runners, and obese women will fall in this category. However, recent studies evaluating the link between obesity and prolapse have yielded conflicting results. Nygaard et al. found no association between BMI or waist circumference and pelvic organ prolapse. They did find that women reporting past heavy labor were more likely to have uterine prolapse than those without this history. In contrast, results from the Women's Health Initiative have suggested that being overweight (BMI 25–30 kg/m^2) or obese (BMI > 30 kg/m^2) was associated with a significantly increased risk of POP. Waist circumference of ≥88 cm had an associated significant increase in risk of 17% for rectocele and cystocele.[33] Current physical activity appeared to have no substantial impact on the risk for any of the forms of pelvic organ prolapse.

Iatrogenic

Prior surgery for pelvic organ prolapse is another important risk factor for POP, and Some have said have said that the risk the risk of recurrent POP among these women is 500% greater than that of the general population.[36] However, the role of hysterectomy as a risk factor for POP in unclear. The POSST study[35] found no association between prior hysterectomy and POP, and some of its authors have suggested that hysterectomy may offer a protective effect for the development of POP caused by defects such as those often being concurrently repaired at the time of the hysterectomy. However, the majority of studies do find an increased risk of vault prolapse and enterocele after a hysterectomy. Mant reported that the annual incidence of prolapse requiring surgical correction after a hysterectomy was 3.6 per 1000.[37] The risk rises from 1% by 3 years after a hysterectomy to 5% after 15 years.

Pelvic Floor Muscle Strength

Many authors believe that decreased pelvic floor muscle (PFM) strength may be the single most important risk factor leading to POP. Pelvic floor muscle strength decreases with age and parity. An intact levator plate acts as a "flap-valve," keeping the walls of the vagina closed, and supports the vagina over the levator muscles in the standing position, thereby preventing prolapse. Samuelsson reported that in a 35-year-old woman with two children, the probability of having prolapse was 25% if the PFMs were strong and 58% if the PFMs were poor.[32] Techniques to improve pelvic floor muscle tone are reviewed in Chapters 6 and 8.

Familial

Rinne reported from a case control study in Finland that the familial incidence of prolapse was

30%.[38] Certain congenital disorders of connective tissue (Marfan's syndrome, Ehrlers Danlos syndrome) as well as neurological conditions have also been associated with prolapse, especially in young women.

Female Sexual Dysfunction (FSD)

Female sexual dysfunction (FSD) is characterized by psychogenic and organic problems with sexual desire, arousal, orgasm, or dyspareunia that cause personal distress.[39]

Prevalence and Risk factors for FSD

Since few patients volunteer this information and since physicians do not routinely screen for these complaints, accurate prevalence estimates for FSD are limited. A prevalence rate of 40% to 50% is routinely quoted.[40, 41]

Women's sexuality is discontinuous throughout their life cycles and is dependent on personal, current contextual, and relationship variables as well as on medical factors. The US National Health and Social Life Survey (NHSLS) in 1992[42] has provided important data on the prevalence and risk factors for sexual dysfunction among both sexes. This study was a national probability sample study that included men and women between the ages of 18 and 59 years who had at least 1 sexual partner in the past 1 year. In this study, low libido was the most common sexual complaint, affecting 51% of women, followed by arousal disorders in 33%, and pain disorders in 16%, of women.

Age

FSD seems to be age related and progressive, affecting up to 20% to 43% of women in their fertile years[42] and 46% to 81% of the elderly women who are still sexually active.[43] All of the major studies that have been done by the National Council on Aging and the Association of Reproductive Health Professionals (ARHP) show that at age 60 years, approximately half of the women are sexually active and by 80-plus years of age, the figure is barely 20%.

Gender and Ethnicity

The NHSLS study[42] also noted that sexual dysfunction occurs more frequently in women than in men (43% vs 31%). African American women tend to report higher rates of low sexual desire, whereas white women are more likely to report sexual pain. Hispanic women, in contrast, consistently self-report lower rates of sexual problems.

Psychosocial Factors and General Health

The NHSLS data[42] indicate that emotional and stress-related problems generate an elevated risk of experiencing sexual difficulties in all phases of the sexual response cycle. Premarital and postmarital (divorced, widowed, or separated) status is associated with an elevated risk of experiencing sexual problems. Good health and general well-being are generally associated with fewer FSD problems.

Women with pelvic floor dysfunction (i.e. pelvic organ prolapse, urinary and fecal incontinence) report fairly high rates of sexual dysfunction. Handa et al. have reported that sexual complaints were significantly more common among women with pelvic floor disorders (53.2% vs 40.4%) than among women in the control group.[44]

When evaluating female patients for pelvic floor symptoms, asking an open-ended question about sexual function can help to identify substantial numbers of women in need of help. A full approach to diagnosing and treating sexual dysfunction is reviewed in Chapter 11.

Menopause

As our population ages, the number of postmenopausal women with FSD is certainly bound to increase. US Census data indicate that in the year 2000, more than 42 million (1 out of 3) American women were of or over the age of 50, and an additional 2 million women annually reach the age of 50. The transition from premenopause to peri/-postmenopause has a negative impact on sexual health. Estrogen deprivation is associated with certain physiological changes that may lead to FSD in postmenopause, including delay in reaction time of the clitoris, diminished vaginal lubrication, decreased duration of contractions with orgasm, and decreased vaginal congestion. Among postmenopausal women under the age of 55, nearly half have a decrease in sexual desire with the onset of menopause, whereas 10% have an increase and approximately 37% are unchanged.[45]

The role of estrogen replacement therapy in alleviating the symptoms of FSD is controversial.[46] Androgen insufficiency—due to declining ovarian stromal function during menopause as well as oophorectomy—has long been recognized as playing a role in FSD. Androgen levels in the postmenopausal period are usually one half those seen in women in their thirties and forties.[47] Surgical menopause is known to have a profound impact on serum testosterone levels and, in one study, testosterone levels dropped to approximately 40% of the baseline value after an oophorectomy.[48]

Conclusion

Pelvic floor dysfunction—including urinary incontinence, fecal incontinence, pelvic organ prolapse, and female sexual dysfunction—is an incompletely understood clinical condition with multiple risk factors. These risk factors can be associated with various stages of a woman's normal life cycle. With the aging of the general population, primary care providers will encounter large numbers of symptomatic women. As our understanding of the pathophysiology and treatment of these conditions improves, we will, hopefully, begin to see a greater emphasis on prevention. It is generally accepted that most pelvic floor dysfunction is caused by pelvic floor trauma associated with childbirth, aging, menopause, surgical injury, and/or chronic Valsalva. Other factors may include obesity, anatomy, tissue properties, and concurrent medical conditions. Strategies to reduce the risk and progression of pelvic floor dysfunction and to ameliorate existing symptoms are outlined in the chapters ahead.

Key Points

- *Rough Prevalence of Female Pelvic Disorders*
  - Urinary Incontinence 20%–50%
  - Fecal Incontinence 5%
  - Flatal Incontinence 25%
  - Sexual Dysfunction 15–25%
- Major Risk Factors
  - Childbirth, Pregnancy, Aging
  - Obesity, Neuromuscular Injury/Disease
- Lifetime Risk of Undergoing Major Pelvic Surgery: 11%
- Women with Incontinence or Prolapse Reporting FSD: 53%

References

1. Thom, D. Variation in estimates of urinary incontinence prevalence in the community: effects of differences in definition, population characteristics, and study type. *J Am Geriatr Soc.*, 1998; 46:473.
2. Diokno AC, Brock BM, Brown MB et al. Prevalence of urinary incontinence and other urological symptoms in the noninstitutionalized elderly. *J Urology.* 1986;136:1022–1025.
3. Hunskaar S, Burgio K, Clark A et al. Epidemiology of faecal and urinary incontinence and pelvic organ prolapse. In: *Incontinence. 3rd International Consultation on Incontinence*, 3rd ed. Abrams P, Cardozo L, Khoury S, Wein A (ed). Plymouth, UK: Health Publication, Ltd., 2005.
4. Hampel C, Wienhold D, Benken N et al. Prevalence and natural history of female incontinence. *Eur Urol.* 1997;32(Suppl 2):3–12.
5. Melville Jl, Katon W, Delaney K et al. Urinary incontinence in US women: a population-based study. *Intern Med.* 2005;165:537–542.

5a. Fultz NH, Herzog AR. Prevalence of urinary incontinence in middle-aged and older women: a survey—based methodological experiment. *J Aging Health.* 2000;12(4):459–469.

6. Sampselle CM, Harlow SD, Skurnick J et al. Urinary incontinence predictors and life impact in ethnically diverse perimenopausal women. *Obstet Gynecol.* 2002;100:1230–1238.
7. Viktrup L, Lose G, Rolff M et al. The symptom of stress incontinence caused by pregnancy or delivery in primiparas. *Obstet Gynecol.* 1992;79:945–49.
8. Allen RE, Hosker GL, Smith ARB et al. Pelvic floor damage and childbirth: a neurophysiological study. *Br J Obstet Gynaecol.* 1990;97:770–779.
9. Persson J, Wolner-Hanssen P, Rydhstroem H. Obstetric risk factors for stress urinary incontinence: a population-based study. *Obstet Gynecol.* 2000;96:440–445.
10. Foldspang A, Mommsen S, Lam GW et al. Parity as a correlate of adult female urinary incontinence prevalence. *J Epidemiol Commun Health.* 1992;46: 595–600.

11. Milsom I, Ekelund P, Molander U et al. The influence of age, parity, oral contraception, hysterectomy, and menopause on the prevalence of urinary incontinence in women. *J Urol.* 1993;149:1459–1462.
12. Goldberg RP, Abramov Y, Botros S et al. Delivery mode is a major environmental determinant of stress urinary incontinence: results of the Evanston-Northwestern Twin Sisters Study. *Am J Obstet Gynecol.* 2005;193:2149–2153.
13. Rortviet G, Hannestad YS, Daltveit AK et al. Age- and type-dependent effects of parity on urinary incontinence: the Norwegian EPINCONT study. *Obstet Gynecol.* 2001;98:1004–1010
14. Thom DH, Brown JS. Reproductive and hormonal risk factors for urinary incontinence in later life: a review of clinical and epidemiologic literature. *J Am Geriatric Soc.* 1998;46:1411–1417
15. Hendrix SL, Cochrane BB, Nygaard IE et al. Effects of estrogen with and without progestin on urinary incontinence. *JAMA.* 2005;23(293):935–948.
16. Minassian VA, Drutz HP, Al-Badr A. Urinary incontinence as a worldwide problem. *Int J Gynaecol Obstet.* 2003;82:327–338.
17. Peyrat L, Haillot O, Bruyere F et al. Prevalence and risk factors of urinary incontinence in young and middle-aged women. *BJU Int.* 2002;89:61–66.
18. Macmillan AK, Merrie AEH, Marshall RJ et al. The prevalence of fecal incontinence in community-dwelling adults: a systematic review of the literature. *Dis Colon Rectum.* 2004;47:1341.
19. Talley NJ; O'Keefe EA; Zinsmeister AR et al. Prevalence of gastrointestinal symptoms in the elderly: a population-based study. *Gastroenterology.* 1992;102: 895–901.
20. Nelson R; Furner S; Jesudason V. Fecal incontinence in Wisconsin nursing homes: prevalence and associations. *Dis Colon Rectum.* 1998;41:1226–1229.
21. Eva UF, Gun W, Preben K. Prevalence of urinary and fecal incontinence and symptoms of genital prolapse in women. *Acta Obstet Gynecol Scand.* 2003;82:280–286.
22. Drossman DA; Li Z; Andruzzi E et al. US householder survey of functional gastrointestinal disorders. Prevalence, sociodemography, and health impact. *Dig Dis Sci.* 1993;38:1569–1580.
23. Haadem K, Dahlstrom JA, Lingman G. Anal sphincter function after delivery: a prospective study in women with sphincter rupture and controls. *Eur J Obstet Gynecol Reprod Biol.* 1990;35:7
24. Sultan AH; Kamm MA; Hudson CN et al. Anal-sphincter disruption during vaginal delivery. *N Engl J Med.* 1993;23(329):1905–1911.
25. Ryhammer AM, Laurberg S, Hermann AP. Long-term effect of vaginal deliveries on anorectal function in normal perimenopausal women. *Dis Colon Rectum.* 1996;39:852–859.
26. Pollack J, Nordenstam J, Brismar S et al. Anal incontinence after vaginal delivery: a five-year prospective cohort study. *Obstetrics & Gynecology.* 2004;104:1397–1402.
27. Haadem K, Dahlstrom JA, Ling L. Anal sphincter competence in healthy women: clinical implications of age and other factors. *Obstet Gynecol.* 1991;78(5 Pt 1): 823–827.
28. Nelson R, Norton N, Cautley E et al. Community-based prevalence of anal incontinence. *JAMA.* 1995 16(274):559–561.
29. Quander CR, Morris MC, Melson J et al. Prevalence of and factors associated with fecal incontinence in a large community study of older individuals. *Am J Gastroenterol.* 2005;100:905–909.
30. Swift SE. The distribution of pelvic organ support in a population of female subjects seen for routine gynecologic health care. *Am J Obstet Gynecol.* 2000;83:277–285.
31. Hendrix SL, Clark A, Nygaard I et al. Pelvic organ prolapse in the Women's Health Initiative: gravity and gravidity. *Am J Obstet Gynecol.* 2002;186:1160–1166.
32. Samuelsson EC, Victor FT, Tibblin G et al. Signs of genital prolapse in a Swedish population of women 20 to 59 years of age and possible related factors. *Am J Obstet Gynecol.* 1999;180:299–305.
33. Hendrix SL, Clark A, Nygaard I et al. Pelvic organ prolapse in the Women's Health Initiative: gravity and gravidity. *Am J Obstet Gynecol.* 2002;186:1160–1166.
34. Nygaard I, Bradley C, Brandt D. Women's Health Initiative. Pelvic organ prolapse in older women: prevalence and risk factors. *Obstet Gynecol.* 2004; 104:489–497.
35. Swift S, Woodman P, O'Boyle A et al. Pelvic Organ Support Study (POSST): the distribution, clinical definition, and epidemiologic condition of pelvic organ support defects. *Am J Obstet Gynecol.* 2005; 192:795-806
36. Swift SE, Pound T, Dias JK. Case-control study of etiologic factors in the development of severe pelvic organ prolapse. *Int Urogynecol J Pelvic Floor Dysfunct.* 2001;12:187–192.
37. Mant J, Painter R, Vessey M. Epidemiology sexual dysfunction: definitions and classifications. *J Urol.* 2000;183:888–893.
38. Rinne KM, Kirkinen PP. What predisposes young women to genital prolapse? *Eur J Obstet Gynecol Reprod Biol.* 1999;84:23–25.

39. Basson R, Berman J, Burnett A et al. Report of the international consensus development conference on female sexual dysfunction: definitions and classifications. *J Urol.* 2000;163:888–893.
40. Geiss IM, Umek WH, Dungl A et al. Prevalence of female sexual dysfunction in gynecologic and urogynecologic patients according to the international consensus classification. *Urology.* 2003;62:514–518.
41. Nazareth I, Boynton P, King M. Problems with sexual function in people attending London general practitioners: cross sectional study. *BMJ.* 2003;23;327:423–426.
42. Laumann EO, Paik A, Rosen RC. Sexual dysfunction in the United States: prevalence and predictors. *JAMA.* 1999;281:537–544.
43. Graziottin A, Koochaki P. Distress associated with low sexual desire in women in four EU countries. *Maturitas.* 2003;44(Suppl 2):S116.
44. Handa VL, Harvey L, Cundiff GW et al. Sexual function among women with urinary incontinence and pelvic organ prolapse. *Am J Obstet Gynecol.* 2004;191:751–756.
45. Sexuality Information and Education Council of the United States. Sexuality in middle and later life. Available at: http://www.siecus.org/pubs/fact/fact0018.html.
46. Pauls R, Kleeman S, Karram M. Female sexual dysfunction: principles of diagnosis and therapy. *Obstet Gynecol Surv.* 2005;60:196-205.
47. Davis SR. When to suspect androgen deficiency otherthanatmenopause.*FertilSteril.*2002;77(Suppl 4):S68–71.
48. Judd HL, Lucas WE, Yen SS. Effect of oophorectomy on circulating testosterone and androstenedione levels in patients with endometrial cancer. *Am J Obstet Gynecol.* 1974;118:793–798.
49. Keshavarz H, Hills SD, Kieke BA et al. Hysterectomy surveillance – United States, 1994–1999. *MMWR CDC Surveill Summ.* 2002;51:1–8.
50. Walters MD, Karram MM, eds. *Urogynecology & Reconstructive Pelvic Surgery.* 2nd ed. St. Louis: Mosby, 1999.

2
Pelvic Floor Anatomy: Made Clear and Simple

Robert M. Rogers, Jr.

The Female Pelvis

The intent of this chapter is to give the primary care provider, to women of all ages, a clinical appreciation of the anatomy in the female pelvis that currently explains the mechanisms of pelvic organ suspension and support, as well as urinary and fecal continence. Though this chapter describes the current thinking in the "average normal" patient, the reader must realize that each woman is unique in her anatomic makeup. Her pelvic support anatomy is dependent upon the genetic composition of her visceral connective tissues and various muscles—both somatic and visceral—and their adaptations to her aging process and upon the many variables of her lifestyle. Lifestyle conditions that affect the functioning of her pelvic organs and their support include:

- habits of physical activities and the various mechanical stresses that weigh on her pelvic structures
- dietary habits and her state of nutritional balance and adequacy
- social habits such as cigarette smoking and drug use
- her state of health and use of some medications
- habits of urinary control and voiding, and habits of bowel control and defecation
- sexual activities and childbirth and their possible mechanical and infectious consequences
- previous gynecologic surgeries.[1]

The female pelvis includes the organs of storage and elimination of urine and feces—the bladder and urethra, and the rectum and anal canal. The vagina is the organ of vaginal sexual intercourse, elimination of menstrual discharge, and childbirth. These functions are best sustained when the organs are well suspended and supported within the pelvis, with a specific anatomic relationship to each other. Though each organ functions independently of the others, it is anatomically oriented and dependent upon that orientation. The urethra, lower third of the vagina, and anal canal are parallel and almost vertical in the standing nulliparous young woman.[2] These lower vertical structures are supported directly by their attachments to the levator hiatus muscles, perineal body and the anatomic urogenital and anal triangles. (Figure 2.1).

The bladder rests upon the upper two-thirds of the vagina and lower uterine segment. The upper vagina rests upon the rectum. The bladder, upper vagina, and rectum are approximately horizontal in orientation in the young, standing woman and overlie the muscular *levator plate*.[3] These horizontal relationships are especially apparent when the young woman puts stress on her pelvis during a Valsalva moment such as coughing, sneezing, lifting, exercising, and so on.

The levator plate is a dynamic backstop which contracts and strongly supports the upper vagina and rectum in the horizontal position, acting as a "flap valve" to close their walls and prevent their prolapse during moments of physical force.

Damage to the levator muscles and the levator plate compromises the capability of the pelvic suspensory structures to support these organs and is believed to represent a seminal event that often leads to prolapse. Such damage to the pelvic floor muscles usually occurs during vaginal childbirth

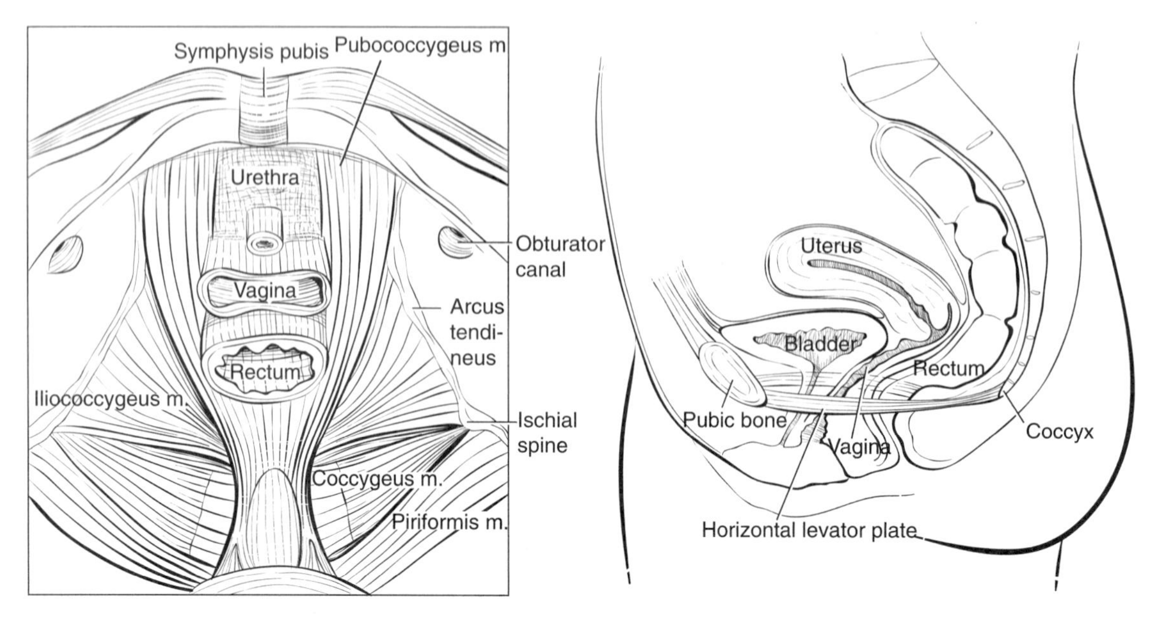

Figure 2.1. Levator muscles: the foundation of pelvic support. (**Left**) The Vagina, Rectum and Urethra rest on a firm "shelf" of levator muscle support. The platform of levator muscle support spans from the pubic bone back to the tailbone and side-to-side from one arcus tendineus to the other. (**Right**) The upper vagina is oriented horizontally when a woman is in the standing position. The strong horizontal levator muscle plate—seen here spanning from pubic bone back to tailbone—is the key to maintaining this normal anatomic position.

and in patients with chronic mechanical stress states such as chronic straining with chronic constipation, sustained heavy lifting over time, and heavy physical exercise.

The anatomic relationships between the pelvic organs and the tissue reactions to various physical stresses depend on the structures that house, suspend, and support the female pelvic organs. These pelvic structures are the bones and ligaments, the skeletal muscles and parietal fascia, and the various visceral connective tissues.

Bones and Ligaments

The bones and ligaments of the female pelvis form the outer structure, which surrounds, protects, suspends and supports the pelvic organs and their suspensory tissues.[4] The *coxal bone* consists of three parts that have fused during a woman's teenage years and into her early twenties. These are the ilium, the ischium and the pubis. The *ilium* is the upper portion and consists of an alar, or upper wing, that is slightly concave on its inner surface. The muscles of hip flexion—iliacus and psoas—course on the medial surface. The crest of the ilium is the upper portion of the hip and serves as the attachment for the abdominal wall muscles. This crest also contains the anterior superior iliac spine and the anterior inferior iliac spine, both of which are attachments for hip girdle muscles. The inner inferior border of the ilium is the arcuate line, or linea terminalis, which is the line that defines entry into the true pelvis. The posterior edges of each ilium and ischium form the border of the greater sciatic notch, through which course the piriformis muscle and sciatic nerve out of the pelvis and into the hip.

The inferior and posterior part of the coxal bone is the *ischium*. When seated, the woman sits on her two ischial tuberosities. The hip extensor muscles, hamstrings, and gluteus muscles originate here. The sacrotuberous ligament also courses from the ischial tuberosity to the posterior part of the lower sacrum. This ligament defines and stabilizes the outlet to the pelvis.

The important *ischial spine* is the point within the pelvis central to learning and understanding female pelvic support anatomy. The ischial spine can, from patient to patient, vary in physical characteristics such as size, shape, bluntness or sharpness, and prominence on palpation. The distance from ischial spine to ischial spine is approximately 10 cm and is the narrowest diameter in the pelvis. This has important implications during childbirth, where the infant's head diameter is also approximately 10 cm. (Figure 2.2)

The ischial spine points posteromedially and is the prominence that demarcates the upper greater sciatic notch and foramen from the lower lesser sciatic notch and foramen. Through the lesser sciatic foramen courses the tendon of the obturator internus muscle, as well as the internal pudendal vessels and pudendal nerve as they course into the pudendal canal on the lateral border of the ischioanal fossa. The ischial spine is best known as the bony landmark that the obstetrician uses to determine the progression of fetal vertex descent during labor. However, it is a key reference point during gynecologic surgery, as well, providing a fixed bony indicator of the level at which the upper vagina (and cervix) should be suspended. This landmark is easily palpated by the examiner, both through the vagina or rectum and during abdominal surgery. This fact is important and assists the operating reparative vaginal surgeon in determining the adequate length of the vagina for sexual intercourse. That satisfactory length should be approximately 8 cm–10 cm from the hymenal ring, which correlates to the level of the ischial spines.

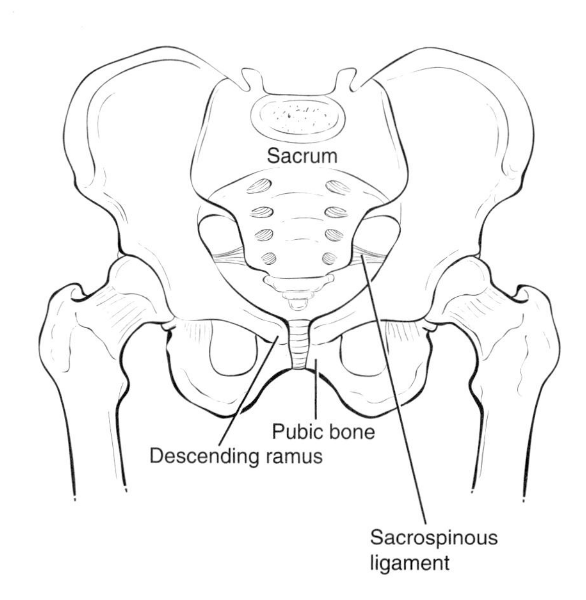

FIGURE 2.2. Bony pelvis.

The ischial spine is located 2 cm to 3 cm above the horizontal level of the pubic crest in the properly standing young woman, and is 7.5 cm to 9.5 cm from the back of the pubic bone. This distance and line also define the arcus tendineus fasciae pelvis (fascial white line), which is the anatomic structure important for understanding the lateral supports to the bladder and urethra, the vagina, and the rectum. One procedure for repairing a vaginal prolapse is a sacrospinous ligament colpopexy (fixation of the top of the vagina to the sacrospinous ligament). The sacrospinous ligament tapers and inserts onto the ischial spine laterally, while broadening out medially as it inserts onto the inner aspect of the lower part of the sacrum. The sacrospinous ligament frames the sciatic notches to form the greater and lesser sciatic foramina. The pelvic muscles and visceral connective tissues have important anatomic relations and attachments to the ischial spines.

The inferior but anterior part of the coxal bone is the *pubis or pubic bone*. The inferior pubic ramus fuses posteriorly with the ramus of the ischium, while the superior pubic ramus fuses laterally with the ilium at the iliopubic (iliopectineal) eminence. The inferior and superior pubic rami fuse medially to form the central body of each pubic bone. These bodies fuse centrally with the cartilaginous symphysis pubis. Located on the upper aspect of each pubic body is the pubic tubercle. The inguinal ligament is derived from the inferior edge of the aponeurosis of the external oblique muscle and courses from the anterior superior iliac spine to the pubic tubercle. Running laterally along the upper aspect of the superior pubic ramus, beginning at the pubic tubercle, is the pectineal line. On the pectineal line is found a thickened ridge of parietal fascia called Cooper's ligament. For surgeons performing a Burch retropubic colposuspension (a bladder neck suspension procedure employed to address stress urinary incontinence), Cooper's ligament is the site of suture attachment. (Figure 2.3)

The superior and inferior pubic rami, fusing posteriorly with the ischium, form a ring of bony edges that results in a large hole in the lower pelvis

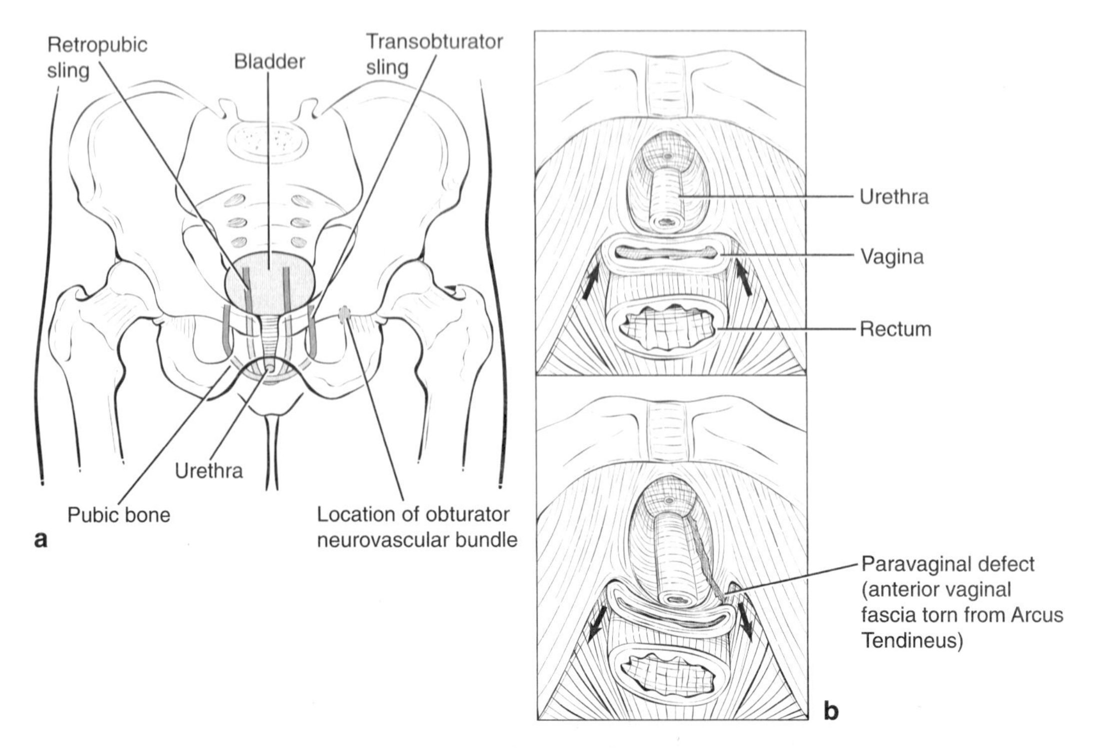

FIGURE 2.3. Two incontinence sling types, in the bony pelvis. The transobturator sling is seen passing from one obturator foramen to another, at a safe distance from the obturator neurovascular bundle. The retropubic sling is seen passing in, a u-shaped configuration, behind the pubic bone. **(b)** Paravaginal defect: tear in the lateral vaginal support.

called the obturator foramen. The obturator foramen is covered with a tough, fibrous membrane that attaches all around to its inner bony borders, except in its anterior and lateral portion, where the obturator artery, vein, and nerve pass from the obturator canal into the inner thigh region. The obturator canal is a groove on the underneath surface of the superior pubic ramus. The canal transmits the obturator vessels and nerve from the retropubic space (of Retzius) through the obturator foramen and membrane to the inner thigh. The FDA has recently approved the passage of instruments and various surgical tapes and meshes through the obturator foramen for surgical treatment of stress urinary incontinence and certain vaginal prolapse problems.

The bony *sacrum* is located centrally in the back of the pelvis and articulates with each coxal bone via the ilium at each sacroiliac joint. These joints are firm but partially synovial, allowing very little rotational movement.[5] The sacral promontory and the upper sacral vertebrae are nearly horizontal or parallel to the floor. Therefore, in the standing position, the weight of the abdominal and pelvic cavity pressure column rests primarily upon the backs of the pubic bodies and symphysis, not upon the muscles and the suspensory visceral connective tissues. This is important to realize because the pelvic muscles and the visceral connective tissue network that suspends the pelvic organs over the muscular levator plate are meant for "light" work or sporadic heavier loads. Chronic heavy workloads, such as chronic constipation, heavy lifting, and other physical stresses can overwhelm this soft-tissue suspensory network and cause "breaks" in its frame, decreasing the effective functioning of the "flap-valve" mechanism. As a result, the cervix and upper vagina slide off the levator plate and evaginate down the vaginal tube towards the introitus, causing tearing in the lateral vaginal supports. (Figure 2.3A) The bones of the pelvis are shaped like a wide funnel with a large, rounded entry; straight sidewalls formed by the sides of the ischii and the obturator foramina and membranes; and the diamond-shaped outlet. To this bony frame is attached the muscles of the female pelvis.

Pelvic Floor Muscles

The pelvis is a basin formed by muscles.[6] The entry is open and round. The back wall is formed by the sacrum centrally and the piriformis muscles laterally, the sidewalls are the right and left obturator internus muscles, and the front wall is formed by the backs of the pubic bodies and pubic symphysis. The floor is formed by the levator ani muscle complexes and the coccygeus muscles covering the sacrospinous ligaments. (Figure 2.4)

Through the floor of the pelvis—also called pelvic diaphragm—course the urethra, the lower third of the vagina, and the anal canal. These pass through the levator hiatus, or central opening between the levator ani muscles of the pelvic diaphragm. Passively resting on top of the posterior portion of the levator ani muscles, named the levator plate, are the upper two thirds of the vagina and the rectum. These orientations are crucial in maintaining pelvic organ support in the physically active woman. Just below or inferior to the pelvic diaphragm is the perineum anteriorly, and the ischioanal fossa posteriorly. The perineum, containing important muscles and fascia, is important in the maintenance of the vertical orientation of the urethra, the lower third of the vagina and the anal canal.

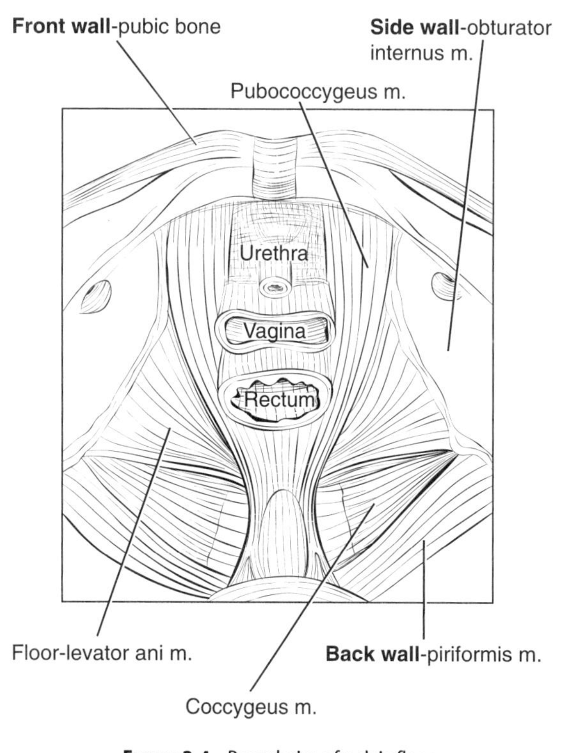

FIGURE 2.4. Boundaries of pelvic floor.

The *piriformis muscle* courses from the upper half of the sacrum, straight outward through the greater sciatic foramen, to insert onto the greater trochanter of the femur. The obturator internus muscle originates from the bony edges of the obturator foramen and the entire inner surface of the obturator membrane to form a wide, fan-shaped muscle. This muscle tapers into a strong tendon, which then turns 120 degrees to exit the pelvis through the lesser sciatic foramen to insert onto the greater trochanter with the piriformis tendon. These two muscles externally rotate the hip. Overlying the piriformis muscle is the sacral plexus of somatic nerves. The sacral plexus is the origin of the sciatic nerve, the pudendal nerve, and the nerves that innervate the pelvic musculature. Therefore, no surgical dissection or sutures should ever be placed near the piriformis muscles. However, the obturator internus muscles of the pelvic sidewall are readily available to guide surgical dissections and to accept sutures for repairing pelvic support problems.

The floor of the pelvis is formed by the upper, or pelvic, surfaces of the levator ani complex of muscles and the coccygeus muscles. The *coccygeus muscle* is a very thin, nonfunctional covering of the strong sacrospinous ligament. In fact, when using this ligament for vaginal support in the older woman, the coccygeus muscle is very fibrotic and not seen after dissection in this area. The *levator ani muscles* are traditionally described as the pubococcygeus and puborectalis anteriorly, and the iliococcygeus muscles posteriorly. The *pubococcygeus and puborectalis muscles* originate from the back of the pubic bone and the anterior part of the obturator internus muscle, along the arcus tendineus levator ani. These muscles form the levator hiatus and allow passage of the urethra, lower third of the vagina, and anal canal through the pelvic diaphragm and perineum to the outside

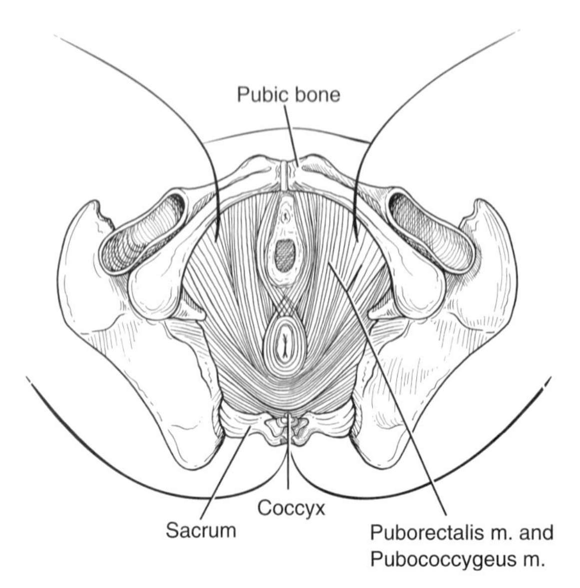

FIGURE 2.5. The sling-like pelvic floor muscles: pubococcygeus and puborectalis.

of the body. The pubococcygeus surrounds and is fused with the lower third of the vagina and inserts into the apex of the perineal body between the vagina and anorectal juncture. The puborectalis muscle is the medial and inferior portion of the pubococcygeus muscle and meets its sister puborectalis muscle behind the anorectal junction. (Figure 2.5)

The anatomic relationship of the puborectalis muscles with the anorectal junction is very important for fecal continence. The puborectalis muscles form the "right angle" of the anorectal junction, which is responsible for solid stool control. These muscles are innervated by branches from the sacral plexus that, in some cases, may be compressed, stretched, and significantly injured during vaginal childbirth. Surrounding the outlet of the anal canal is the sphincter ani muscle. The proper functioning of this muscle is responsible for continence of watery stool and flatus. This muscle is innervated by the inferior rectal nerves from the pudendal nerves, which also can be stretched and injured by childbirth.

The *iliococcygeus muscle* originates from the pelvic sidewall from the arcus tendineus levator ani. The arcus tendineus levator ani is a thickening of the parietal fascia overlying each obturator internus muscle and is directed from the back of the pubic bone to a point near the ischial spine. The iliococcygeus muscles then slope down in a horizontal manner to fuse into the *levator plate*, which runs from the anorectal junction to the coccyx and sacrum and is approximately 4 cm long. Inserting into the levator plate is also the puborectalis muscle. Lying passively on top of the levator plate and lower part of the sacrum is the rectum, cervix, and upper two thirds of the vagina. When the woman increases intrapelvic pressure with a Valsalva maneuver such as straining, coughing or laughing, the pressure generated pushes the upper vagina and rectum down against the contracted, firm levator plate. This "flap-valve" mechanism is responsible for prevention of pelvic organ prolapse in the "**normal**" woman. The other crucial mechanism for preventing pelvic organ prolapse is the contraction and closure of the pelvic diaphragm and levator hiatus by the pubococcygeus and puborectalis muscles.

The *perineum* is located inferior to the levator ani floor of the pelvis and is diamond shaped. Its major muscular components are illustrated in Figure 2.6. The sidewalls are the obturator internus muscles below the two arcus tendineus levator ani. The outer part of the perineum is bordered by the outlet of the pelvic bones. The perineum is anatomically divided into two triangles described by drawing a line through the two ischial tuberosities. The anterior portion towards the pubic arch

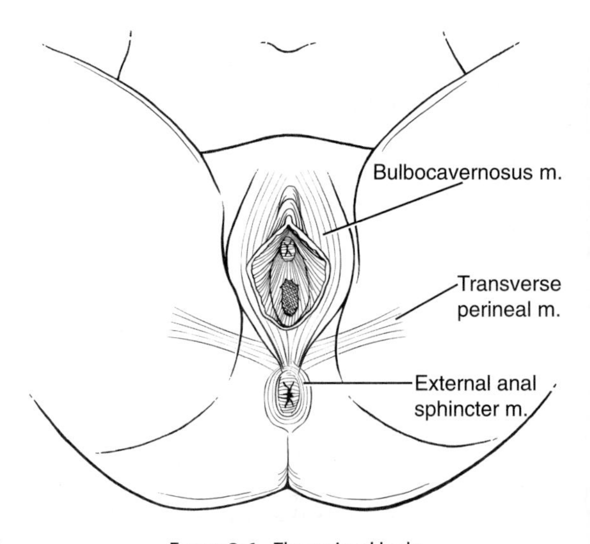

FIGURE 2.6. The perineal body.

is the urogenital triangle, while the posterior or anal triangle contains the anus and points towards the coccyx. The anal triangle also contains the fa-filled ischioanal fossa. The urogenital triangle has two layers described – the superficial space and the deep compartment. The boundary between these two spaces is the perineal membrane, a tough, fibrous membrane that stretches between the ischiopubic rami. Through the perineal membrane passes the lower third of the urethra and the lower third of the vagina. The posterior edge of the perineal membrane is the anterior border of the anal triangle.

The muscles in the superficial space are the superficial transverse perinei, the bulbocavernosus, and the ischiocavernosus. They overlie the vascular erectile bulbs and assist in clitoral erection and the woman's sexual response. These muscles are innervated by the perineal branches of the pudendal nerve. The muscles of the deep compartment apply to the urinary continence mechanism. On top of the perineal membrane are the compressor urethrae and urethrovaginal muscles. These small muscles run over the lower third of the urethra and are part of the external urethral sphincter, along with the sphincter urethrae, which surrounds the urethra from the urethrovesical junction down to the perineal membrane. All these muscles, as well, are innervated by perineal branches of the pudendal nerve. The pudendal nerve is also exposed to the injurious forces of compression and stretching during vaginal childbirth. Some women are then left with residual damage to their continence mechanisms.

Anchoring the urogenital and anal triangles centrally is the perineal body, found between the vaginal introitus and the anus. The lower third of the vagina is fused with the perineal body anteriorly, while the anal canal is fused with the perineal body posteriorly. The square base is located 1 cm–2 cm above, or superior to, the level of the ischial tuberosities. The apex of the perineal body, roughly shaped like a pyramid, is located at the transition of the lower third of the vagina with the middle third and at the 90° angulation of the anal canal with the rectum at the anorectal junction. The perineal body and pubic bones anchor the closure mechanisms of the vaginal introitus and anal canal. (Figure 2.6)

Pelvic Organ Suspension—Visceral Connective Tissues

The crucial mechanisms of pelvic organ support are the flap valve of the upper vagina and rectum against the levator plate, and the closure of the vaginal introitus by the contraction of the pubococcygeus/puborectalis muscles around the lower third of the vagina and anorectal junction. The flap-valve mechanism is dependent upon the visceral connective tissue network that suspends the upper vagina, cervix, and rectum over the levator plate. The closure of the lower third of the vagina is the result of the direct fusion of the pubococcygeus/puborectalis muscles with the lower third of the vagina, perineal body, and anorectal junction.

Think of the suspensory function of the pelvic visceral connective tissues as a three-dimensional scaffold that is somewhat flexible, yet anchored to the muscular pelvic basin.[7,8] (Figure 2.7)

The scaffold is constructed of a tight webbing, and occasional fusion, of a meshwork of collagen and elastin. Histologically, visceral connective tissue is a three-dimensional meshwork composed predominantly of collagen fibers intermingled with some elastin and smooth muscle. It is located along the back wall and the sidewalls of the pelvic basin and then tapers down to the vaginal introitus and perineal body. The visceral

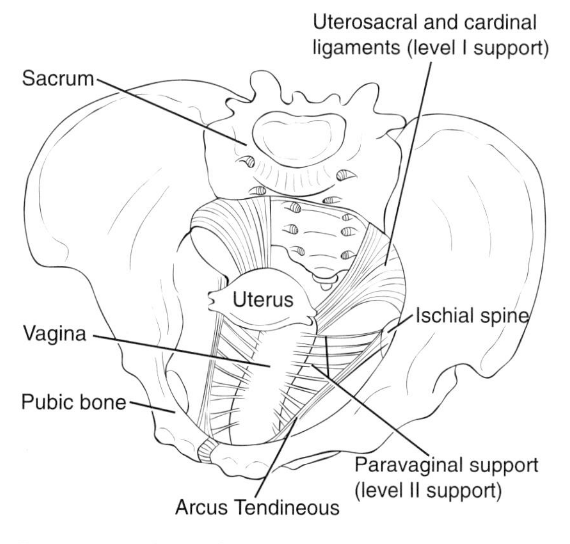

FIGURE 2.7. Endopelvic fascia: "scaffolding" for the pelvic organs.

connective tissues, or endopelvic fasciae, that form this scaffolding are attached to the parietal fasciae from the pelvic inlet and piriformis muscles posteriorly; the anterior border of the greater sciatic foramen, the obturator internus, and the levator ani muscles laterally; and the perineal membrane and perineal body inferiorly. These tissues surround and envelop the visceral arteries and veins, the lymph nodes and channels, and the visceral nerves that service the pelvic organs and tissues. This network of visceral connective tissues suspends the pelvic organs—bladder, urethra, vagina, and lower rectum—over the levator plate, while giving physical support to the many anatomic structures that travel through it. The visceral connective tissues are actually many sheets that fuse into sheaths, or further thicken into stronger septa, depending on the mechanical stress requirements of a particular segment of the visceral suspensory network.

The suspensory network is continuous and interdependent throughout the pelvis and is found beneath the parietal peritoneum and overlying the parietal fascia of the pelvic basin muscles. DeLancey has described three levels of pelvic organ suspension for the purposes of our understanding and visualization.[9]

The "DeLancey Levels" of Pelvic Connective Tissue Support

Level I: Connective tissues include the cardinal and uterosacral ligaments, suspending the cervix and upper vagina into the hollow of the sacrum and over the levator plate

Level II: Suspends each side of the vagina and rectum to the pelvic sidewall. Defines passive support of the bladder, mid- vagina, and rectum beneath the vagina.

Level III: Fusion of the lower third of the vagina and anal canal with the pubococcygeus muscles and perineal body. Secures the vertical orientation of the urethra, lower third of the vagina, and the anal canal in the standing woman.

The *cardinal ligament-uterosacral ligament complexes* (Level I) are formed by multiple sheets of visceral connective tissue that fuse around the internal iliac artery and vein and artery leading to the uterine vessels, and then to the cervix. The supravaginal portion of the cervix is encircled by thicker visceral connective tissue, called the *pericervical ring*. These fused sheets form stronger sheaths and are anchored to the parietal fascia of the piriformis muscles and posterior part of the obturator internus muscles. The inferior and medial part of this sheath is the *uterosacral ligament*, which runs from the posterolateral aspect of the pericervical ring of visceral connective tissue to the tough presacral fascia overlying the edge of the middle sacrum. Running within the cardinal ligament sheath, but anterior to the uterosacral portion, is the ureter.

To explain uterine prolapse and vaginal relaxation, gynecologists, in prior years, felt and taught that these visceral suspensory ligaments became stretched or attenuated. However, observations in the 1970s and 1980s have been incorporated into present day concepts of uterine and vaginal prolapse. We now speak of pelvic organ support defects and site-specific repairs. The visceral connective tissues can be observed to stretch to a point, but then break, or form multiple breaks, to allow the pelvic organs to prolapse down, away from the supporting levator plate. The goal of reparative vaginal surgery is to find the defects in the suspensory network and repair them, usually with permanent suture material.

The Level II axis is oriented horizontally in the standing woman and forms passive platforms. The anterior platform passively supports the bladder and prevents anterior vaginal wall prolapse, better known as cystocele. The posterior platform passively restrains the rectum from protruding into the vagina and, thus, prevents a posterior vaginal wall prolapse, better known as rectocele. These platforms of visceral connective tissues are attached laterally to the sidewalls of the pelvis and posteriorly (proximally) to the pericervical ring. Therefore, these suspensory platforms are anchored posteriorly to the cardinal-uterosacral ligament complexes via their common attachments to the pericervical ring. This is an important concept for the reparative vaginal surgeon. This important junction at the pericervical ring occurs consistently at the anatomic location of the ischial spines, deep within the female pelvis. The anterior horizontal platform between the vagina and the bladder is the pubocervical fascia. The posterior horizontal platform between the vagina and rectum is the rectovaginal fascia, or septum.

The *pubocervical fascia* is the common surgical term for the fibromuscular coat surrounding the vaginal epithelium. This anterior vaginal connective tissue is thickened and attached to each pelvic sidewall by a wing or septum of thickened, visceral connective tissue that forms each anterolateral sulcus found in the vagina of the nulliparous woman. This lateral vaginal septum is anchored to the sidewall by a linear thickening of the parietal fascia overlying the levator ani muscles. This linear structure—named the arcus tendineus fasciae pelvis, or fascial white line—runs from the pubic arch along the pelvic sidewall, ending at the ischial spine. This is a length of approximately 7.5 cm to 9.5 cm. The bladder passively rests upon and is supported by the hammock of pubocervical fascia.

Observed surgically in the retropubic space, the pubocervical fascia and lateral vaginal septum are continuous and appear as a horizontal hammock upon which the bladder passively rests. The proximal or posterior edge of the pubocervical fascia is attached to the pericervical ring at the level of the ischial spines. Thus, the upper edge is pulled back towards the hollow of the sacrum by its attachment to the cardinal-uterosacral ligament complexes. These attachments prevent anterior vaginal wall prolapse or *cystocele* formation. Observations indicate that most cystoceles are the result of upper transverse tears of the pubocervical fascia from one of two structures. The first tear is from the front of the pericervical ring. The second is where the pericervical ring itself transversely tears away from the cardinal-uterosacral ligament complexes. These support defects occur most commonly during vaginal childbirth.

As the anterior vaginal wall prolapse (cystocele) evolves, the pubocervical fascia progressively tears away from the lateral attachments to the fascial white lines, and the anterior vaginal wall progressively falls.

Degrees of Prolapse

These days, many pelvic surgeons use the quantitative "POP-Q" prolapse grading system, which is reviewed in Chapter 5. However, in most primary care settings the following simplified grading scale will suffice:

First Degree: Prolapse bulge extends into the vagina, below the halfway point to hymenal ring
Second Degree: Extends to hymenal ring
Third Degree: Extends beyond the hymenal ring and vaginal introitus (externally visible)
Fourth Degree: Complete prolapse with no visible support remaining

Present-day reparative vaginal surgeons most commonly find transverse tears and paravaginal tears in most anterior vaginal wall prolapses (cystoceles). Therefore, surgical repair entails the reattachment of these connective tissue breaks to their "normal" anatomic attachments—to each arcus tendineus fasciae pelvis laterally and to an apical fixation point at the level of the ischial spines.

Likewise, the urethra has a hammock of pubocervical fascia underneath it, which is attached to each arcus tendineus fascia pelvis. When the woman increases the intrapelvic pressure by Valsalva, the urethra rotates back against the hammock of pubocervical fascia and is compressed. This is an important mechanism of urinary incontinence. A break, or breaks, of this hammock from the lateral pelvic sidewalls, as can occur in vaginal childbirth, produces a hypermobile urethra and stress urinary incontinence. Repair entails the restoration of this suburethral hammock. There are various surgical means to do this. Reflections of the pubocervical fascia around the middle third of the urethra to the underside of the pubic arch are modified histologically and called the pubourethral ligaments

Concerning the posterior vaginal wall and prevention of a prolapse or rectocele, the intact rectovaginal fascia or septum is found in the rectovaginal space and is attached to the pelvic sidewalls laterally, and then posteriorly, to the uterosacral ligaments and cervix. Likewise, vaginal childbirth can cause detachment of the rectovaginal fascia from its attachments, thus resulting in posterior vaginal wall prolapse or varying degrees of *rectocele*. Prolapse to the mid-vagina is a first-degree rectocele; to the introitus, second-degree; and outside the vagina, third-degree. Complete posterior vaginal wall prolapse is a fourth-degree rectocele. Most posterior defects are a transverse tear of the upper edge of the rectovaginal fascia from the uterosacral ligaments, with progression to lateral tears away from the sidewalls.

Occasionally, the transverse defect can occur from the apex of the perineal body. Repair entails finding and suturing the fascial defects to their "normal" anatomic positions. Many rectoceles are also accompanied by an enterocele.

Richardson has defined *enterocele* as a detachment of the pubocervical fascia from the rectovaginal septum, thus allowing the peritoneum to push the vaginal apex down into the vaginal canal.[10] Therefore, surgical repair of an enterocele now entails the reconstruction of the pericervical ring by attaching the pubocervical fascia to the rectovaginal fascia and, then, attaching this to each uterosacral ligament at the level of the ischial spines. This can be accomplished through either the vaginal route or an abdominal approach.

Conclusion

The restoration of "normal" vaginal and pelvic anatomic relationships is the goal of the vaginal surgeon. Surgical placement of the upper vagina and rectum over the levator plate is paramount. This is done by finding and repairing the defects in the suspensory network of visceral connective tissues found in the female pelvis. Reconstruction of the perineal body is just as important. Repair of prolapse can be accomplished vaginally, abdominally, or laparoscopically. We continue to study and better understand the science of pelvic organ prolapse and dysfunction and to improve the art of surgical repair of vaginal support defects.

For primary care practitioners, an improved understanding of female pelvic anatomy will allow for more accurate identification of problems and more opportunities to provide relief.

Key Points

- The foundation of "normal" female pelvic anatomy includes a strong horizontal orientation to the levator muscle plate. The intact levator plate acts as a "flap valve", supporting the upper two-thirds of the vagina and the rectum in a horizontal position. In many cases, loss of the horizontal levator plate may be the seminal event leading to prolapse.
- The *ischial spine* is a key landmark for learning and understanding female pelvic support anatomy. Vaginal suspension surgeries strive to support the vaginal apex to the depth of the ischial spine, using a variety of nearby muscular and ligamentous structures (e.g. sacrospinous, iliococcygeus, uterosacral).
- The pelvic connective tissue "scaffolding" consists of collagen, elastin and smooth muscle. This network of visceral connective tissue suspends the pelvic organs—bladder, urethra, vagina, and lower rectum—and tethers these organs to fixed pelvic sidewall structures.
- Anatomic boundaries of the female pelvis are *pubic bone* (front wall), *obturator internus* (side wall), *levator ani* (floor), and *piriformis* (back wall).

References

1. Bent AE. Pathophysiology. In: Bent AE, Ostergard DR, Cundiff GW et al., eds. *Urogynecology and Pelvic Floor Dysfunction, 5th ed.* Philadelphia: Lippincott Williams & Wilkins; 2003:43–50.
2. DeLancey JOL. Vaginographic examination of the pelvic floor. *Int Urogynecol J.* 1994;5:19–24.
3. DeLancey JOL. Standing anatomy of the pelvic floor. *J Pelvic Surg.* 1996;2:260–263.
4. Retzky SS, Rogers RM, Richardson AC. Anatomy of female pelvic support. In: Brubaker LT, Saclarides TJ, eds. *The Female Pelvic Floor: Disorders of Function and Support.* Philadelphia: FA Davis; 1996: 3–21.
5. Williams PL, Bannister LH, Berry MM et al., eds. *Gray's Anatomy: The Anatomical Basis of Medicine and Surgery*, 38th ed. New York: Churchhill Livingstone; 1995:678.
6. Rogers RM. Anatomy of pelvic support. In: Bent AE, Ostergard DR, Cundiff GW et al., eds. *Urogynecology and Pelvic Floor Dysfunction,* 5th ed. Philadelphia: Lippincott Williams & Wilkins; 2003;19–33.
7. Uhlenhuth E, Day EC, Smith RD et al. The visceral endopelvic fascia and the hypogastric sheath. *Surg Gynecol Obstet.* 1948;86:9–28.
8. Peham HV, Amreich J. *Operative Gynecology.* Vol 1. Philadelphia: JB Lippincott Company; 1934;166–242.
9. DeLancey JOL. Anatomic aspects of vaginal eversion after hysterectomy. *Am J Obstet Gynecol.* 1992; 166:1717–1728.
10. Richardson AC. The anatomic defects in rectocele and enterocele. *J Pelvic Surg.* 1995;1:214–221.

3 Effects of Pregnancy and Childbirth on the Pelvic Floor

Roger P. Goldberg

Childbirth and the Pelvic Floor

For many women, pregnancy, as well as labor and delivery, represent the key physiological events predisposing to incontinence and pelvic floor dysfunction. Our knowledge of obstetrical pelvic floor injuries, and their connection to incontinence and pelvic floor disorders later on, has vastly increased in recent years. Primary care clinicians addressing urogynecology problems should be aware of the potential effects of pregnancy and childbirth on the pelvic floor.

The basic foundation of female pelvic support consists of the paired levator ani muscles,[1,2] whose position is maintained by endopelvic connective tissue, and tone preserved by nerves arising from the lumbosacral roots. All of these components—muscular anatomy, connective tissue supports, and nerve supply—are exposed to acute physical strains during childbirth, as well as to chronic "wear and tear" resulting from intraperitoneal forces.

Injury to the pelvic floor commonly accompanies even a seemingly uneventful childbirth, and perhaps this should come as little surprise. After all, a woman's first vaginal birth routinely involves soft tissue compression lasting for hours. The second ("pushing") stage of labor generates pressure between the fetal head and vaginal wall averaging 100 mmHg and reaching as high as 230 mmHg. When applied over many hours, these obstetrical forces often result in permanent physical and functional changes. (Figure 3.1)

Perineum and Anorectum

Injury to the perineum, whether from episiotomy or spontaneous laceration, may result in loss of vaginal or rectal tone and/or anal incontinence. External anal sphincter defects can be identified by endoanal ultrasound in 20% to 53% of women after normal vaginal delivery,[3–7] a possible risk factor for anal incontinence that will be subsequently reported in 4% to 50% of cases.[8–13] Flatal incontinence is reported six times more often by women who have experienced an anal sphincter injury during delivery.[8] The risk of anal incontinence is increased with prolonged labor, forceps use, and episiotomy.[14] The *internal* anal sphincter, extending an additional 12 mm cranial to the external sphincter margin, is prone to disruption by perineal lacerations and may be commonly overlooked during primary obstetrical repair.[15] Using transanal ultrasonography, internal anal sphincter lacerations have been identified in 17% of primiparas experiencing no visible perineal injury at delivery.[16]

Neurological injury to the anal sphincter may also play a role, explaining why normal function may not always be restored by surgical repair. Prolonged motor latencies may persist in the internal (upper) anal sphincter for up to five months after vaginal delivery.[17] Because of the limitations associated with the surgical repair of severe perineal and anorectal injuries, primary prevention of obstetrical trauma at the time of delivery should be considered the best approach for reducing chronic post-reproductive dysfunction in these areas. (Figure 3.2)

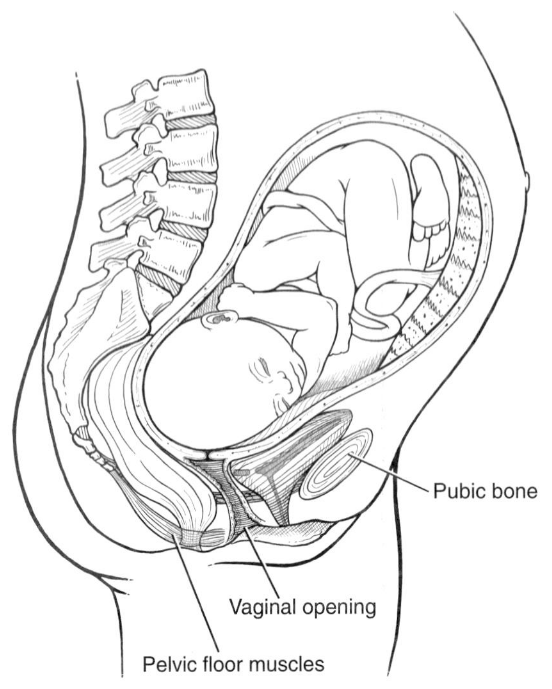

FIGURE 3.1. Pelvic organs and pelvic floor during pregnancy.

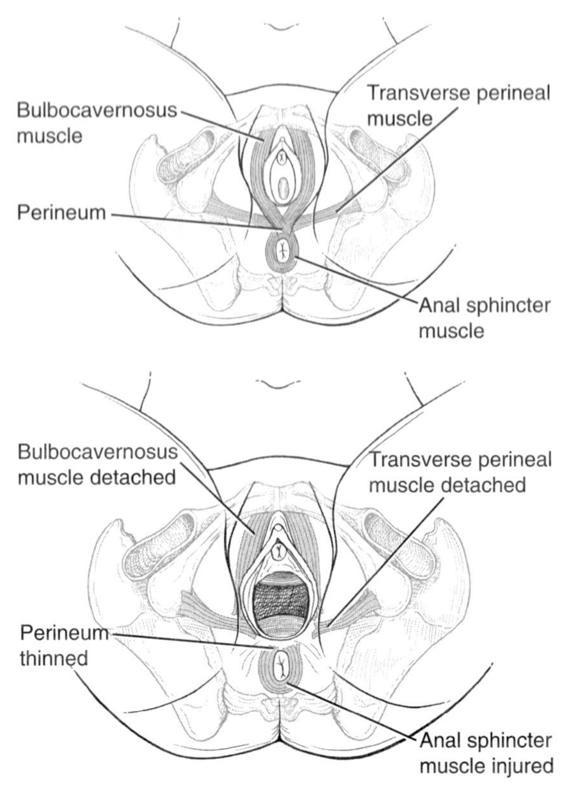

FIGURE 3.2. Perineal anatomy before and after childbirth.

Episiotomy

The routine use of episiotomy was once thought to provide an array of maternal benefits including preservation of pelvic muscle tone and sexual function, improved perineal healing, and reduced rates of anal sphincter injury. However, the bulk of modern evidence strongly suggests that episiotomies increase, rather than decrease, the risk of pelvic floor dysfunction.

Midline episiotomy has been associated with a sharply elevated risk of severe lacerations into the vagina, perineum, and rectum.[18–20] Mediolateral episiotomies carry a much lower (1% to 2%) likelihood of anorectal injury. (Figure 3.3)

Episiotomies are associated with slower and less complete recovery of pelvic floor muscle strength than is experienced with either an intact perineum after delivery or spontaneous perineal lacerations.[19,21] Pain and healing complications are more common when episiotomies are performed routinely rather than selectively, according to one randomized trial of selective episiotomy (RCT).[22] A separate RCT[23] found that nearly all

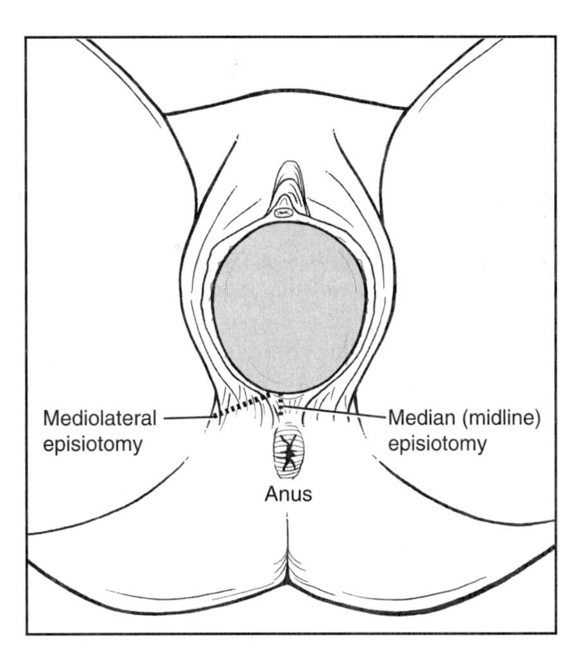

FIGURE 3.3. Episiotomy types: Median and mediolateral.

perineal lacerations involving the anal sphincter were associated with midline episiotomy (46 of 47 in primiparous women and 6 of 6 among multiparous women). The authors concluded that restriction of episiotomy use among multiparous women results in significantly less perineal injury. A retrospective cohort study[24] found midline episiotomy to be associated with an elevated risk of fecal incontinence at three (odds ratio 5.5) and six (3.7) months postpartum compared with women with an intact perineum. Compared to spontaneous laceration, episiotomy tripled the risk of fecal incontinence at three months (95% confidence interval 1.3 to 7.9) and six months (0.7 to 11.2) postpartum, and doubled the risk of flatal incontinence at three (1.3 to 3.4) and six months (1.2 to 3.7).

The relationship between episiotomy and sexual function is not fully clear although, at three months postpartum, sexual satisfaction appears to be highest among women without perineal injury, and lowest among women with an episiotomy that had extended during birth.[19] One other study demonstrated the highest level of satisfaction among women whose perineum remained intact during delivery, but found no difference between women who had undergone episiotomy and those who had experienced spontaneous perineal laceration.[25]

Although selective episiotomies have a significant place in obstetrical practice, their routine use is not justified. A Cochrane report[26] concluded that the practice of routine episiotomy increases the overall risk of maternal trauma and complications during vaginal birth. The American College of Obstetricians and Gynecologists (ACOG) has formally stated that routine episiotomy should not be considered a part of current obstetrical practice.

Levator Ani Muscles and Childbirth

The levator ani muscles represent the core of pelvic floor support, providing a muscular buffer against the constant downward force of the pelvic and abdominal organs. Obstetrical injuries to the levator ani muscles and their nerve supply may, in many instances, represent the seminal events eventually leading to pelvic prolapse or incontinence. Trauma to the levator ani may include detachment of individual muscle components from their insertion points along the pelvic sidewalls. Generalized atrophy of these levators may result from pudendal nerve trauma.

Peschers et al.[27] evaluated levator ani function before and after childbirth, and found that muscle strength was significantly reduced three- to eight-days postpartum following vaginal birth, but not after cesarean, and returned to normal values within two months for most women. Allen and Hosker[28] also demonstrated a persistent reduction in muscle contraction strength. Using MRI to compare levator ani anatomy in nulliparous women against those after their first vaginal birth, DeLancey et al.[29] found no levator ani defects in the nulliparas. Twenty percent of primiparous women had a visible defect in the levator ani muscle, with the majority of defects seen in the pubovisceral ("Kegel") portion of the levator ani.

Pudendal Nerve Changes

Pelvic floor neuropathy is a common repercussion of childbirth—less often recognized than vaginal and perineal injury, but arguably more significant as a risk factor for subsequent pelvic floor dysfunction. The pudendal nerve, arising from the S2-S4 nerve roots, supplies most of the anatomic structures maintaining pelvic support and continence—including the perineum and vagina, levator muscle complex, and anus. Compression and stretching of the pudendal nerve during childbirth appears to be a major risk factor associated with subsequent diminished levator muscle function. As a result of neuropathic changes, the sling-like components of the levator complex, such as the pubococcygeus muscle, may fail to reflexively contract and elevate sphincter pressure during a cough or sneeze. Likewise, the resting tone of the shelf-like levator plate and perineal body may diminish.

Stretching and compression of the pudendal nerve appears to be particularly vulnerable as the fetus descends past the ischial spine in the midpelvis. Snooks and Swash[30] reported that partially reversible pudendal nerve injury occurs commonly with vaginal birth, an effect that appears to be prevented by cesarean delivery.[77] Rates of nerve injury are increased with forceps delivery, multiparity, longer second-stage labor, third-degree perineal tear, and macrosomia.[28,31] Denervation within the pubococcygeus and anal sphincter muscles accompanies 42% to 80% of vaginal deliveries.[30] Although some reinnervation by surrounding nerves may occur, permanent loss of muscle function is common.[32,33] Cesarean delivery appears to effectively prevent denervation injuries when performed electively, but does not confer full protection if performed after the onset of labor.

For many women, pelvic neuropathy will have no clinical consequences; for others, these nerve injuries initiate a pathophysiologic sequence eventually leading to incontinence, prolapse and pelvic floor dysfunction. Pudendal conduction abnormalities[34,35] and denervation of the pelvic floor after childbirth have been associated with both genital prolapse and urinary incontinence.[36] Snooks et al.[33] demonstrated that denervation–reinnervation patterns on electromyography may become more pronounced with increased passage of time from delivery and indicate higher risks of urinary and fecal incontinence. Anal incontinence is associated with pelvic floor neuropathy in up to 75% to 80% of cases.[30,37] Among multiparas, levator denervation occurs in up to 50% of women with symptomatic pelvic organ prolapse.[39,40] To what extent these changes to the levator ani musculature represent a direct cause or consequence of pelvic organ prolapse is not fully certain. (Figure 3.4)

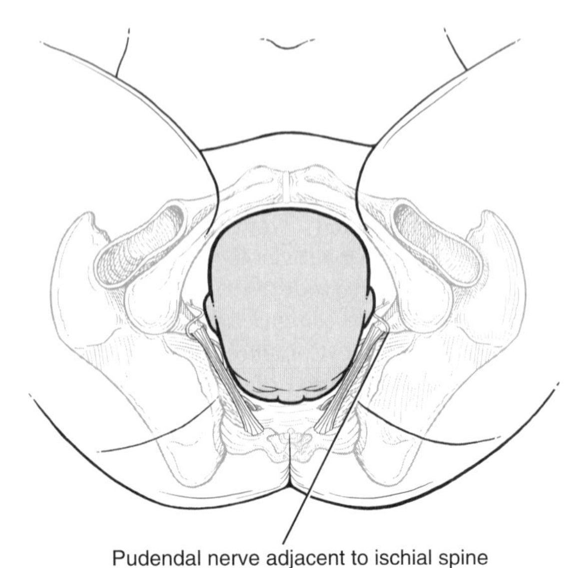

FIGURE 3.4. Compression of pudendal nerve during labor.

Connective Tissues and Ligaments

In the etiology of post-childbearing pelvic floor disorders, endopelvic connective tissue injuries have an established role.[41] Recent efforts have been focused on identifying "site specific" breaks and detachments of the endopelvic connective tissue from their anatomical insertion sites, as the origins for pelvic organ prolapse.[42] These include paravaginal defects in the anterior vaginal compartment, site-specific defects in the rectovaginal (Denonvilliers) fascia, and ligamentous/fascial detachments of the vaginal apex. Stretch injuries to the endopelvic connective tissue during childbirth may account for various other forms of prolapse outlined in other chapters.

Urinary Incontinence and Childbirth: The Connection

Stress urinary incontinence occurs symptomatically in 32% to85% of pregnant women, peaking in the third trimester.[43–45] Francis[43] showed an intrapartum prevalence of 85% in multiparas and 53% in nulliparas, with nearly half of these patients noting some degree of incontinence before the observed pregnancy. When SUI arises with pregnancy and childbirth, it may often fail to resolve. Stanton et al.[46] found 38% of nulliparas had SUI during the third trimester and 6% had persistent postpartum leakage. Among 98 multiparas, 10% had SUI prior to pregnancy, 42% had SUI in the third trimester and 11% had persistent postpartum incontinence. Meyer et al.[47] found that 22% of patients with stress incontinence during pregnancy had persistence after delivery.

Mode of delivery may have a significant impact on the persistence of incontinence. Viktrup et al.[43] prospectively studied incontinence symptoms before, during, and after pregnancy in 305 primiparous women. The multivariate analysis identified the length of labor pushing, fetal head circumference, episiotomy, and birth weight as risk factors for postpartum SUI, whereas cesarean birth was protective against incontinence. Among women with SUI during pregnancy, 21 of 167 women (13%) had persistent incontinence postpartum compared to none of the 35 delivered by cesarean ($p < 0.05$). At three months postpartum only 4% had persistent stress incontinence complaints; after one year, only 3% still had leakage. However, in subsequent pregnancies it appears that these patients are at greater risk for more severe incontinence, with earlier onset and persistence beyond the puerperium. Viktrup and Lose[48] questioned 91% of their cohort five years later and found a 30% prevalence of SUI. Nineteen percent of women who were not incontinent in the original trial developed SUI during that time period. Again, cesarean delivery was found to significantly decrease the risk of incontinence.

Anatomically speaking, urethral hypermobility is an important change associated with SUI[49,50] and is significantly increased after vaginal delivery when compared to cesarean delivery in both primiparous and multiparous women ($p < 0.001$).[51] Vaginal delivery is also associated with decreased urethral closure pressure and functional urethral length[52]; the absence of these changes after cesarean delivery highlights the importance of birth mode rather than of only pregnancy.

One common question is whether the risk of incontinence and pelvic floor dysfunction increases with subsequent deliveries or whether the majority of damage occurs with the first birth. Some work[53] has suggested that childbearing beyond the first delivery has minimal impact on pelvic floor neurophysiology and that most pudendal nerve damage occurs during the first vaginal delivery. Hojberg et al.[54] reported that the first vaginal delivery was the major risk factor for incontinence, and subsequent deliveries had little effect. However, other population-based observational studies and prospective trials have shown strong associations between SUI and increasing parity.[55] Moller et al,[56] for instance, found an association of parity and stress incontinence with an odds ratio of 2.2 after one vaginal delivery, 3.9 after a second vaginal delivery, and 4.5 after a third delivery. Marshall et al.[45] studied 7771 women early in puerperium and found a strong association between parity and stress incontinence. A 1989 consensus conference of the National Institutes of Health identified parity as an established risk factor for urinary incontinence.[58]

Sexual Function

Female sexual problems after childbirth—those occurring during the postpartum period and others presenting years later—receive little attention in clinical practice, even in the "age of Viagra." But various studies indicate that approximately one in four childbearing women report adverse sexual changes persisting beyond six months postpartum, with 17% reporting painful intercourse. Among women with overactive bladders, 23.8% report that this bladder condition impacts their sex lives.[59] Coital incontinence (leakage during sex) is reported by one in four sexually active women in a urogynecologic setting, and 72% report that it adversely affects their sexual enjoyment.

The physiological changes accounting for loss of sexual function may include pudendal nerve injury, poor perineal healing, vaginal laxity, and loss of levator ani muscle tone. One study found that persistent dyspareunia at 6 months was least likely after cesarean birth (3.4%), and most likely after operative vaginal delivery (14%).[60] However, a recent study comparing 562 identical twin sisters (the first study comparing parous and nonparous women) found that total parity—and not the mode of delivery—was the primary determinant of sexual dysfunction as measured by the validated "PISQ" (Pelvic Organ Prolapse-Incontinence) sexual quality-of-life questionnaire.[60a] The good news? Twenty-five percent of women enjoy sex *more* after their first childbirth than before conception—perhaps due to loss of psychological inhibition or in some cases, perineal and vaginal relaxation providing relief of entry dyspareunia or vaginismus.

Validated questionnaires now exist for primary care providers interested in screening for these conditions and assessing their impact on quality of life. But in fact, asking a few pointed questions *(such as "do you have any problems with sexual function that you wish to discuss?")* can be a very effective means of identifying patients in your practice who would benefit from referral. Female sexual disorders and associated treatment strategies are discussed in Chapter 11.

Preventing Obstetrical Pelvic Floor Injury

It could be argued that pelvic floor disorders are "inevitable" consequences of childbirth just as skin cancer is an "inevitable" consequence of sun exposure. Both are associated with identifiable risk factors, both can greatly affect quality of life, and both are preventable in many cases. Primary care clinicians are in a unique role to dispel the myth that incontinence and pelvic disorders are unavoidable costs of motherhood and to encourage strategies for reducing the risk of these disorders.

During Pregnancy

Daily pelvic floor exercises may consist of 20 to 30 daily repetitions throughout pregnancy and are discussed in Chapter 6. Improved tone and effective isolation of the pelvic floor muscles may enhance the patient's ability to voluntarily relax them during labor and delivery. Prenatal pelvic floor exercises may reduce the likelihood of incontinence symptoms after delivery.[61,62] Perineal massage is another low-tech modality that involves gentle stretching of the lubricated perineum in preparation for delivery. Two studies of perineal massage begun during the third trimester have reported a modestly decreased risk of perineal laceration, ranging from 9% to 12%.[63,64]

Patients should be encouraged to avoid excessive weight gain—not only for the sake of their general health maintenance, but also to reduce the strain of pregnancy and childbirth on the pelvic floor. One study demonstrated that, although the postpartum improvement of transient urinary incontinence during pregnancy is common, *persistent* leakage is more likely among women who gain more weight before delivery. Body mass index ≥30 has been identified as a risk factor for postpartum SUI and urgency.[65,66] A reasonable target for weight gain is roughly 2 lbs to 4 lbs during the first trimester and one pound per week thereafter, translating into 25 lbs to 35 lbs for a full-term pregnancy. For women with preexisting obesity, significantly less weight gain is acceptable. Exercise during pregnancy should be tailored to specific considerations including changes in posture, balance, and coordination; altered respiratory patterns; increased joint and ligament mobility due to relaxin; and increased vulnerability of the pelvic floor beneath the gravid uterus.

Avoiding constipation is another important strategy for minimizing pelvic floor strain during pregnancy, as gastrointestinal motility decreases due, in part, to increased progesterone and iron supplementation. Valsalva straining during defecation increases stress on pelvic floor supports and should be discouraged as a chronic habit. Dietary fiber should be accompanied by adequate hydration, exercise, and stool softeners.

Labor and Delivery: The Pelvic Floor Perspective

Pushing Positions & Techniques

The most common labor strategy in modern obstetrical settings involves pushing in the lithotomy position, starting right after full cervical dilation is determined by vaginal examination. However, a number of approaches actually exist, and their potential effects on the pelvic floor should be considered. Full dilation, it should be understood, refers exclusively to the cervix; from the standpoint of the major pelvic floor supports discussed in this and other chapters, an enormous degree of tissue dilation has yet to occur for most women.

As mentioned, lithotomy is a common labor position, with the lower extremities flexed and abducted during each contraction. Although some practitioners suspect that the "uphill" orientation of this position may increase the difficulty of delivery, specific disadvantages for pelvic floor function have not been proven. Squatting is purported to increase the diameter of the pelvic outlet and help shift the tailbone posteriorly and has been associated with reduced rates of forceps delivery and perineal lacerations when compared with a semi-recumbent position.[67,68] (Figure 3.5)

Sitting has been associated with quicker labor; however, studies evaluating birthing chairs have

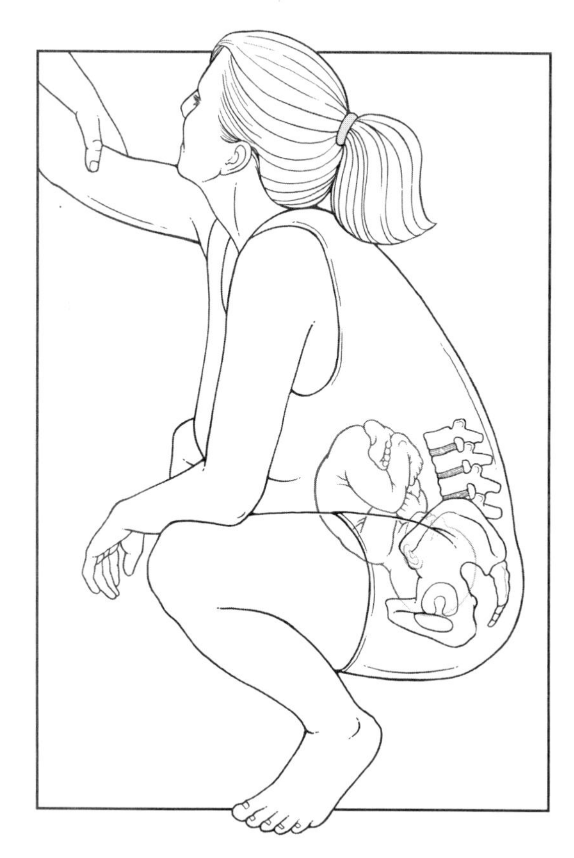

FIGURE 3.5. Woman squatting during labor.

shown a greater likelihood of perineal swelling and labial lacerations, as well as increased blood loss. Lateral positioning ("side lying") may be useful for multiparous women with an already-relaxed introitus by improving control over the speed of fetal expulsion at the end of second stage labor, thereby helping to avoid perineal injury caused by a precipitous delivery. Upright ("stand and deliver") positioning has been advocated as a means to shorten labor and reduce the need for forceps or vacuum assistance. Randomized trials have found lower rates of perineal injury and postpartum pain, with a decreased risk of undergoing episiotomy, in upright positioning as compared with lithotomy.[69] A Cochrane analysis concluded similar benefits of upright or lateral, compared with supine, positioning.[70] The upright, sitting, and squatting positions should be avoided if significant perineal swelling develops.

Immediate versus Delayed Pushing

Advocates of early pushing (beginning at full cervical dilation) argue that the duration of labor grows too long in the absence of a constant maternal expulsive effort, introducing more stress for the baby and a greater likelihood of maternal neuromuscular injury. Critics of active pushing, on the other hand, maintain that early or aggressive pushing shortens labor to a lesser degree than is often assumed, while increasing maternal exhaustion, stressing the pelvic floor supports, and possibly increasing the risk for pelvic injury. Among primigravid women, active pushing for longer than one hour has been shown to confer an increased risk of pudendal neuropathy and denervation injury.

"Delayed" pushing usually means resisting the urge to push while allowing the fetus to passively descend past the pelvic supports. One multicenter study[71] evaluated a delayed pushing strategy among 1862 nulliparous women, all with epidural analgesia, randomized to either immediate pushing at full dilation or delayed pushing for up to two hours before pushing. Difficult deliveries were less likely in the delayed pushing group, and forceps assistance was less often necessary. A more recent randomized controlled trial of delayed pushing found no increase in adverse events, despite prolongation of second stage of up to 4.9 hours.[72] Physiologic (or spontaneous) pushing is similar to the delayed approach, involving a delay until the onset of an overwhelming physical urge. One comparative study found that advanced perineal lacerations were less likely, and an intact perineum more likely, with spontaneous rather than directed pushing[73]. In contrast, another RCT of 350 women found no differences between active or spontaneous pushing with respect to perineal injury or duration of labor.[74]

Longer pushing stages appear to be associated with higher rates of pelvic floor injury and neuropathy. Pushing longer than 2 hours has been associated with higher rates of new-onset flatal incontinence (73% vs 44%).[75] A prolonged pushing stage may also predispose to maternal exhaustion. If this results in a greater likelihood of operative delivery by forceps or vacuum, the increased risk for pelvic floor injury resulting from these interventions should be recognized.

Forceps and Vacuum: Impact on Pelvic Function

Although in years past both forceps and vacuum procedures were advocated as a means to avoid pelvic injury and provide a more controlled delivery, today it is widely accepted that operative delivery tends to increase, rather than decrease, the risk of perineal injury and often has a negative impact on other pelvic floor structures.[76] Although vacuum and forceps procedures retain a valuable role in obstetrical care, they should not be routinely performed.

Forceps delivery markedly increases the risk of advanced perineal lacerations[77] as well as pelvic neuropathy—perhaps not surprising, since the average force of forceps against the surrounding pelvic tissues has been estimated at 75psi. Up to 80% of women who undergo forceps delivery will have anal sphincter injuries detectable by transanal ultrasound.[4] Forceps use also confers an elevated risk of urinary incontinence. In fact, one study indicated the odds of SUI seven years after childbirth may be up to 10 times higher among women with a previous forceps delivery.[78] Compared with spontaneous vaginal delivery, urinary incontinence after forceps delivery is more likely to persist compared with cases presenting after spontaneous vaginal or vacuum delivery.[79] Women have significantly weaker levator and anal strength after forceps delivery compared with those who had a spontaneous vaginal birth.[80]

There is evidence to suggest that, compared with forceps, vacuum delivery is generally associated with lower rates of severe perineal lacerations and anal injury.[81–83] A Cochrane report concluded that vacuum delivery is associated with significantly less risk of perineal injury compared with forceps.[84]

Pelvic Risks of Macrosomia

Macrosomia is associated with a variety of potential fetal problems, including birth trauma, shoulder dystocia, and lower Apgar scores. On the maternal side, potential complications include higher rates of spontaneous perineal injury and episiotomies and increased risk of perineal injuries involving the anorectum,[20,85–87] pudendal nerve injury,[88] and significantly weaker anal squeeze pressures.[89] Vaginal delivery of one or more babies weighing at least 4000 grams raises the risk of long-term stress incontinence.[90] A decision analysis of elective cesarean delivery for macrosomia determined that a policy of elective cesarean delivery would prevent one case of anal incontinence for every 539 such performed. The expected quality of life associated with the elective cesarean delivery policy was also greater.[91]

Elective Cesarean Delivery to Protect the Pelvic Floor

The use of cesarean delivery for the prevention of pelvic injury is a divisive issue and the subject of much ongoing debate. In a 1996 survey of obstetricians published in the Lancet,[92] 31% of female obstetricians reported that for an ordinary full-term pregnancy they would personally select cesarean over vaginal delivery, and 80% of this subgroup cited concern over perineal injury as their main rationale. A similar survey conducted among 135 midwives, in contrast, found that only 6% would choose cesarean delivery to protect their pelvic floor. Whether this reflects the fact that midwives provide care only to women before and during childbirth, and are not usually exposed to their pelvic floor problems later in life, is unclear.

Medically, it is important to emphasize that pregnancy itself may for some women be enough to cause pelvic floor injury, with the route of delivery playing only a minor role. Nonetheless, cesarean birth clearly appears to reduce the likelihood of several different pelvic floor disorders. Pelvic nerve and muscle function are generally protected by cesarean delivery,[88] with the timing of intervention largely determining the degree of protection. When cesareans were performed before the onset of first labor, pudendal nerve injury is effectively prevented.[93] Clearly, the most protective cesarean deliveries appear to be those performed before the onset of a woman's first labor.

Stress urinary incontinence is less common after cesarean delivery compared with vaginal birth, although it is not fully eliminated.[43,95] A recent study of 542 identical twin sisters[96] provided new insight into the relationship between obstetrical delivery mode and stress urinary incontinence among younger post-reproductive women (mean age 47 years). By comparing genetically identified individuals, the identical twin study design offered a unique biological control group that facilitated the analysis of environmental determinants. The major environmental predictors of stress urinary incontinence were parity ($P = .001$), obesity ($P = .002$), and birth mode, with vaginal delivery conferring a considerable increase in the risk of SUI relative to cesarean birth (odds ratio 2.28, 95% confidence interval 1.14 to 4.55, $P = .019$). It was concluded that among premenopausal childbearing women, vaginal delivery mode represents a potent determinant of stress urinary incontinence, carrying more than twice the risk of cesarean delivery.

Anal sphincter lacerations are nearly nonexistent after cesarean deliveries that are performed before the onset of labor.[97] And yet, since anal incontinence is a relatively uncommon outcome, it remains uncertain under which circumstances an elective cesarean delivery would be an appropriate consideration for preventing anal injury.

Even if the likelihood of pelvic floor dysfunction could be decreased by elective cesarean for some women, in this debate it is essential to factor the broad medical impact and costs that would be required to achieve this narrow gain. Cesarean birth is by no means always in the best interest of mother or baby. Thus, despite the fact that up to 31% of British female obstetricians would personally choose a cesarean birth for themselves, most societies remain appropriately ambivalent regarding each woman's right to choose cesarean birth.

Postpartum Strategies

Surprisingly little attention is devoted to recuperation of the pelvic floor after delivery, despite the remarkable level of physical stress it has just endured. Immediately postpartum, strategies for pelvic floor recuperation should be discussed. Perineal care may include ice packs and lower extremity elevation to counteract swelling. Perineal hygiene is important to avoid infection and early suture breakdown. Lotions and ointments, and direct scrubbing of the perineal area, should be avoided. Breastfeeding may contribute to vaginal discomfort, as hypoestrogenic changes throughout the vagina and lower urinary tract result in dryness and atrophy, diminished urethral function, and occasionally increased severity of stress and urge incontinence. Estrogen-dependent symptoms will improve after the cessation of breastfeeding as normal ovarian function resumes.

Pelvic floor exercises should be resumed during the postpartum period. An appropriate postpartum Kegel exercise routine may consist of 2 to 5 daily sessions of 10 to 20 slow levator contractions for up to 10 seconds, as outlined in Chapter 6. Exercising in the recumbent position may help to minimize caudal traction on the pelvic floor supports before full involution of the uterine fundus. Several studies have demonstrated the potential efficacy of postpartum pelvic floor exercises in preventing incontinence and other pelvic floor symptoms.[98–101] Morkved and Bo demonstrated that postpartum urinary incontinence could be reduced by eight weeks of structured group training, combined with home exercises three times weekly, and that benefits are still present at one year postpartum. When pelvic floor exercises are combined with biofeedback and electrostimulation, stress incontinence is reduced for up to 19% of women.[98] For any exercise-based regimen, it is important to consider that sustained symptom relief will require a long-term daily commitment, which becomes unrealistic for many women to maintain. If incontinence or pelvic symptoms persist beyond 3 to 6 months postpartum, referral should be strongly considered.

Constipation and straining should be avoided to protect the integrity of perineal sutures and to minimize stress against the pelvic floor. For multiparas with descent of the perineal body, perineal branches of the pudendal nerve may be particularly prone to cumulative stretch injury during physical straining. Dietary fiber and stool softeners, along with occasional laxatives or suppositories, should be used as needed. Women returning to exercise and physical activity should take into consideration the vulnerability of pelvic floor supports, with limited weight bearing for the first several months to reduce abdominopelvic straining. Bracing the pelvic floor (quick flexion of the pelvic floor muscles) during sudden physical stress may be useful for reducing leakage episodes and repetitive strain on the pelvic floor supports.

Conclusions

Primary care clinicians are in the unique position of encountering women before, during, and long after their childbearing; and at all stages, attention to pelvic floor issues can positively influence a woman's quality of life. In some cases, postreproductive problems can be prevented. In other cases, early recognition can allow an affected individual to avoid long-term incontinence and pelvic floor dysfunction—conditions that generations of women have suffered in silence. The basic connections between childbirth and the pelvic floor—indeed, between obstetrics and gynecology—should be familiar to all practitioners interested in treating these important female disorders.

Key Points

- Whether childbirth is long or short, easy or difficult, millions of women experience physical sequelae in the years and decades that follow. Pudendal nerve abnormalities, and levator muscle injuries, are relatively common.
- Mode of delivery appears to play an important role in the risk of stress incontinence in premenopausal women. Differences in SUI rates diminish after menopause, and with the great equalizer of advancing age.
- Risk factors for various types of injury include vaginal birth mode, episiotomy, macrosomia, and operative delivery.
  - Strategies for improving pelvic health, and avoiding injury, exist for before, during, and after childbirth. Examples include pelvic floor conditioning, avoidance of routine episiotomy and operative vaginal delivery, avoidance of prolonged second stage labor, and attention to pelvic floor rehabilitation during the postpartum period.

References

1. DeLancey JO. Anatomy and biomechanics of genital prolapse. *Clin Obstet Gynecol.* 1993;36:897–909.
2. Wall LL. The muscles of the pelvic floor. *Clin Obstet Gynecol.* 1993;36:910–925.
3. Burnett SJ, Spence-Jones C, Speakman CT, Kamm MA, Hudson CN, Bartram CI. Unsuspected sphincter damage following childbirth revealed by anal endosonography. *Br J Radiol.* 1991;64:225–227.
4. Sultan AH, Kamm MA, Hudson CN, Thomas JM, Bartram CI. Anal sphincter disruption during vaginal delivery. *N Engl J Med.* 1993;329:1905–1911.
5. Rieger N, Schloithe A, Saccone G, Wattchow D. A prospective study of anal sphincter injury due to childbirth. *Scand J Gastroenterol.* 1998;33:950–955.
6. Campbell DM, Behan M, Donnelly VS, O'Herlihy C, O'Connell PR. Endosonographic assessment of postpartum anal sphincter injury using a 120 degree sector scanner. *Clin Radiol.* 1996;51:559–561.
7. Zetterstrom J, Mellgren A, Jensen LL et al. Effect of delivery on anal sphincter morphology and function. *Dis Colon Rectum.* 1999;42(10):1253–1260.
8. Crawford LA, Quint EH, Pearl ML, DeLancey JO. Incontinence following rupture of the anal sphincter during delivery. *Obstet Gynecol.* 1993;82:527–531.
9. Bek KM, Laurberg S. Risks of anal incontinence from subsequent vaginal delivery after a complete obstetric anal sphincter tear. *Br J Obstet Gynaecol.* 1992;99:724–726.
10. Go PM, Dunselman GA. Anatomic and functional results of surgical repair after total perineal rupture at delivery. *Surg Gynecol Obstet.* 1988;166:121–124.
11. Mellerup Sorenson S, Bondesen H, Istre O, Vilmann P. Perineal rupture following vaginal delivery: long-term consequences. *Acta Obstet Gynecol Scand.* 1988;67:315–318.
12. Faltin DL, Sangalli MR, Roche B, Floris L, Boulvain M, Weil A. Does a second delivery increase the risk of anal incontinence? *Br J Obstet Gynaecol.* 2001;108:684–688.
13. Fornell EK, Berg G, Hallbook O, Matthiesen LS, Sjodahal R. Clinical consequences of anal sphincter rupture during vaginal delivery. *J Am Coll Surg.* 1996;183:553–558.
14. Groutz A, Fait G, Lessing JB, David MP, Wolman I, Jaffa A, Gordon D. Incidence and obstetric risk

factors of postpartum anal incontinence. *Scand J Gastroenterol.* 1999;34:315–318.

15. DeLancey JO, Toglia MR, Perucchini D. Internal and external anal sphincter anatomy as it relates to midline obstetric lacerations. *Obstet Gynecol.* 1997;90:924–927.
16. Sultan AH, Kamm MA, Hudson CN, Thomas JM, Bartram CI. Anal sphincter disruption during vaginal delivery. *N Engl J Med.* 1993;329:1905–1911.
17. Sato T, Konishi F, Minakami H et al. Pelvic floor disturbance after childbirth: vaginal delivery damages the upper levels of sphincter innervation. *Dis Colon Rectum.* 2001;44:1155–1161.
18. Shiono P, Klebanoff MA, Carey JC. Midline episiotomies: more harm than good? *Obstet Gynecol.* 1990;75:765–770.
19. Klein MC, Gauthier RJ, Robbins JM et al. Relationship of episiotomy to perineal trauma and morbidity, sexual dysfunction, and pelvic floor relaxation. *Am J Obstet Gynecol.* 1994;171:591–598.
20. Green JR, Soohoo SL. Factors associated with rectal injury in spontaneous deliveries. *Obstet Gynecol.* 1989;73:732–738.
21. Rockner G, Jonasson A, Olund A. The effect of mediolateral episiotomy at delivery on pelvic floor muscle strength evaluated with vaginal cones. *Acta Obstet Gynecol Scand.* 1991;70:51–54.
22. Argentine Episiotomy Trial Collaborative Group. Routine vs selective episiotomy: a randomised controlled trial. *Lancet.* 1993;342(8886–8887):1517–1518.
23. Klein MC, Gauthier RJ, Jorgensen SH et al. Does episiotomy prevent perineal trauma and pelvic floor relaxation [published correction appears in *Online J Curr Clin Trials.* 1992 Sep 12;doc 20]? *Online J Curr Clin Trials.* 1992 Jul 1;doc 10.
24. Signorello LB, Harlow BL, Chekos AK, Repke JT. Midline episiotomy and anal incontinence: retrospective cohort study. *BMJ.* 2000;320(7227):86–90.
25. Signorello LB, Harlow BL, Chekos AK, Repke JT. Postpartum sexual functioning and its relationship to perineal trauma: a retrospective cohort study of primiparous women. *Am J Obstet Gynecol.* 2001;184:881–888.
26. Carroli G, Belizan J. Episiotomy for vaginal birth. *Cochrane Database Syst Rev.* 2000;CD000081.
27. Peschers UM, Schaer GN, DeLancey JO, Schuessler B. Levator ani function before and after childbirth. *Br J Obstet Gynecaecol.* 1997;104:1004–1008.
28. Allen RE, Hosker GL, Smith AR, Warrell DW. Pelvic floor damage in childbirth: a neurophysiological study. *Br J Obstet Gynaecol.* 1990;97:770–779.
29. DeLancey JO, Kearney R, Chou Q, Speights S, Binno S. The appearance of levator ani muscle abnormalities in magnetic resonance images after vaginal delivery. *Obstet Gynecol.* 2003;101:46–53.
30. Snooks SJ, Swash M, Setchell M, Henry MM. Injury to innervation of pelvic floor sphincter musculature in childbirth. *Lancet.* 1984;2:546–550.
31. Snooks SJ, Swash M, Henry MM, Setchell M. Risk factors in childbirth causing damage to the pelvic floor innervation. *Int J Colorectal Dis.* 1986;1:20–24.
32. Mallett VT, Hosker G, Smith ARB, Warrell DW. Pelvic floor damage and childbirth; a neurophysiologic follow-up study. *Neuro Urodyn.* 1993;12:357–358.
33. Snooks SJ, Swash M, Mathers SE, Henry MM. Effect of vaginal delivery on the pelvic floor: a 5-year follow-up. *Br J Surg.* 1990;77:1358–1360.
34. Snooks SJ, Barnes PR, Swash M. Damage to the innervation of the voluntary anal and periurethral sphincter musculature in incontinence: an electrophysiological study. *J Neurol Neurosurg Psychiatry.* 1984;47:1269–1273.
35. Smith AR, Hosker GL, Warrell DW. The role of pudendal nerve damage in the aetiology of genuine stress incontinence in women. *Br J Obstet Gynaecol.* 1989;96:29–32.
36. Smith ARB, Hosker GL, Warrell DW. The role of partial denervation of the pelvic floor in the aetiology of genitourinary prolapse and stress incontinence of urine. A neurophysiological study. *Br J Obstet Gynaecol.* 1989;96:24–28.
37. Snooks SJ, Henry MM, Swash M. Faecal incontinence due to external anal sphincter division in childbirth is associated with damage to the innervation of the pelvic floor musculature; a double pathology. *Br J Obstet Gynecol.* 1985;92:824–828.
38. Gilpin SA, Gosling JA, Smith AR, Warrell DW. The pathogenesis of genitourinary prolapse and stress incontinence of urine. A histological and histochemical study. *Br J Obstet Gynaecol.* 1989;96:15–23.
39. Sharf B, Zilberman A, Sharf M, Mitrani A. Electromyogram of pelvic floor muscles in genital prolapse. *Int J Gynaecol Obstet.* 1976;14:2–4.
40. Norton PA. Pelvic floor disorders: the role of fascia and ligaments. *Clin Obstet Gynecol.* 1993;36:926–938.
41. Richardson AC, Lyon JB, Williams NL. A new look at pelvic relaxation. *Am J Obstet Gynecol.* 1976;126:568–571.
42. Viktrup L, Lose G, Rolff M, Barfoed K. The symptom of stress incontinence caused by pregnancy or delivery in primiparas. *Obstet Gynecol.* 1992;79:945–949.

43. Francis WJ. The onset of stress incontinence. *J Obstet Gynaecol Br Emp.* 1960;67:899–903.
44. Marshall K, Thompson KA, Walsh DM, Baxter GD. Incidence of urinary incontinence and constipation during pregnancy and postpartum: survey of current findings at the Rotunda Lying-in Hospital. *Br J Obstet Gynecol.* 1998;105:400–402.
45. Stanton SL, Kerr-Wilson R, Harris VG: The incidence of urological symptoms in normal pregnancy. *Br J Obstet Gynaecol.* 1980;87:897–900.
46. Meyer S. Schreyer A, De Grandi P, Hohlfeld P. The effects of birth on urinary continence mechanisms and other pelvic floor characteristics. *Obstet Gynecol.* 1998;92:613–618.
47. Viktrup L, Lose G: The risk of stress incontinence 5 years after first delivery. *Am J Obstet Gynecol.* 2001;185:82–87.
48. Bergman A, McCarthy TA, Ballard CA, Yanai J. Role of the Q-tip test in evaluating stress urinary incontinence. *J Reprod Med.* 1987;32:273–275.
49. Peschers U, Schar G, Anthuber C, Schussler B. Postpartal pelvic floor damage: is connective tissue impairment more important than neuromuscular changes? *Neuro Urodyn.* 1993;12:376–377.
50. Peschers U, Schaer G, Anthuber C, DeLancey JO, Schuessler B. Changes in vesical neck mobility following vaginal delivery. *Obstet Gynecol.* 1996;88: 1001–1006.
51. Van Geelen JM, Lemmens WA, Eskes TK, Martin CB. The urethral pressure profile in pregnancy and after delivery in healthy nulliparous women. *Am J Obstet Gynecol.* 1982;144:636–649.
52. Hojberg KE, Salvig JD, Winslow NA, Lose G, Secher NJ. Urinary incontinence: prevalence and risk factors at 16 weeks of gestation. *Br J Obstet Gynaecol.* 1999;106:842–850.
53. Persson J, Wolner-Hanssen P, Rydhstroem H. Obstetric risk factors for stress urinary incontinence: a population-based study. *Obstet Gynecol.* 2000;96:440–445.
54. Moller LA, Lose G, Jorgensen T. Risk factors for lower urinary tract symptoms in women 40 to 60 years of age. *Obstet Gynecol.* 2000;96:446–451.
55. Rowe JW. The NIH consensus development panel: urinary incontinence in adults. *JAMA.* 1989;261: 2685–2690.
56. Sand PK, Dmochowski R, Goldberg RP, McIlwain M, Lucente VR. Does overactive bladder impact interest in sexual activity? Baseline results from the MATRIX study. Paper presented at: 30th Annual Meeting of the International Urogynecology Society; August 11, 2005; Copenhagen, Denmark.
57. Buhling KJ, Schmidt S, Robinson JN, Klapp C, Siebert G, Dudenhausen JW. Rate of dyspareunia after delivery in primiparae according to mode of delivery. *Eur J Obstet Gynecol Reprod Biol.* 2006;124:42–46.
58. Sampselle CM, Miller JM, Mims BL, DeLancey JO, Ashton-Miller JA, Antonakos CL. Effect of pelvic muscle exercise on transient incontinence during pregnancy and after birth. *Obstet Gynecol.* 1998;91: 406–412.
59. Reilly ET, Freeman RM, Waterfield MR, Waterfield AE, Steggles P, Pedlar F. Prevention of postpartum stress incontinence in primigravidae with increased bladder neck mobility: a randomised controlled trial of antenatal pelvic floor exercises. *Br J Obstet Gynaecol.* 2002;109:68–76.
60. Labrecque M, Eason E, Marcoux S et al. Randomized controlled trial of prevention of perineal trauma by perineal massage during pregnancy. *Am J Obstet Gynecol.* 1999;180(3 Pt 1):593–600.
60a. Goldberg RP, Abramov, Y, Botros S, et al. Delivery mode is a major environmental determinant of stress urinary incontinence: results of the Evanston *Northwestern Twin Sisters Study.* AJOG 2005;193(6):2149–2153.
61. Labrecque M, Eason E, Marcoux S. Randomized trial of perineal massage during pregnancy: perineal symptoms three months after delivery. *Am J Obstet Gynecol.* 2000;182(1 Pt 1):76–80.
62. Rasmussen KL; Krue S; Johansson LE; Knudsen HJ; Agger AO. Obesity as a predictor of postpartum urinary symptoms. *Acta Obstet Gynecol Scand.* 1997;76(4):359–362.
63. Elia G, Dye TD, Scariati PD. Body mass index and urinary symptoms in women. *Int Urogynecol J Pelvic Floor Dysfunct.* 2001;12(6):366–369.
64. Gardosi J, Hutson N, B-Lynch C. Randomised, controlled trial of squatting in the second stage of labour. *Lancet.* 1989;2(8654):74–77.
65. Golay J, Vedam S, Sorger L. The squatting position for the second stage of labor: effects on labor and on maternal and fetal well-being. *Birth.* 1993;20: 73–78.
66. de Jong PR, Johanson RB, Baxen P, Adrians VD, van der Westhuisen S, Jones PW. Randomised trial comparing the upright and supine positions for the second stage of labour. *Br J Obstet Gynaecol.* 1997;104:567–671.
67. Gupta JK, Nikodem VC. Woman's position during second stage of labour. *Cochrane Database Syst Rev.* 2000;CD002006.
68. Fraser WD, Marcoux S, Krauss I, Douglas J, Goulet C, Boulvain M. Multicenter, randomized, controlled trial of delayed pushing for nulliparous women in the second stage of labor with continuous epidural analgesia. The PEOPLE (Pushing Early or Pushing Late with Epidural) Study Group. *Am J Obstet Gynecol.* 2000;182(5):1165–1172.

69. Hansen SL, Clark SL, Foster JC. Active pushing versus passive fetal descent in the second stage of labor: a randomized controlled trial. *Obstet Gynecol.* 2002;99(1):29–34.
70. Sampselle CM, Hines S. Spontaneous pushing during birth. Relationship to perineal outcomes. *J Nurse Midwifery.* 1999;44:36–39.
71. Parnell C, Langhoff-Roos J, Iversen R, Damgaard P. Pushing method in the expulsive phase of labor. A randomized trial. *Acta Obstet Gynecol Scand.* 1993;72:31–35.
72. Janni W, Schiessl B, Peschers U et al. The prognostic impact of a prolonged second stage of labor on maternal and fetal outcome. *Acta Obstet Gynecol Scand.* 2002;81(3):214–221.
73. Combs CA, Robertson PA, Laros RK. Risk factors for third-degree and fourth-degree perineal lacerations in forceps and vacuum deliveries. *Am J Obstet Gynecol.* 1990;163:100–104.
74. Donnelly V, Fynes M, Campbell D, Johnson H, O'Connell PR, O'Herlihy C. Obstetric events leading to anal sphincter damage. *Obstet Gynecol.* 1998;92:955–961.
75. Van Kessel K, Reed S, Newton K, Meier A, Lentz G. The second stage of labor and stress urinary incontinence. *Am J Obstet Gynecol.* 2001;184:1571–1575.
76. Arya LA, Jackson ND, Myers DL, Verma A. Risk of new-onset urinary incontinence after forceps and vacuum delivery in primiparous women. *Am J Obstet Gynecol.* 2001;185:1318–1323.
77. Meyer S, Hohlfeld P, Achtari C, Russolo A, De Grandi P. Birth trauma: short and long term effects of forceps delivery compared with spontaneous delivery on various pelvic floor parameters. *Br J Obstet Gynaecol.* 2000;107:1360–1365.
78. Combs CA, Robertson PA, Laros RK Jr. Risk factors for third-degree and fourth-degree perineal lacerations in forceps and vacuum deliveries. *Am J Obstet Gynecol.* 1990;163(1 Pt 1):100–104.
79. Sultan AH, Kamm MA, Bartram CI, Hudson CN. Anal sphincter trauma during instrumental delivery. *Int J Gynaecol Obstet.* 1993;43:263–270.
80. Wen SW, Liu S, Kramer MS et al. Comparison of maternal and infant outcomes between vacuum extraction and forceps deliveries. *Am J Epidemiol.* 2001;153:103–107.
81. Johanson RB, Menon BK. Vacuum extraction versus forceps for assisted vaginal delivery. *Cochrane Database Syst Rev.* 2000;CD000224.
82. Jander C, Lyrenas S. Third and fourth degree perineal tears. Predictor factors in a referral hospital. *Acta Obstet Gynecol Scand.* 2001;80:229–234.
83. Handa VL, Danielsen BH, Gilbert WM. Obstetric anal sphincter lacerations. *Obstet Gynecol.* 2001;98: 225–230.
84. Riskin-Mashiah S, O'Brian Smith E, Wilkins IA. Risk factors for severe perineal tear: can we do better? *Am J Perinatol.* 2002;19:225–234.
85. Snooks SJ, Swash M, Henry MM, Setchell M. Risk factors in childbirth causing damage to the pelvic floor innervation. *Int J Color Dis.* 1986;1:20–24.
86. Groutz A, Gordon D, Keidar R et al. Stress urinary incontinence: prevalence among nulliparous compared with primiparous and grand multiparous premenopausal women. *Neurourol Urodyn.* 1999; 18:419–425.
87. Culligan PJ, Myers JA, Goldberg RP, Blackwell L, Gohmann SF, Abell TD. Elective cesarean section to prevent anal incontinence and brachial plexus injuries associated with macrosomia—a decision analysis. Int Urogynecol J Pelvic Floor Dysfunct. 2005;16:19–28; discussion 28.
88. Al-Mufti R, McCarthy A, Fisk NM. Obstetricians' personal choice and mode of delivery. *Lancet.* 1996;347:544.
89. Sultan AH, Kamm MA, Hudson CN. Pudendal nerve damage during labour: prospective study before and after childbirth. *Br J Obstet Gynaecol.* 1994;101:22–28.
90. Faundes A, Guarisi T, Pinto-Neto AM. The risk of urinary incontinence of parous women who delivered only by cesarean section. *Int J Gynaecol Obstet.* 2001;72:41–46.
91. Goldberg RP, Abramov Y, Botros S et al. Delivery mode is a major environmental determinant of stress urinary incontinence: results of the Evanston-Northwestern Twin Sisters Study. *Am J Obstet Gynecol.* 2005;193:2149–2153.
92. Fynes M, Donnelly VS, O'Connell PR, O'Herlihy C. Cesarean delivery and anal sphincter injury. *Obstet Gynecol.* 1998;92(4 Pt 1):496–500.
93. Meyer S, Hohlfeld P, Achtari C, De Grandi P. Pelvic floor education after vaginal delivery. *Obstet Gynecol.* 2001;97(5 Pt 1):673–677.
94. Reilly ET, Freeman RM, Waterfield MR, Waterfield AE, Steggles P, Pedlar F. Prevention of postpartum stress incontinence in primigravidae with increased bladder neck mobility: a randomised controlled trial of antenatal pelvic floor exercises. *Br J Obstet Gynaecol.* 2002;109:68–76.
95. Morkved S, Bo K. The effect of post-natal exercises to strengthen the pelvic floor muscles. *Acta Obstet Gynecol Scand.* 1996;75:382–385.
96. Morkved S, Bo K. Effect of postpartum pelvic floor muscle training in prevention and treatment of urinary incontinence: a one-year follow up. *Br J Obstet Gynaecol.* 2000;107:1022–1028.

4
Pathophysiology of Incontinence and Pelvic Floor Dysfunction

Paul Tulikangas

Introduction

The female pelvis has many diverse, and sometimes contradictory, functions. Its bony structure and muscles are responsible not only for ambulation but also for support of the internal organs. The urethra and bladder are meant to dependably store urine until it is time to urinate. The rectum stores stool and gas until there is a socially appropriate time for release. The pelvis is also a passageway for childbirth—perhaps the most challenging of all of its functions, especially since we expect a normal return of physiological functioning after a significant degree of neuromuscular and connective tissue trauma.

In this chapter we will review what is known about the pathophysiology of incontinence and prolapse, the two most common female pelvic disorders. The goal is to be able to provide intelligent answers to the patient in your office who asks, *"Why did this happen to me?"*

Normal Bladder Function

The bladder is responsible for the storage and timely release of urine. Most problems with urinary tract function can be classified as ones of either storage or emptying.

The bladder is a mucosa-lined smooth muscle with multiple nerve endings. To store urine, it increases its size dramatically without increasing its internal pressure. It is arguably the most compliant organ in the body.

The female urethra is approximately 4 cm long and has internal smooth muscle and external striated muscle components. The internal sphincter has primarily autonomic innervation, and the external sphincter has primarily somatic innervation. The compression of the internal and external sphincters and the pressure from the vascular plexus in the wall of the urethra keep urine in the bladder.

During bladder filling, the pudendal nerve activates the striated external urethral sphincter, increasing its pressure. A spinal sympathetic reflex also occurs that inhibits detrusor contractions (by stimulating beta receptors in the bladder) and further increases urethral sphincter tone (by stimulating alpha receptors in the urethra).

If there is an episode of increased intra-abdominal pressure during storage (e.g. exercise, cough, laugh, or sneeze), the pressure will also rise in the bladder. If the urethra is correctly positioned under the pubic bone and the urethra and bladder neck are supported by a strong underlying "floor" of anterior vaginal support, then urethral pressure will also increase and there will be no loss of urine.

Recent studies also suggest that there may be an active contraction of the external urethral sphincter and increase in its pressure before an increase in intra-abdominal pressure. This closure mechanism is mediated through the pudendal nerve from motor neurons in the spinal cord. The closure mechanism appears to be activated by serotonin agonists and depressed by serotonin antagonists.

Urinary Urgency, Frequency and Urge Incontinence: "Overactive Bladder"

Many conditions can lead to urinary urgency, frequency and urge incontinence, and the number of women seeking help for "overactive bladder" symptoms continues to dramatically increase. Underlying causes include behavioral, inflammatory, neuromuscular, endocrine, and anatomic, as summarized in Table 4.1. It should be emphasized that the disorder is idiopathic, without a discrete underlying disease state, in over 90% of cases.

Patients who consume large volumes of fluid will obviously void more frequently. Other patients develop frequent voiding habits despite normal physiologic bladder function. Inflammatory conditions such as urinary tract infections and some chemotherapy agents lead to inflammation of the bladder lining and urinary urgency, frequency, and urge incontinence. Bladder cancer can present with irritative bladder symptoms but is typically accompanied by microscopic or gross hematuria.

TABLE 4.1. Causes of Urinary Urgency and Frequency

Behavioral
excess fluid intake excess caffeine intake habitual increased voiding frequency anxiety
Inflammatory
urinary tract infection interstitial cystitis radiation cystitis chemical cystitis (some chemotherapy agents) bladder cancer urinary stones or benign urothelial growths
Neurologic
multiple sclerosis cerebrovascular disease involving the central nervous system Parkinson's disease dementia tumors involving the central nervous system spinal cord injury
Endocrine
genital urinary atrophy diabetes
Anatomic
bladder outlet obstruction pelvic mass urethral diverticulum pregnancy

Interstitial cystitis, a commonly diagnosed condition, presents with urinary urgency, frequency, and bladder pain. The preferred term for this condition is painful bladder syndrome. This condition is defined by the patients' symptoms and not necessarily by the underlying pathophysiology related to their disease. Painful bladder and interstitial cystitis are discussed in more detail in Chapter 13.

Urinary urgency, frequency, and urge incontinence often occur in women who have involuntary contractions of the detrusor muscle at inappropriate times. When these contractions are documented on urodynamic testing, the condition is called *detrusor overactivity (DO)*. Congenital DO is a disorder in children characterized by daytime urge incontinence and nocturnal enuresis. It is thought to be secondary to delayed maturation of the central nervous system control of the bladder.

The incidence of DO in adults may occasionally result from underlying neurologic dysfunction. For instance, after a cerebral vascular accident, it is common to develop DO (termed neurogenic detrusor overactivity if there is a known neurologic lesion) as a result of an interruption of the cortical inhibition of the pontine micturition center. After a spinal cord injury, DO often occurs because of the autonomous function of the sacral voiding reflex. It is possible that more subtle injuries to the central nervous system account for the DO seen in many adults. Peripheral neuropathies could also play a role in the development of bladder spasms. Diabetics have a high rate of DO, which might be attributed to peripheral nerve injury affecting the sensation in the bladder that is needed to suppress minor bladder contractions. Spinal stenosis can cause bladder instability. Back injuries such as disc disease and compression factors can cause bladder instability, but this is uncommon.

What about a patient with overactive bladder symptoms who has no underlying disease or obvious cause of the symptoms? These patients are common, and there are many theories about what causes idiopathic detrusor overactivity.

Table 4.2. Changes with aging that lead to urinary frequency and incontinence

Increasing collagen within the detrusor muscle
Decreased nocturnal production of anti-diuretic hormone
Increased lower extremity edema
Disease states
Parkinson's disease
autonomic neuropathies
cerebral vascular accidents
Alzheimer's Disease
multiple sclerosis
diabetes mellitus
diabetes insipidus
congestive heart failure
urinary tract infections
obstructive sleep apnea

Some evidence supports a neurogenic cause of uninhibited bladder contractions. There are neurologic reflexes that promote bladder storage by depressing the detrusor contractions and pathways that promote bladder emptying and stimulate detrusor contractions. A disruption in this balance could lead to detrusor overactivity.

Recent research has demonstrated, in patients with overactive bladder symptoms, abnormalities in the detrusor muscle that suggest a myogenic etiology for detrusor instability. In patients with detrusor overactivity, the detrusor muscle cells had abnormal junctions that would lead to more rapid bladder contractions and difficulty suppressing unintended contractions.

Several age-dependent changes also play a role in the development of urinary frequency and urge incontinence. These are summarized in Table 4.2.

Stress Urine Incontinence

Stress urinary incontinence occurs when increased intra-abdominal pressure is associated with urine loss in the absence of a detrusor contraction. Typically, a rapid rise in abdominal pressure is associated with a concurrent increase in urethral pressure **and there** is no loss of urine. If the urethra is not positioned correctly under the pubic bone, and/or if the underlying vaginal and pubocervical fascia weakens or detaches, there can be a decrease in urethral pressure and urine loss. Also, if the urethral sphincter itself does not function correctly, there can be urine loss—regardless of its position.

Loss of urethral support is most commonly associated with vaginal childbirth. MRI imaging of women before and after vaginal delivery has demonstrated injury to the levator muscles that act to provide pelvic support. Levator muscle strength decreases after vaginal delivery. When the levator muscles do not function well, there is loss of pelvic support, including abnormal mobility of the urethra. Chapter 3 includes more detailed information regarding the potential problems associated with childbirth.

Factors that increase intra-abdominal pressure also contribute to stress urine incontinence. Patients with chronic obstructive pulmonary disease are more likely to have stress urine incontinence, and patients with higher BMIs tend to have more severe SUI.

Elegant studies of pudendal nerve function in women before and after vaginal delivery have demonstrated neuropathy in many women. This might ultimately lead to poor urethral sphincter function and stress urine incontinence.

Pelvic Organ Prolapse

The etiology of pelvic organ prolapse is multifactorial. In most women, there is likely neuromuscular injury to the levator muscles in the pelvis, followed by connective tissue injury to the tissues that support the bladder, uterus, rectum, and vagina.

Most women who present for treatment of pelvic organ prolapse are in their fifties and sixties. The greatest risk factor for pelvic organ prolapse is vaginal delivery. What happens in the 20 to 30 years between the time of vaginal delivery and the development of pelvic organ prolapse?

In healthy women, the pelvic floor is closed by the levator ani muscles. The connective tissue in the pelvis (uterosacral ligaments, endopelvic fascia, perineal membrane) supports the pelvic organs at rest. With increased intra-abdominal pressure, the levator muscles contract to hold the pelvic organs in place. If there is nerve injury or muscle dysfunction, the levator muscles don't contract appropriately and there is often connective tissue injury.

The most common cause of neuromuscular injury in women is vaginal childbirth. When pelvic floor muscle function is impaired, increased stress is put on the connective tissue supports of the pelvic organs. The uterosacral ligaments, vaginal walls, endopelvic fascia, and perineal membrane are injured. When these supports fail, prolapse occurs.

In patients with pelvic organ prolapse there is always a failure of the connective tissue supports. These supports are repaired in surgery for pelvic organ prolapse. Unfortunately, for many women there is also pelvic floor muscle injury that we often cannot treat, with the underlying pelvic floor muscle dysfunction likely leading to recurrent prolapse.

Normal Anorectal Function

The anorectal complex includes the rectum, which acts as a reservoir for the storage of stool, and the anal canal, which acts as part of the continence mechanism. Stool is stored in the rectosigmoid colon. The rectum is typically 12 cm in length. It is an easily distensible, low-pressure segment of colon. At rest, the anorectal angle is formed by the ventral contraction of the puborectalis muscle which is important for continence of solid stool. The internal anal sphincter is a circular band of smooth muscle that is controlled primarily by reflex arcs at the spinal level. The external anal sphincter is a striated muscle that encircles the internal sphincter and is responsible for continence when there is distension of the anal canal. Soft tissue around the anus improves coaptation of the anal mucosa to aid incontinence of gas and soft stool.

Anal Incontinence

For a patient to be continent of stool and gas she must have a compliant rectal reservoir, a functioning puborectalis sling, and an intact anal sphincter complex. The rectum should be compliant to store stool until one is able to defecate. Complex afferent nerves sense rectal distension and signal the cerebral cortex of the need to defecate. If the rectum is not compliant, fecal urgency and loss of stool is often the result. Rectal storage issues are most common in patients with ulcerative or radiation proctitis.

Loss of gas or liquid or solid stool is referred to as anal incontinence. This typically represents a breakdown in the continence mechanism. There are three components to the continence mechanism—the internal anal sphincter, the external anal sphincter, and the puborectalis portion of the levator muscles. The internal anal sphincter is under involuntary control and is nearly always in a state of contraction. It contributes approximately 85% of the resting tone of the anal sphincter. The external anal sphincter is a striated muscle that is voluntarily contracted. The puborectalis is part of the levator ani muscles that close the opening in the pelvic floor. When it is contracted it pulls the anorectal junction anteriorly, increasing the angle between the anus and the rectum. This movement, in conjunction with the contraction of the external anal sphincter, closes the anal canal.

Fecal incontinence often occurs from disruption of the anal sphincter. This disruption can involve the internal and/or external anal sphincter. Some studies have found that at least one third of women undergoing vaginal delivery will have a disruption in their anal sphincter. Some of these tears occur in women who do not even have a perineal skin laceration. In addition to anatomic disruption of the sphincter, there can also be pudendal nerve injury, which can lead to atrophy and poor sphincter function.

Constipation

Constipation is difficult to define and can mean different things to different people. For research purposes, it is typically defined as bowel movements occurring less than three times a week or a need to strain for more than 25% of bowel movements. Constipation is typically divided into issues of motility and defecation. Colonic motility is complex. An average meal may take only 1 to 2 hours to pass through the small intestines but up to 30 hours to pass through the colon.

The colon is responsible for absorption of water and nutrients from the stool as well as for motility. Colonic motility is a result of a series of intermittently timed peristaltic contractions. Constipation is observed in patients with both normal- and slow-transit time. Table 4.3 lists a number of possible causes of constipation.

Normal-transit constipation is often referred to as "functional" constipation. Some patients with normal transit constipation have increased rectal compliance or reduced rectal sensation. Most of these patients have improved function with increased dietary fiber intake and occasional laxative use.

Slow-transit constipation is usually documented by colonic transit studies. It is most common in young women. Evaluation of these women reveals fewer peristaltic contractions after meals, which might delay the transit of stool through the colon. Biopsies have demonstrated changes in the myenteric plexus neurons and neurotransmitters that regulate colonic motility.

TABLE 4.3. Causes of Constipation

Functional causes
depression low activity level inadequate toilet facilities
Dietary causes
low fiber intake low fluid intake low caloric intake
Endocrinologic disorders
diabetes hypothyroid hypercalcemia
Metabolic disorders
hypokalemia
Colonic obstruction
tumors volvulus
Neuromuscular disorders
Hirschsprung's disease scleroderma muscular dystrophy spinal cord lesions intestinal pseudo-obstruction

In Hirschsprung's disease the ganglion cells in the distal bowel are absent, leading to abnormal colonic development and severe constipation in children.

Defecatory Dysfunction

Difficulty with defecation is typically secondary to anorectal outlet obstruction. This obstruction can be either anatomic or physiologic.

Many patients will avoid defecation secondary to painful hemorrhoids or anal fissures. This may lead to constipation and ultimately more severe defecation disorders.

The most common cause of anatomic outlet obstruction is a rectocele. This is a form of pelvic organ prolapse in which the anterior wall of the rectum herniates into the posterior wall of the vagina. With defecation, stool can be trapped in this hernia and passed only with mechanical assistance (e.g. pushing on the herniated posterior vaginal wall or perineum with a finger). Although less common, rectal prolapse can also occur. This involves intussusception of the rectum either internally (above the anal sphincter) or externally. Rectal masses, such as rectal cancer, could also obstruct defecation.

Physiologic obstructions to defecation include paradoxical contraction of the puborectalis muscle and anal sphincter dyssynergia. Both of these muscles relax during normal defecation. The inability to relax these muscles can lead to obstructed defecation. These dysfunctions can be seen radiologically as a reduced descent of the perineum and an inability to straighten the anorectal angle.

Urinary Retention and Problems with Voiding

Voiding dysfunction occurs when there is difficulty emptying the bladder. This can occur if there is either impaired detrusor pressure or an obstruction to the urethra.

A common cause of bladder outlet obstruction in women is pelvic organ prolapse. If the anterior vaginal wall prolapses and the bladder drops down, the urethra can "kink" and obstruct. This typically happens in women with more advanced prolapse—usually beyond the vaginal opening. Less common causes of obstruction include pelvic masses or foreign objects in the vagina. All surgeries for urine incontinence can also potentially cause obstruction and voiding dysfunction.

The voiding reflex is normally triggered in the cerebral cortex. This activates the pontine micturition center, which stimulates a detrusor contraction through the intermediolateral gray columns and, then, the pelvic nerve. The most common neurologic problems associated with voiding dysfunction are peripheral neuropathies. Other etiologies for detrusor dysfunction include chronic urinary tract obstruction, pelvic radiation, and pelvic muscle dysfunction.

Key Points

- Urinary urgency, frequency, and urge incontinence are often caused by involuntary bladder contractions. In some women there is an underlying neurologic problem, but most cases are idiopathic.
- Stress urine incontinence is usually caused by poor urethral support or a poorly functioning urethral sphincter.
- Voiding dysfunction is caused by an obstruction to urine flow or poor detrusor muscle contraction.
- Pelvic organ prolapse, in most women, is caused by neuromuscular dysfunction of the pelvic floor. When the muscles do not function correctly, the connective tissue supports to the pelvic organs are exposed to increased risk of injury, and prolapse occurs.
- Anal incontinence is most commonly caused by poor rectal storage or dysfunction of the anal sphincter mechanism.
- Constipation can occur in women with either normal or slow colonic transit times.
- Women with slow colonic transit times often have abnormalities in the colonic nerves and neurotransmitters.
- Defecatory dysfunction is commonly caused by obstruction ("pocketing") of stool within a rectocele. Neuromuscular dysfunction of the pelvis can also interfere with the defecation process.

References

1. DeLancey JO. Stress urinary incontinence: where are we now, where should we go? *Am J Obstet Gynecol.* 1996;175:311–319.
2. DeLancey JO. Anatomy and biomechanics of genital prolapse. *Clin Obstet Gynecol.* 1993;36:897–909.
3. Brubaker L. Urinary urgency and frequency: what should a clinician do? *Obstet Gynecol.* 2005;105:661–667.
4. Lembo A, Camilleri M. Chronic constipation. *N Engl J Med.* 2003;349:1360–1368.
5. Rudolph W, Galandiuk S. A practical guide to the diagnosis and management of fecal incontinence. *Mayo Clin Proc.* 2002;77:271–275.

5 Diagnosing Incontinence and Pelvic Floor Problems: An Efficient, Cost-Effective Approach for Primary Care Providers

Peter L. Rosenblatt and Eman Elkadry

Introduction

Primary care clinicians often wonder whether they should be involved in the evaluation and management of urogynecologic issues, such as urinary and fecal incontinence, voiding dysfunction, and pelvic organ prolapse. Referring patients with urogynecologic complaints to specialists such as urogynecologists or urologists is certainly an option for those clinicians who are unfamiliar with the evaluation and management of these problems. As will be covered in this chapter, however, a basic evaluation including a directed history and physical, combined with a few simple tests, is all that is required in most patients in order to arrive at a presumptive diagnosis and initiate a well-structured, conservative treatment plan.

Urinary incontinence affects up to 30% of the entire adult female population, and the prevalence increases among older age groups.[1,2] Of the estimated 1.5 million nursing home residents in the U.S., urinary incontinence affects over one half and is often a contributing factor when deciding to admit an elderly person to a nursing home.[3] Population studies have estimated that the proportion of postmenopausal women in the U.S. will increase dramatically over the next 50 years and that the proportion of women over the age of 85 will triple, from 2% to 6%.[4] Contributing factors include the aging baby-boomer population and improved health care, leading to improved longevity. It has become clear that there are simply not enough specialists available at the present time to handle the urogynecologic problems that will become increasingly prevalent among these women. It is, therefore, imperative that primary care clinicians become familiar with the basic evaluation and first-line treatment options for women with these disorders.

Evaluation of women with urogynecologic complaints may vary in complexity from a simple history and physical examination, which can be performed by any physician, to complex multichannel urodynamic testing performed by specialists. Primary care physicians should routinely screen their patients for these problems and provide the first-line management as described below.

Screening for Urinary Incontinence

Telephone survey studies have demonstrated that urge incontinence and overactive bladder symptoms are extremely prevalent, occurring in 17% of all adult women.[5] This finding would rank these disorders among the most common problems facing women today. Unfortunately, it has been estimated that over one half of the women affected by overactive bladders do not seek medical attention, because of either embarrassment or the impression that incontinence is an inevitable part of the aging process. Physicians should keep in mind that women are often reluctant to volunteer their symptoms of urinary and fecal incontinence. Therefore, it is important to incorporate a few key questions regarding these issues into the standard history of any new or annual patient visit. One key, open-ended question might be, *"Do you ever leak urine or have any other bladder problems that are bothersome to you?"* Avoid questions that use the phrase "incontinence", as many women who leak urine and are bothered by their symptoms nevertheless do not consider themselves "incontinent". A patient questionnaire that includes questions about urinary incontinence and overactive bladder is a useful tool that can be completed by the patient at home or in the waiting room (Table 5.1).

Fortunately, in recent years there has been growing acceptance among women that incontinence is a topic that can be discussed with their physicians, thanks, in part, to increased public awareness driven by pharmaceutical and medical device companies involved in the development of incontinence treatments. Additional questions should focus on symptoms that may suggest the etiology of the problem, and efforts should be made to quantify the problem, as well as to determine the effect the condition has on the woman's lifestyle. The clinician should try to determine activities that precipitate urine loss. For example, leakage that occurs coincident with sudden increases in abdominal pressure such as coughing, sneezing, laughing, and lifting is strongly suggestive of stress incontinence, while symptoms such as urgency, frequency, nocturia, and leakage associated with a strong urge suggest overactive bladder syndrome, which may be associated with the urodynamic diagnosis of detrusor overactivity. In addition, small urine loss quantity is more often associated with stress incontinence, while large urine volume loss usually suggests uncontrollable detrusor muscle overactivity. The greater the number of symptoms of overactive bladder, the more likely is the diagnosis of urge incontinence. Overactive bladder symptoms accompanied by dysuria or gross hematuria suggest a urinary tract infection. It should be kept in mind that some women with lower urinary tract infections do not present with the classic symptom of dysuria and may be falsely diagnosed with overactive bladder if a urinalysis is not obtained. Approximately one third of women present with "mixed" symptoms of incontinence, with a combination of overactive bladder and stress urinary incontinence. Questions about absorbent pads should include the type used and the quantity used on a daily basis. It is also useful to attempt to identify when the problem began and whether the woman perceives her condition as stable or worsening over time. Any relationship to prolapse symptoms should be determined. Many women with stress incontinence have coincident loss of support for the anterior vaginal wall (cystocele); and, in fact, severe degrees of prolapse may lead to paradoxical improvement in stress incontinence symptoms

TABLE 5.1. Urinary symptoms questionnaire

Symptoms of an Overactive Bladder	Yes	No
Do you frequently have a strong, sudden urge to urinate?	☐	☐
Do you sometimes not make it to the bathroom in time?	☐	☐
Do you frequently go to the bathroom 8 or more times per 24 hours?	☐	☐
Do you get up 2 or more times during the night to go to the bathroom?	☐	☐
How long have you had these symptoms?	☐	☐
Symptoms of Stress Incontinence	**Yes**	**No**
Do you experience a loss of urine when you are doing physical activities, such as lifting heavy objects or exercising?	☐	☐
Do you sometimes have a slight loss of urine when you sneeze, cough, or laugh?	☐	☐
Mixed Incontinence	**Yes**	**No**
Do you have symptoms of both an overactive bladder and stress incontinence?	☐	☐
Symptoms of a Urinary Tract Infection	**Yes**	**No**
Do you experience a burning sensation when you urinate?	☐	☐
Do you frequently have a strong, sudden urge to urinate?	☐	☐
Do you go to the bathroom 8 or more times per 24 hours?	☐	☐
Did your symptoms come on suddenly?	☐	☐

resulting from anatomic kinking of the urethra. This is an important consideration when counseling women prior to placement of a vaginal pessary or when contemplating surgical correction of pelvic organ prolapse. For example, patients should be informed that a pessary can uncover occult incontinence, which may require switching to a pessary that provides additional support to the bladder neck, such as an incontinence dish or ring.

The Urogynecologic History

A standard medical history should be taken. Medical problems that might impact on urinary symptoms—such as diabetes, neurologic disorders, congestive heart failure, and COPD—should be sought. Transient or reversible causes of incontinence should be sought out and treated, as indicated (Table 5.2). The physician should inquire about the patient's obstetrical history, including number of vaginal deliveries and any operative deliveries (e.g. forceps and vacuum deliveries), which may suggest pelvic floor muscle, fascial, or nerve injury. Birth weight and duration of the second (pushing) stage of labor can be useful information for the same reason. Multiparous women have been shown to be at greater risk of urinary and fecal incontinence, as well as of pelvic organ prolapse. A thorough gynecologic history should include any pelvic surgery, including hysterectomy, oophorectomy, and any pelvic floor defect procedures, including "bladder suspension" procedures for urinary incontinence. Since many women do not remember the specifics of the surgery they had, it is often very useful to obtain operative reports from these previous procedures. A history of previous failed incontinence surgery may indicate injury to the urethral sphincter mechanism, which results in a condition known as intrinsic sphincter deficiency. Inquiries regarding previous evaluations, including urodynamic testing and treatments for incontinence, should be made.

Table 5.2. Transient (Reversible) Causes of Urinary Incontinence

Condition	Management
Detectable by history	
Drug side effects (e.g. diuretics, anticholinergics, psychotropics, narcotics, alpha-adrenergic agents)	Discontinue or change medication, if clinically possible
Delirium	Treat underlying cause
Excessive fluid intake	Reduction of fluid intake
Restricted mobility	Physical therapy or environmental changes (e.g., bedside commode)
Detectable by physical examination	
Atrophic vaginitis	Local estrogen therapy
Stool impaction	Disimpaction and implement bowel regimen (stool softeners, fiber, laxatives)
Detectable by urinalysis	
Urinary tract infection	Antibiotic therapy
Glycosuria	Control diabetes

Table 5.3. Medications that can affect the lower urinary tract system

Type of Medication	Lower Urinary Tract Effects
Diuretics	Polyuria, frequency, urgency
Anticholinergics	Urinary retention, overflow incontinence
Narcotic analgesics	Urinary retention, fecal impaction, sedation
Psychotropic agents	
antidepressants	Anticholinergic actions, sedation
antipsychotics	Anticholinergic actions, sedation
sedatives/hypnotics	Sedation, muscle relaxation, confusion
Alpha-adrenergic blockers	Stress incontinence
Beta-adrenergic agonists	Urinary retention
Calcium-channel blockers	Urinary retention, overflow incontinence

The clinician must obtain a complete list of medications used by the patient—both prescription as well as over-the-counter—as many medications have significant effects on the function of the lower urinary tract (Table 5.3). Previous medications used to treat the bladder symptoms, such as anticholinergics, should be recorded, including the dose used, duration of treatment, perceived effectiveness, and side effects experienced.

Voiding Diary

A voiding diary, or "urolog", is another useful tool for diagnosing and objectively quantifying urinary incontinence. The simplest method is to have the patient keep a written log of her fluid intake and her voids, leaks, and urge episodes over a period of one to five days. Most urogynecologists go one step further by having their patients measure and record voided volume with a collection hat placed on the toilet (Figure 5.1).

VOIDING & SYMPTOM DIARY

TIME	FOOD	DRINKS		URINATED		LEAKED URINE				WHAT WHERE YOU DOING AT THE TIME?
		What Kind?	How Much?	# of Times this Hour	Amount (ounces)	# of Times this Hour	Amount (S/M/L)	With Urge?	With Stress?	
(Sample)	Bagel	Tea	½ Cup	1	8	2	M	Yes	No	Washing Dishes
6-7 am										
7-8 am										
8-9 am										
9-10 am										
10-11 am										
11-12 am										
12-1 pm										
1-2 pm										
2-3 pm										
3-4 pm										
4-5 pm										
5-6 pm										
6-7 pm										
7-8 pm										
8-9 pm										
9-10 pm										
10-11 pm										
11-12 pm										
12-1 am										
1-2 am										
2-3 am										
3-4 am										
4-5 am										
5-6 am										

* Stress: Physical exertion or sudden straining (for example coughing, sneezing, exercising, lifting, or bending)
* Urge: Sudden strong desire to empty your bladder ("I've gotta go!")

FIGURE 5.1. Voiding Diary. Reduced average voided volume may be seen in both overactive bladder syndrome as well as in patients with stress incontinence, who often void frequently to reduce the likelihood of leakage with activities.

This is extremely valuable information for several reasons. First, average voided volume and functional bladder capacity (usually the first morning void) can be estimated. Second, total daily fluid intake can be estimated by adding up voided volumes, which is a much more reliable estimate than adding up the reported fluid intake volumes. Women with significant urinary frequency who have normal voided volumes should be counseled that their problem will resolve with a reduction of their fluid intake to normal levels. These women should be reassured that they do not have an overactive bladder and that anticholinergics are not indicated. This has been a common problem among women who have increased their water intake for dieting or other health reasons. Voiding diaries are also useful tools for constructing a schedule for timed voiding or bladder retraining drills.

Physical Examination

A general physical examination should be performed, with special attention given to several areas. During the abdominal examination, the clinician should inspect for previous surgical incisions and inquire about those that may not have been mentioned in the surgical history. The clinician should also palpate for abdominal masses, such as fibroids or other tumors that may be causing lower urinary tract symptoms by a "mass" effect. A neurologic examination of the lower extremities is important, as the innervation of the bladder originates from the same sacral nerve roots (S_2 – S_4), and such testing may uncover an underlying neurologic etiology of lower urinary tract dysfunction. For example, while approximately 95% of women with multiple sclerosis will develop urinary incontinence or other bladder symptoms during the course of their disease, 10% of women with multiple sclerosis will present with urinary incontinence or voiding dysfunction as the initial symptom of their neurologic disease.[6] Other neurologic conditions that may cause lower urinary tract symptoms include cerebral vascular accidents and Parkinson's disease. Therefore, clinicians should screen for these conditions in their evaluation of patients with urinary incontinence. Bilateral testing for patellar and ankle reflexes as well as a determination of lower extremity strength should be performed routinely on these patients. A broken-off wooden cotton swab can be used to test for sharp versus dull sensation over the S3 – S4 dermatomes (Figure 5.2). The wooden side can also be used to test for the bulbocavernosus reflex (or "anal wink") by gently stroking down on the labia minora or perianal area and observing for contracting of the external anal sphincter. Although a positive finding is reassuring, a negative result does not necessarily imply neurologic dysfunction and should not be a cause for alarm in an otherwise healthy woman.

A pelvic examination starts with inspection of the external genitalia for signs of atrophy, dermatitis, and masses such as pelvic prolapse or distal suburethral diverticula. Significant reduction in the size of the labia minora or a pale or shiny appearance of the labia suggests hypoestrogenism, which occurs in menopausal women. Inspection of the vaginal walls may reveal the same types of atrophic changes, with a loss of the normal rugae (or folds) of the epithelium. Although a bivalve speculum should be used to observe the cervix, the speculum should then be taken apart and the posterior blade alone used for the remainder of the speculum examination. This allows for analysis of the anterior and posterior vaginal walls for evidence of prolapse or other

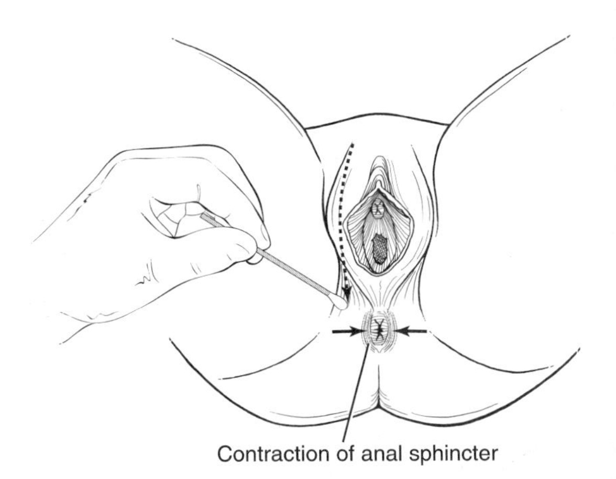

FIGURE 5.2. Bulbocavernosus reflex.

abnormalities. With a posterior blade gently retracting the posterior vaginal wall, the extent of the anterior wall prolapse may be determined by asking the patient to perform a Valsalva maneuver (Figure 5.3).

The posterior speculum blade is then rotated 180 degrees, so that it gently displaces the anterior vaginal wall. Once again, the woman is asked to bear down, and the extent of the posterior wall defect is assessed. (Figure 5.4) Evaluating prolapse of the apex (either cervix or vaginal "vault" after hysterectomy) may require use of the entire bivalve speculum. Alternatively, a Scopette or tongue depressor may be placed at the apex of the vagina. The patient is asked to bear down, and the movement of the instrument is used to determine the extent of her prolapse.

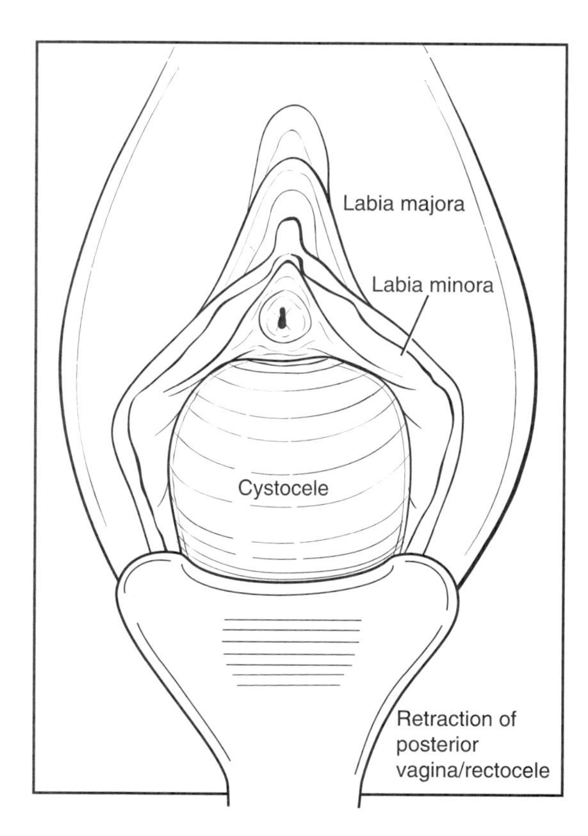

FIGURE 5.3. Examination of cystocele: Retractor or speculum blade is used to retract the posterior vaginal wall, bringing the anterior wall and cystocele into view.

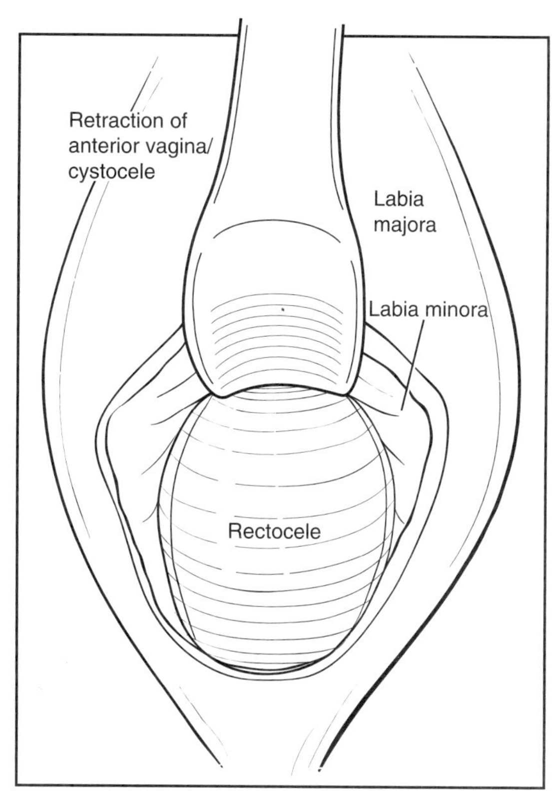

FIGURE 5.4. Examination of rectocele: "With the anterior vaginal wall retracted, the posterior prolapse (rectocele) can now be appreciated."

Bimanual Examination

In addition to palpating the size, shape, and contour of the uterus and adnexa, the pelvic floor (levator ani) muscles should be palpated bilaterally. The patient is then asked to squeeze around the examiner's fingers in order to allow a determination of the strength of her pubococcygeal muscle (or "Kegel") squeeze. It is extremely helpful for the examiner to place his or her other hand on the patient's lower abdomen so that abdominal straining can be detected, and feedback may be given to the patient in an effort to prevent this counterproductive contraction of the abdominal muscles. This simple type of examination not only provides essential biofeedback to the patient (which is significantly more effective than verbal or written instructions) but also reassures the clinician that the patient is performing this exercise correctly. Women who have difficulty isolating their pelvic floor muscles during the pelvic examination may be referred for formal pelvic floor physical therapy and biofeedback.

During the bimanual examination, the examiner should pay attention to the presence of any masses or tenderness along the anterior vaginal wall, which may represent a suburethral diverticular cyst or abscess. Diverticula may present with dysuria (with recurrent urinary tract infections), dyspareunia, or post-void dribbling, and usually require referral for surgical excision.

Finally, rectovaginal examination is then performed, as described later in more detail (see evaluation of fecal incontinence).

Urinalysis and Culture

A clean catch urine specimen should be obtained and a dipstick analysis performed to screen for evidence of infection by testing for leukocytes, blood, and nitrites. If leukocytes or nitrites are positive, a separate specimen may be sent for culture and sensitivity. Alternatively, if the patient has no history of recurrent urinary tract infections, a course of antibiotics may be prescribed without sending the specimen for culture. Microscopic hematuria without leukocytes or nitrites may be a sign of urinary tract pathology, including nephrolithiasis, glomerulonephritis, or tumor of the urinary tract. A more extensive workup, including urine cytology, abdominal CT (or renal ultrasound), and referral for cystoscopy, should be considered if microscopic hematuria is discovered. Microscopic hematuria is defined as three or more red blood cells per high-power microscopic field in urinary sediment from two of three properly collected urinalysis specimens on three separate occasions. The presence of glycosuria should raise the possibility of diabetes, which, if unrecognized, may be responsible for polydipsia and/or polyuria, mimicking the symptoms of overactive bladder.

Urine Cytology

As mentioned above, patients presenting with recurrent microscopic or gross hematuria in the absence of signs or symptoms of urinary tract infection should be assessed with urine cytology. In addition, women over the age of 65 who present with overactive bladder symptoms should be screened with urine cytology. Cytology is most accurate when performed as a clean catch, first morning void. Abnormal cytology warrants referral for further evaluation, which usually includes cystoscopy and abdominal CT.

Optional Tests Used in the Diagnosis of Urinary Incontinence

Urethral Hypermobility

Measurement of urethral mobility is a useful, though optional, test in the evaluation of urinary incontinence, especially when there is a significant stress component. This is most easily performed using a sterile cotton swab. The external urethral meatus is first cleaned with an antiseptic solution, such as Betadine on a Scopette or sponge. An anesthetic jelly is applied to the end of a sterile cotton swab, and the swab is gently placed through the urethra and into the bladder. Slight traction on the cotton swab will bring the cotton end to the bladder neck; at this point, slight resistance is usually appreciated. The "resting" angle (the angle between the cotton swab and the floor) is measured with a goniometer, or similar instrument, and recorded. The patient is then asked to perform a Valsalva maneuver, and the "straining" angle is measured (Figure 5.5).

Urethral hypermobility is considered to be present when the straining angle exceeds 30 degrees and represents a deficiency in the fascial support for the urethra. The presence of urethral hypermobility supports the diagnosis of genuine stress incontinence, although it is certainly not diagnostic, as urethral hypermobility may occur with overactive bladder, as well as in asymptomatic continent women. As the test is not very specific, it might be asked why one should bother performing the test at all? A negative cotton-swab test (straining angle less than 30 degrees) in the presence of stress incontinence suggests that the patient has intrinsic sphincter deficiency, also known as a "lead-pipe" or "drain-pipe" urethra. This diagnosis has some important management implications, since pelvic floor exercises are rarely

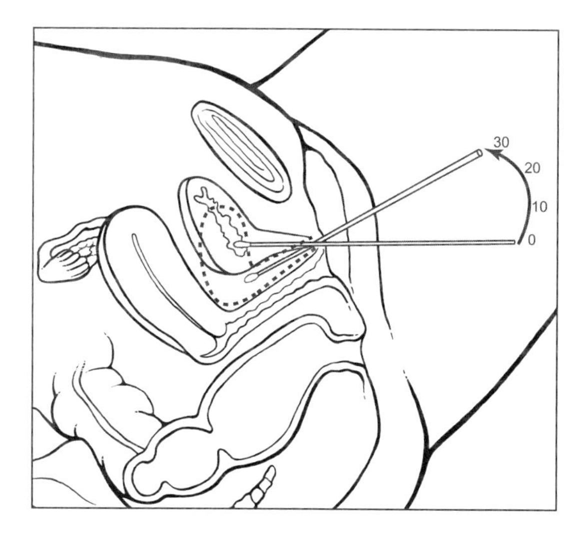

FIGURE 5.5. Q-tip testing for urethral mobility: A cotton swab lubricated with 2% Xylocaine is gently inserted into the urethra. While the patient Valsalva straining, the degree of deflection from the horizontal axis is measured with a simple protractor.

effective in this group of patients and surgical treatment with periurethral injections or suburethral slings is usually needed.

Post-void Residual Measurement

There is some controversy regarding the necessity of measuring post-void residual (PVR) in all women who present with urinary incontinence. Overflow incontinence is a very unusual cause of incontinence in women, compared with men. When overflow incontinence does occur, there are usually obvious risk factors present, such as recent incontinence surgery (causing iatrogenic urethral obstruction), neurologic disease, or diabetes (with peripheral neuropathy). In these patient populations, it is recommended that PVR be determined before initiating treatment. PVR should also be determined in women with overactive bladder who fail to improve or who worsen with anticholinergic treatment, since occasionally these medications will increase PVR to a point where the woman may become symptomatic from high residual volumes. In most women, however, it is acceptable to initiate conservative treatments, such as behavioral modification and pharmacotherapy, without measuring the PVR.

PVR measurement may be easily obtained by straight catheterization and should be performed shortly after the patient voids. The external urethra is cleaned with an antiseptic solution and a catheter (such as the Mentor 14 FR straight female catheter) is inserted into the urethra. The sterile sample can be divided for dipstick analysis and sent for culture and sensitivity, if indicated. PVR values of less than 100 cc are considered normal while values of more than 200 cc are abnormally elevated. Values between 100 cc and 200 cc are borderline and may warrant further investigation or, at least, repeated sampling to determine whether the value is accurate. PVR may also be determined noninvasively by ultrasound. A specialized instrument (BladderScan®, Diagnostic Ultrasound, Bothell, WA) can determine the PVR within 10%, although the presence of uterine fibroids or large adnexal cysts may reduce the accuracy of the test. Estimating PVR based on bimanual examination has been shown to be inaccurate and should not be used for this indication.

Cough Stress Test

Although a presumptive diagnosis of stress incontinence can be made based on history, a definitive diagnosis of stress incontinence can be performed in the office by directly observing urine loss from the urethra during a cough. It is occasionally seen during the pelvic exam with straining alone, or with coughing. A standing cough stress test can also be performed when the patient has a full bladder. The patient may be asked to come to the office with a full bladder or, alternatively, her bladder can be filled through a catheter. It is important to observe urine loss coincident with the cough in order to correctly diagnose genuine stress incontinence. A delayed or prolonged urine leak following the cough may actually indicate the presence of "cough-induced detrusor overactivity".

Simple Cystometry

Simple cystometry evaluates the ability of the bladder to fill with, and store, urine and is one of the most useful tests for diagnosing the etiology of urinary incontinence. It may be performed in the office with minimal equipment. After the patient voids, the external urethral meatus is cleaned with an antiseptic solution; a lubricated red-rubber catheter is inserted into the bladder; and a straight catheterized specimen is obtained for post-void residual measurement. A 60 cc catheter-tipped syringe with the plunger removed is placed on the end of the catheter, and **50 cc aliquots** of room-temperature sterile water or saline is slowly poured into the syringe (Figure 5.6).

The patient is asked to report various sensations experienced during filling, and these volumes are recorded. The volume at which a first desire to void is normally experienced is between 150 cc and 250 cc. A normal desire to void is usually felt at 300 cc to 400 cc, and a strong desire to void at 400 cc to 600 cc. During the test, the water level (meniscus) within the syringe should be carefully inspected, as an increase in the level may indicate an involuntary bladder contraction, which is diagnostic of detrusor overactivity. It should be kept in mind, however, that abdominal straining will

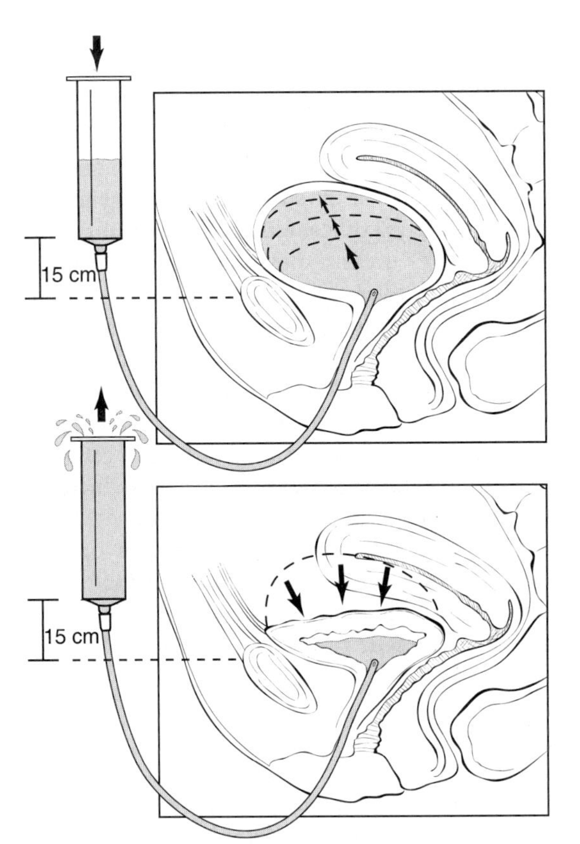

FIGURE 5.6. Eyeball Cystometry. Bladder filling is evaluated in the office setting by placing a straight catheter and filling the bladder with sterile water through a 60 cc syringe with the plunger removed.

produce a false positive rise in the meniscus; therefore, the patient should be asked not to strain during the procedure, and an examiner's hand may be placed gently on the lower abdomen during filling in order to detect such a response. When the patient reaches capacity, the catheter is removed and the patient is asked to perform a cough stress test. If the results of this test are negative, she is asked to stand and repeat the same maneuver, since there is a greater likelihood of stress incontinence occurring in the standing position. In this manner, simple cystometry can be used to make the diagnosis of both detrusor overactivity and stress incontinence.

There are, of course, several potential pitfalls with this test. There is a relatively high false-negative rate for detecting detrusor overactivity on simple cystometry, since contractions of the detrusor muscle may occur infrequently. In order to increase the likelihood of detecting these contractions, a number of techniques have been utilized to provoke involuntary bladder contractions, including instilling the fluid relatively quickly (approximately 100 cc per minute), at a relatively cold (room) temperature, and using environmental stimuli, such as dipping the woman's hand in cold water or having her listen to the sound of running water during the test. Detrusor contractions are also more likely to occur in the standing position, although it is technically more difficult to perform the test in this manner. Of course, it is also possible to provoke a detrusor contraction in an otherwise asymptomatic woman. Therefore, management should be guided by clinical correlation with the findings on cystometry rather than by simply reacting to the results of the test.

Voiding Dysfunction

Voiding dysfunction is a term that describes the patient's subjective report of some type of difficulty with voiding. She may describe symptoms of decreased urinary stream, incomplete bladder emptying, hesitancy, post-void dribbling, or the need for straining to initiate or to completely empty her bladder. Certainly, obtaining a history of recent gynecologic surgery—such as a sling procedure for stress incontinence or repair of a cystocele—is essential, as these procedures may both lead to partial or complete urethral obstruction. Medications, especially those with anticholinergic side effects, are common culprits that lead to symptoms of voiding dysfunction. Pelvic examination should concentrate on the presence of prolapse or other masses, such as suburethral diverticula or vaginal cysts, which may also cause obstruction or dribbling. The two most important tests that screen for voiding dysfunction problems are (1) measurement of post-void residual and (2) uroflowmetry.

Simple Uroflowmetry

Uroflowmetry studies evaluate the voiding phase of bladder function. This is most useful for women presenting with complaints of voiding dysfunction, although specialists may order this test in patients with urinary incontinence to screen for potential problems that may be associated with surgery for stress incontinence. Although sophisticated uroflowmetry equipment that provides specialists with a great deal of voiding parameters can be purchased, a very useful screening uroflowmetry can be performed with nothing more than a collection hat and a stopwatch. The patient is asked to void on a collection hat and the time of her void is measured with the timer. Average flow rate is determined by dividing the voided volume by the voiding time, measured in seconds. (Average flow rate = voided volume [cc]/flow time [seconds].)

A normal average flow rate is >10 cc/sec. Values less than 10 cc/sec may be indicative of a poorly contracting bladder, varying degrees of outlet (urethral) obstruction, or a discoordination between the bladder and the urethra during voiding—a term known as detrusor-sphincter dyssynergia. This condition may be seen with certain neurologic conditions, such as those resulting from spinal cord injuries.

Pelvic Organ Prolapse

Symptoms of Pelvic Organ Prolapse

Women with pelvic organ prolapse may report sensations of bulging or pressure, or they may actually report feeling a mass protruding through their vaginal opening. Symptoms may worsen over the course of the day if the women are ambulatory, due to the effects of gravity, and often improve when they lie down or sleep. Other activities that increase intraabdominal pressure, such as coughing, lifting heavy items, or straining with constipation, may worsen prolapse symptoms. Symptoms tend to be more severe if the prolapse occurs over a relatively short time period (e.g. several months) than if the process occurs more insidiously over years. Many women with pelvic organ prolapse are asymptomatic or have minimal symptoms, even with significant degrees of prolapse.

Grading Systems for Prolapse

In order to properly evaluate and record pelvic organ prolapse, some type of grading scale should be employed. For a basic evaluation of prolapse, some clinicians will refer to the prolapse as mild (prolapse with a leading edge that does not protrude to the level of the hymeneal ring), moderate (prolapse that extends to, or slightly beyond, the hymen), or severe (prolapse that extends well beyond the vaginal opening). It is also helpful to try to determine what tissue is prolapsing. Is it the cervix (uterine prolapse), the anterior vaginal wall (cystocele), or the posterior wall (rectocele or, occasionally, enterocele)? This may not always be clear, and often the prolapse involves a combination of these entities.

More elaborate grading systems exist; and although the primary care clinician does not need to evaluate patients with this much detail, an understanding of the system will enable the clinician to interpret reports from consultants. Many different scoring systems have been proposed, and this has led to some degree of confusion and difficulty when comparing measurements. In an effort to standardize this evaluation, the pelvic organ prolapse quantification (POP-Q) system has been proposed by several medical organizations and is currently the most commonly used system among urogynecologists and other specialists who deal with these disorders. Specific points are measured at the anterior, posterior, and apical compartments of the vagina, using the hymen as a fixed reference point; and these values are used to stage the prolapse using an ordinal system ranging from 0 to 4.

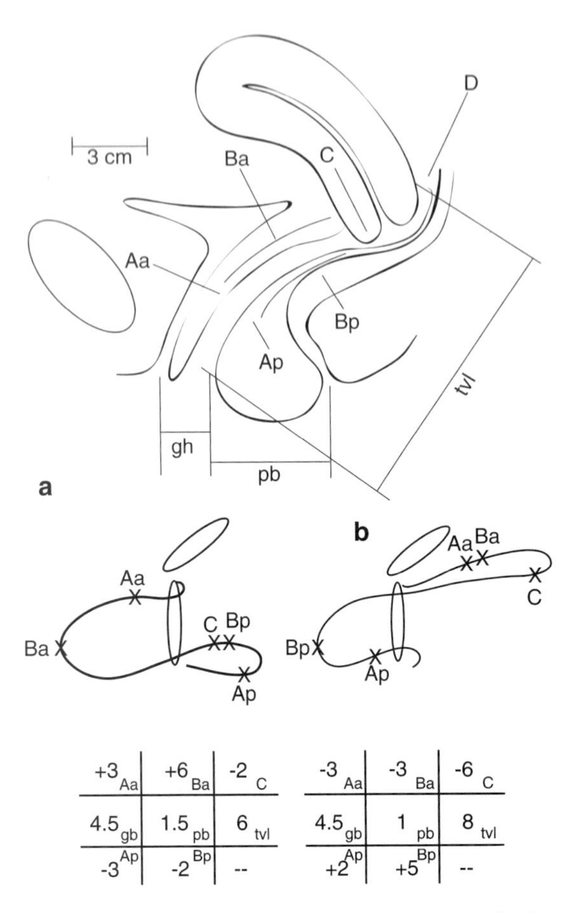

FIGURE 5.7. a. Aa measures +3 (worst possible measure for that point); Ba measures +6 (indicating that anterior wall is "leading edge"); C measures −2 (indicating that the apex comes to within 2 cm from introitus). Ap does not move and is therefore −3; Higher up, the posterior wall has worse support (therefore Bp is −2). **b.** There is no anterior wall prolapse, therefore, Aa and Ba measure −3; The apex is relatively well supported, therefore, C is −6; The posterior wall has poor support.

- Stage 0: No prolapse (the apex can descend with straining no more than 2 cm relative to the total vaginal length—measured without straining)
- Stage 1: The most distal portion of the prolapse descends with straining to a point more than 1 cm above the hymen
- Stage 2: The maximal extent of the prolapse is within 1 cm of the hymen (either outside or inside the vagina)
- Stage 3: The prolapse extends more than 1 cm beyond the hymen, but no more than within 2 cm of the total vaginal length
- Stage 4: complete eversion, defined as extending to within 2 cm of the total vaginal length

The Details of the POP-Q System

The POP-Q system describes nine discrete points that can be measured during a pelvic examination. These measurements are usually recorded in a tic-tac-toe-shaped diagram and can then be used to create a midsagittal image of the vaginal walls in relationship to the hymen (Figure 5.7).

Rather than previous systems that suggested which organ was prolapsing into the vaginal canal (e.g. cystocele, rectocele, enterocele, uterine prolapse), the POP-Q system divides the vagina into an anterior, posterior, and apical component and does not attempt to describe the organ that exists beyond the vaginal wall. All measurements (except for total vaginal length) are measured in centimeters, while the patient is bearing down, in the lithotomy position.

In order to perform POP-Q measurements, the posterior blade of a standard bivalve speculum is used to isolate the anterior, and then posterior, compartments. It is also useful to have a measuring tool that can be used for evaluation of prolapse. A ring forceps that has been scored at various distances is a very useful instrument, although a much simpler approach is to create pen marks on an ordinary cotton swab or tongue depressor (Figure 5.8).

The first two points are measured at the perineum, without the use of a speculum. Point gh (genital hiatus) measures the distance from the external urethral meatus to the posterior

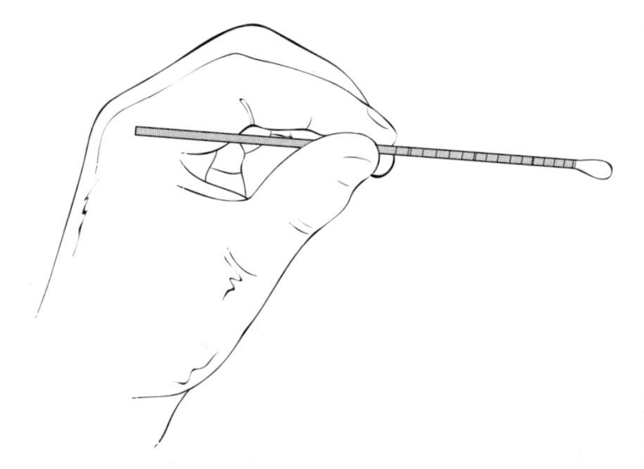

FIGURE 5.8. Demarcated Q-tip for POP-Q evaluation.

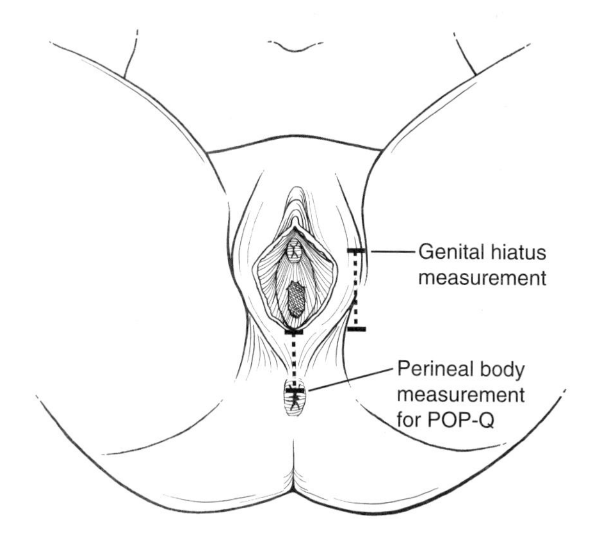

FIGURE 5.9. Illustration of PB and GH measurements of gh and pb: Gh is measured in cm from the external urethral meatus to the posterior fourchette, and pb is the distance from the posterior fourchette to the mid-anal verge.

fourchette. Point pb (perineal body) is measured from the posterior fourchette to the mid-anal verge (Figure 5.9).

The remaining seven points are measured from a fixed point, which is defined as the level of the hymeneal ring. There are two points measured on the anterior vaginal wall—Aa and Ba (where the small "a" stands for "anterior"). Point Aa is measured from a point along the anterior vaginal wall that is 3 cm from the external urethral meatus. With the patient bearing down, the distance between this point and the hymen is determined and recorded. Point Ba is located along the vaginal wall between Point Aa and the top of the vagina and represents the most prolapsed (or distal) point along this segment. Therefore, its specific location is variable, depending on where the most prolapsed portion of the anterior wall is located.

There are another two points, Ap and Bp (where the small "p" stands for "posterior"), measured on the posterior vaginal wall in a manner similar to that performed on the anterior wall. Point Ap is measured from a point along the vaginal epithelium 3 cm from the posterior fourchette, and Point Bp is the most distal point along the posterior vaginal wall between Ap and the vaginal apex.

Point C is the distance from the cervix to the hymen or, if the patient has had a hysterectomy, the distance from the vaginal cuff to the hymen. Point D is only measurable if the uterus is in place, as it represents the distance from the posterior fornix to the hymen.

The final point, TVL, represents the total vaginal length and is the only point measured without the patient bearing down. TVL is best measured with the speculum removed; the ring forceps or tongue depressor is placed at the top of the vagina without pushing it under tension. This last measurement is helpful when determining the prognosis for pessary success, since vaginal length less than 6 cm has been associated with lower success rates.[7]

Other Tests for Prolapse

Occasionally, additional tests may be used to further evaluate pelvic organ prolapse. If the clinician suspects an enterocele is present, a rectovaginal exam is performed. An enterocele is present when a sliding bulge (peritoneum filled with intestines) is palpated between the examiner's fingers. If the enterocele is not appreciated in the lithotomy position, the exam should be performed in the upright position.

Indications for Referral

When should a woman with urinary incontinence or prolapse be referred to a specialist such as a urogynecologist or urologist? The answer to the question lies, to some extent, with the individual clinicians, depending on their training, experience, and comfort level with these patients. Certainly, those women who are interested in surgery for correction of their incontinence and/or prolapse should be referred to an appropriate pelvic surgeon. Those women who fail an initial course of management for incontinence may require referral for urodynamic evaluation in order to confirm or change the diagnosis and subsequent treatment plan. Women with histories of incontinence surgery, or those who have undergone radical pelvic surgery or pelvic irradiation, are generally more difficult to accurately diagnose and manage; these women should undergo a

Table 5.4. Indications for referral of patients with urinary incontinence or prolapse to specialist

Indications for referral of patients with urinary incontinence or prolapse to specialist
Uncertain diagnosis and inability to develop a reasonable management plan
Initial treatment plan unsuccessful
Previous incontinence surgery or history of radical pelvic surgery or pelvic irradiation
Known or suspected neurologic injury
Pre-surgical evaluation for prolapse or stress incontinence
Recurrent microscopic hematuria
Suspected suburethral diverticulum or urinary tract fistula
Continuous or unpredictable incontinence
Symptomatic prolapse or prolapse beyond hymen

more complex evaluation. A complete list of indications for referral to a specialist is shown in Table 5.4.

What You Should Know About Complex Urodynamics

Women with urinary incontinence and/or voiding dysfunction who are referred to specialists often undergo a battery of tests, known as complex or multichannel urodynamics. These tests are designed to evaluate the patient's lower urinary tract function and attempt to determine the cause of her problem. It is important for the referring physician to have some basic knowledge of these tests so as to understand the findings of the tests and better assist a patient in choosing among the treatment options recommended by the specialist.

Subtracted Water Cystometry

Subtracted water cystometry provides a more accurate and sensitive technique for measuring the filling and storage function of the bladder. It can be used to measure the patient's sensations during filling, to look for uncontrollable bladder contractions, and to determine the bladder's compliance. This test is performed in a manner similar to simple cystometry, where the bladder is slowly filled with saline or water through a catheter placed in the urethra. Bladder pressure is measured with a transducer placed at the tip of the catheter and is recorded on a graph during filling. In order to account for increases in abdominal pressure (such as coughing or bearing down), which may be misinterpreted as bladder contractions, the abdominal pressure is recorded separately using a pressure transducer placed in the patient's vagina or rectum. This abdominal pressure is automatically and instantaneously subtracted from the bladder pressure, resulting in a separate graphic representation of the true detrusor pressure. It is this pressure graph that is used in looking for abnormal bladder contractions and compliance problems.

Studies of Urethral Competence

Evaluation of urethral sphincter function is important in determining the cause of stress incontinence and may provide the specialist with information that determines the best management option for the patient. One such test is the *urethral pressure profile*. In this test, a pressure transducer located on a special catheter is pulled through the urethra, at a constant rate, in order to measure pressures along the length of the urethra. The pressure in the bladder is automatically subtracted from the urethral pressure, providing the clinician with the *urethral closure pressure*, which is simply a pressure difference between the bladder and the urethra. If the difference between these pressures is minimal (<20 cm H_2O), then the patient may leak urine with minimal exertion, such as standing up from the sitting position or bearing down slightly. These women are said to have intrinsic sphincter deficiency, a severe form of stress incontinence. Urethral closure pressures >20 cm H_2O are found in most women with stress incontinence. In this situation, while the urethral sphincter may be considered normal, the pathologic condition leading to the incontinence may be a lack of fascial support to the bladder neck and urethra.

The *Valsalva leak point pressure test* is another method used to evaluate the competence of the urethral sphincter. The bladder is filled with a standard volume of fluid, and the patient is asked to slowly bear down in an incremental manner until leakage is noted from the external urethral meatus. The lowest pressure at which leakage occurs is recorded as the leak point pressure. An LPP greater than 90 cm H_2O is considered to represent a normal urethral sphincter, whereas lower LPP values may be indicative of intrinsic urethral sphincter deficiency (ISD). This is an important distinction, as patients with ISD often do not respond well to conservative treatments such as pelvic muscle exercises.

Video Fluorourodynamics

Some specialists will use a combination of multichannel urodynamic testing with fluoroscopic visualization of the bladder and urethra, utilizing a contrast material instilled in the bladder, in order to diagnose certain patients with urinary incontinence or voiding dysfunction. These tests do provide some additional information for the specialist, although they also expose the patient to radiation and are more expensive than traditional multichannel urodynamic testing. In general, this test should be used judiciously when the specialist feels that the diagnosis cannot be made by traditional testing alone.

Cystoscopy

Cystoscopic evaluation of the lower urinary tract may be ordered by a specialist under certain circumstances (Table 5.5). Persistent microscopic hematuria and recurrent urinary tract infections are common indications for referral for cystoscopy. Patients with refractory overactive bladder (OAB) in association with hematuria should undergo cystoscopy to rule out a bladder tumor or stone. Some specialists will perform cystoscopy on patients with stress incontinence in order to visually evaluate the urethra for signs of scarring; this finding may alter their choice of surgical procedure.

Table 5.5. Indications for Cystoscopy

Indications for Cystoscopy
Microscopic hematuria
Recurrent urinary tract infections
Recurrent urinary incontinence after surgery
Suspected urinary tract fistula
Persistent irritative voiding symptoms
Suspected suburethral diverticulum
Suspected interstitial cystitis

Diagnosing Fecal Incontinence and Defecatory Dysfunction

Fecal Incontinence (FI) is a common but underreported problem in women. Often the effects of FI are more devastating than other forms of pelvic dysfunction. Embarrassment prevents two out of three women from discussing symptoms of FI with their physician (Johanson & Lafferty 1996)[11] unless directly asked. Feelings of shame often lead to depression, social isolation, and deterioration in quality of life. For older women, FI may be the final factor pushing caretakers to decide on nursing home placement. Therefore, the first diagnostic step is to ask about symptoms of FI and their effect on a patient's life.

Fecal incontinence can affect all age groups, but the prevalence increases with age. Women at risk include multiparous women, new mothers, perimenopausal women and, particularly, older women The true prevalence in a general population is not known because of varying definitions of FI as well as patient reluctance to report symptoms, but it has been reported to be anywhere from 0.1% to 18%. Twenty-one percent of women who have pelvic organ prolapse and/or urinary incontinence also have fecal incontinence,[8] and 17% of patients presenting to a urogynecology clinic have FI symptoms.

As with urinary continence, multiple components contribute to maintain fecal continence. Anal continence depends on stool consistency and volume, rectal capacity, colonic transit time, anorectal sensation and reflexes, resting anal tone, and ability to resist the fecal bolus coming through the anal sphincter, as well as normal mental function. Therefore, the cause of FI can also be multifactorial, including direct trauma or nerve damage to the continence mechanism from childbirth, prior surgery, radiation, or idiopathic denervation. Central and peripheral nervous system diseases, medical problems, anatomic abnormalities, and stool consistency play a causative role. Some causative factors are listed in Table 5.6.

Table 5.6. Etiology of Fecal Incontinence and Defecatory Dysfunction

Causes of Fecal Incontinence	Defecatory Dysfunction
Anatomic	Anatomic
Prior surgery	**Colonic or Anal outlet obstruction:**
Anal procedures:	Posterior vaginal prolapse (rectocele)
Sphincterotomy	Rectal prolapse
Hemorrhoidectomy	Strictures
Stretch procedure	Nneoplasm
Fistula repair	Fissures (pain)
Trauma	Paradoxical puborectalis contraction
Obstetric:	
Occult or apparent sphincter disruption	Neurologic
	CNS disease
	Parkinson's disease
Neurologic	Multiple Sclerosis
CNS disease	Stroke
Dementia	
Stroke	**PNS disease**
Multiple sclerosis	Aganglionosis (Hirschsprung's disease, Chagas disease
Trauma	Diabetes mellitus
PNS disease	Decreased motility
Diabetes	
	Bowel Habits
Denervation (puborectalis and external anal sphincter)	Poor diet
Vaginal delivery (may not be symptomatic for years)	Sedentary lifestyle
	Change in habits
Radiation	Medications
Chronic constipation	Narcotics
Idiopathic	Anticholinergics
	Antidepressants
Abnormalities of Rectal Storage	Beta blockers
(Causes fecal urgency)	Calcium channel blockers
Inflammatory bowel disease	
Prior bowel resection	**Endocrine**
Neoplasms	Hypothyroidism
Radiation	Hypercalcemia
Rectal prolapse	Hypokalemia
Internal hemorrhoids	Uremia
Fecal impaction	
Diarrhea	**Idiopathic**
	History of Abuse
Decreased sensation/ sampling reflex	**Psychiatric**
Inflammatory bowel disease	
Rectal prolapse	
Neurologic disorders	

The leading cause of fecal incontinence in women remains childbirth injury through pudendal nerve stretch and compression (denervation injury) as well as direct external anal sphincter disruption. Symptoms may occur immediately or may not develop for several years, when weakening pelvic floor muscles can no longer compensate for a weak or disrupted anal sphincter. A weakened pelvic floor also causes FI after chronic constipation or increased intraabdominal pressure. The theory is that habitual straining, especially at defecation, results in traction neuropathy (stretching) of the terminal portion of the pudendal nerve. This, in turn, contributes to weakness of the pelvic floor, leading to more straining, more denervation and, eventually, to fecal incontinence. So, it is important to ask about previous deliveries—especially vaginal deliveries with tears into the rectum or external anal sphincter. Similarly, a history of chronic constipation or other conditions that lead to chronically increased intraabdominal pressure should be identified. If these problems are ongoing, they should be treated.

Symptoms of Fecal Incontinence

The best approach to inquiring about FI symptoms is to ask directly as part of routine screening. There are also questionnaires available that the patient can fill out in the waiting room or at home prior to the visit. A simple screening question is: *Do you ever lose gas or stool without wanting to?* If there is a positive response, then further history is elicited starting with how often accidents occur, how severely, and the duration and progression of symptoms, as well as impact on lifestyle. Important information includes quality of lost stool, ability to control flatus and solid formed stool, and the ability to voluntarily contract the anal sphincter and pelvic muscles to prevent or mitigate loss. Solid stool is the easiest to control, followed by liquid stool, then flatus. Loss of solid stool indicates a more severe problem. Awareness of fecal loss without the ability to stop it indicates anal sphincter or pelvic muscle damage (motor deficiency) with resulting inability to adequately contract those muscles.

It is important to inquire about fecal urgency (sudden urge to evacuate with inability to reach a bathroom in sufficient time), which could indicate impaired rectal compliance or decreased ability to store stool. Fecal urgency can exist in the setting of inflammatory bowel disease, radiation proctitis, coloanal anastomoses, or any inflammatory condition of the rectal mucosa.

Absence of any sensation prior to stool loss indicates sensory deficiency (sensory incontinence). This occurs in the presence of neurologic disease or rectal prolapse. Fecal soiling in the absence of urgency, or other fecal loss, can indicate deformation of the anal canal or presence of fecal mass with seepage (fecal impaction).

In addition to the consistency of lost stool, regular bowel motions should be assessed. Consistency is affected by diet, food intolerance, medications, diverticular disease, inflammatory bowel diseases, and ingested fluid volume. Liquid stool enters the rectum too quickly for normal activity of external anal sphincter and pelvic floor muscles. Therefore, it is important to ask about dietary habits—especially fiber intake. Sometimes simple dietary adjustments and bulkier stool can compensate for motor deficiency.

Asking about a patient's normal bowel habits is also important. Does incontinence occur because of frequent loose stools or only if there is constipation or missed morning evacuation? Establishing a regular bowel pattern with a fixed morning evacuation may also improve symptoms by keeping the rectum empty for the rest of the day.

Medical and Surgical History

In addition to assessing obstetric history, instrument vaginal delivery (forceps or vacuum), and rectal injury, as indicated above, a history of anal or bowel surgery, or pelvic irradiation, should be assessed along with potentially contributing medical problems, back injuries, or physical restrictions.

Physical Examination

A simple physical exam begins by assessment of a woman's functional state. Focusing on the pelvic area, a visual inspection is performed. Fecal soiling and skin irritation can sometimes be observed, especially in older women. The perineum and anal area are inspected for scarring or a widened vaginal or rectal orifice (sign of muscle weakness and loss). A dovetail sign may be present, in which the longitudinal folds heading circumferentially away from the sphincter are missing anteriorly, usually from 10 to 2 o'clock, denoting a disrupted external anal sphincter. Having the patient squeeze as if trying to hold in a bowel movement can visually demonstrate the strength and full circular integrity of the sphincter contraction. Having the patient bear down can demonstrate any rectal prolapse, hemorrhoids, or perineal descent (ballooning down of the perineum). Women with anatomic abnormalities of the perineum, external anal sphincter, or pelvic floor should be referred for further evaluation.

Next, the cutaneo anal reflex is checked by lightly stroking the perineal skin with a finger or Q-tip and looking for a reflex contraction of the external anal sphincter. Sensation response to sharp and soft ends of a Q-tip also gives a crude idea of perineal innervation. Then, digital vaginal examination assesses pelvic floor muscle (Levator ani) strength on a scale of 0 to 5 (0 indicating no palpable contraction, 5, a very strong contraction able to resist force by the examiner's fingers). Occasionally patients recruit accessory gluteal, abdominal, and leg muscles in an effort to contract weakened pelvic floor muscles. These should not be confused with pelvic floor muscle contractions. In women with such inability to contract pelvic floor muscles, a home pelvic floor exercise program (Kegels) is ineffective. Digital examination of the rectum assesses anal sphincter strength, resistance to pressure, and integrity. The resting tone reflects the internal anal sphincter (IAS), while squeeze tone assesses external anal sphincter (EAS). Muscle bulk can also be appreciated, as can any defects or muscle attenuation, especially in the 10 to 2 o'clock position. A digital rectal exam also evaluates for scars, rectocele, fistula, blood or masses.

Based on findings on history and physical, many women can begin conservative dietary, behavioral, and pelvic floor strengthening programs. Further testing can be reserved for those who do not respond to treatment, or if an anatomic problem is suspected (Figure 5.10).

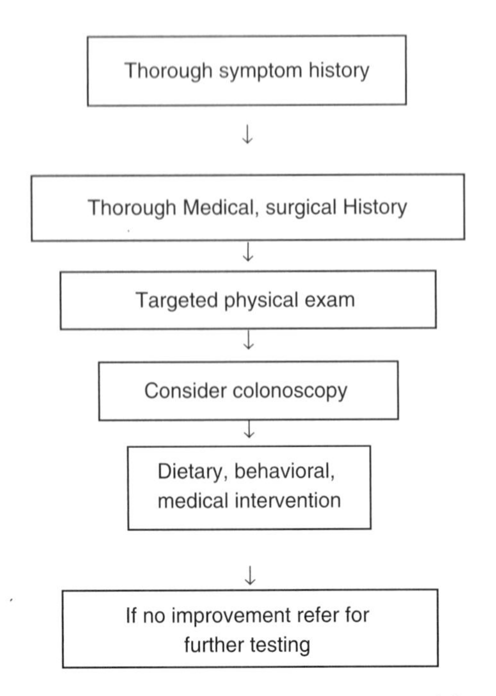

FIGURE 5.10. Assessment of fecal incontinence, defecatory dysfunction.

Diagnostic Testing

Endoscopy

Proctosigmoidoscopy excludes hemorrhoids, fissures, fistula, and abscess as well as malignancy, inflammatory bowel disease, proctitis, or villous adenoma. Colonoscopy is more thorough and evaluates for a partially obstructive colorectal cancer that could also result in a change in bowel habits and incontinence.

Endoanal Ultrasound

If a sphincter disruption is suspected, an ultrasound can clearly demonstrate a defect. The test is performed with a 10 MHz transducer that allows 360-degree visualization. The probe is inserted and gradually withdrawn. Both the IAS and EAS, as well as the puborectalis (levator sling), can be visualized, helping with diagnosis as well as planning of any surgical intervention. Currently, anal ultrasound is limited by scar and fibrous tissue. The IAS is more easily visualized than the EAS.

Magnetic Resonance Imaging (MRI)

It remains to be seen whether MRI will prove more precise than ultrasound for imaging the pelvic floor muscles, especially the puborectalis, EAS, and IAS.

Defecography

Defecography is indicated if a rectal prolapse or intussusception (occult prolapse) is suspected, but is not necessary for most women with FI. This is a dynamic fluoroscopic imaging of a contrast-filled rectum while the patient is sitting on a radiolucent commode. Pictures are taken at rest, while squeezing, and with defecation. Normally, there is rapid and complete evacuation of the barium. Several measurements of the anatomy are then taken. Defecography also reveals rectoceles, rectal deformities and sigmoidoceles.

Anal Manometry

The purpose of manometry is to assess IAS tone (resting pressure), assess the functional length (high pressure zone) of the anal canal, and assess voluntary contraction of the EAS (squeeze pressure). This is a 10-minute outpatient procedure that does not require a bowel preparation. A soft plastic catheter with multiple perfusion ports is paced into the anorectum and is gradually withdrawn, measuring pressure along the way. In incontinent women the resting and squeeze pressures are lower than normal range, and the high-pressure zone is shorter. Manometry can also assess the rectoanal inhibitory reflex, anorectal sensory threshold, rectal capacity, and rectal compliance. Compliance is assessed by inserting a balloon, determining the minimal volume the rectum can sense, and then sequentially inflating the balloon to a volume that cannot be tolerated.

FI symptoms can be present in the setting of normal manometry findings, and abnormal findings can occur in incontinent women. Again, history and physical exam alone are often more helpful than testing for the majority of women.

Neurophysiologic Testing

The purpose of neurophysiologic testing is to assess the neuromuscular integrity of the anal sphincter by measuring the electric activity generated by muscle fibers. This is accomplished by either EMG (electromyography) or pudendal nerve terminal motor latency. EMG uses concentric needle or single fiber electrodes and is able to record electrical activity and to indicate patterns of denervation and reinnervation after injury, as seen in birth injuries. Often the location and severity of injury in the EAS can be mapped out by sequentially moving the needle. This method causes great discomfort for patients. External patch EMG is available but is less sensitive.

Pudendal nerve terminal motor latency is obtained by measuring the latency period from the time the pudendal nerve is stimulated to the time of response of the anal muscle. Both EMG and PNML have been used to predict functional surgical outcomes for repair of a disrupted sphincter. There is less chance of postoperative continence in women with evidence of impaired nerve function, and patients can be accordingly counselled.

Other Diagnostic Tests

Anal mucosal electrosensitivity involves stimulating the anal mucosa with gradually increasing current until the threshold of sensation is reached. This is impaired in instances of neurogenic fecal incontinence.

Thermal sensitivity uses a water-perfused thermode to detect the ability to distinguish between gas, liquid, and solid stool. Spinal latency testing is used to diagnose cauda equine injury as the cause of FI.

Defecatory Dysfunction

As with fecal incontinence, constipation affects more women than men and is often encountered in practice. Again, evaluating constipation starts with a good history and physical. Most importantly, the patient must define what she means by constipation. Is it infrequent bowel movement? Hard, difficult to pass stools? Pain with bowel movements? It is important to ask how many bowel movements a patient has per week, what is their consistency, the degree of difficulty in passing stools, and/or a need to splint (press on vagina or perineum to be able to evacuate). The patient should be asked, as well, about the presence of pain and the ability to relax the pelvic floor. Depending on stool consistency, the patient's dietary habits and fiber and fluid intake should be ascertained. Level of physical activity can also play a role.

Medical problems and medications can also affect bowel function, so medical history should be reviewed. Neurologic, endocrine, and psychiatric problems can be prominently involved. Stressful life changes, new diet or environment, smoking, or caffeine cessation can also play a role. A history of physical or sexual abuse can lead to constipation with dyspareunia or pelvic muscle spasms (Table 5.7).

Physical Examination

Evaluation starts with an abdominal exam to assess for masses or palpable stool. Pelvic examination starts with inspection at rest for hemorrhoids, fissures, or significant vaginal prolapse. Asking a patient to strain can demonstrate rectal prolapse, perineal descent, or posterior vaginal wall prolapse that was not evident at rest.

Table 5.7. Pertinent questions for patients who present with symptoms of fecal incontinence and defecatory dysfunction

Fecal Incontinence	Defecatory dysfunction
Medical history	Medical history
Surgical history	Surgical history
Bowel diseases	Bowel diseases
True incontinence vs. fecal urgency	Bowel movements per week
Frequency of accidents	Excessive straining, digital Support of vagina or perineum
Time of day, related activities	Stool consistency
Duration of problem	Duration of problem
Severity: gas, liquid, solid	Bowel regimen, laxative use
Pad use	Related pelvic symptoms (pain, muscle spasms)
Sensory awareness	Rectal fullness
Bowel habits	Presence of prolapse
Constipation history	Recent change in routine
Diarrhea	History of abuse

Bimanual exam and digital rectal exam will further evaluate for pelvic muscle tone, ability to relax puborectalis, as well as the presence of rectal masses and strictures. A rectovaginal fascial defect (pocketing in anterior rectal wall) can also be assessed.

Diagnostics

Proctosigmoidoscopy evaluates for masses, polyps, ulcer secondary to internal rectal prolapse, and melanosis coli (brown-black discoloration from laxative use). Most patients do not need further workup beyond this point and can begin with dietary, behavioral and medical therapy as outlined in the next chapter. However, if simple interventions do not result in relief, or if the constipation is particularly severe, then further testing might be needed to evaluate for colonic inertia, anatomic abnormality, or pelvic floor spasticity (hypertonic pelvic floor).

Defecography

Performed in a similar to that described for fecal incontinence, defecography can delineate anatomic abnormalities leading to constipation. In the case of defecatory dysfunction—especially with straining and evacuation—rectoceles, internal rectal prolapse, or other abnormalities of the rectal wall can be seen. The normal mechanism of evacuation can also be assessed. The angle between the anal canal and the rectum can be measured at rest, squeeze, and strain. This angle is maintained by the puborectalis muscle (the sling muscle that aids in anal continence). During normal evacuation, this angle increases as the anal canal straightens. However, if the puborectalis does not relax normally, this straightening does not occur and may interfere with passage of the contrast. This is called paradoxical puborectalis contraction and can lead to constipation, obstructing the anal outlet.

Functional Motility Studies

Colonic transit study (Sitz mark study) is performed when slow transit (colonic inertia) is suspected. Patients stop all laxatives 24 hours prior to the study and eat a high-fiber diet (30 grams daily). The patient then consumes a number of radiopaque markers. Serial X-rays are then taken to monitor their progress. Normally, 80% of the markers should be passed by day 5, and all markers should have been evacuated by day 7. Depending on where the markers accumulate, dysfunction can be localized to one area of the large bowel, or diffuse dysfunction can be assessed.

Manometry can assess rectal compliance by measuring the sensitivity and total volume tolerated in a fluid-filled balloon. If the compliance is increased, this can indicate an enlarged or insensitive rectum. Also, the absence of reflex internal sphincter inhibition with rectal distention (the rectal anal inhibitory reflex) can signal Hirschsprung's disease.

EMG studies of the anal sphincter and puborectalis can also demonstrate paradoxical muscle contraction if measured electrical activity does not decrease with straining. This may also be palpable on physical exam, as the patient will be unable to voluntarily relax these muscles. Colonic inertia and paradoxical contractions can coexist, so it is important to look for both.

Conclusions

The initial office evaluation and management of urinary and fecal incontinence may be undertaken by primary care physicians. A detailed history and directed physical examination will, in most cases, lead the physician to a preliminary diagnosis that will allow a conservative and effective plan to be formulated. Patients who have a more complicated history or who do not respond to initial measures may be referred for more complex testing, as outlined above. Even if the primary care physician elects to refer the patient to a specialist, having an understanding of these tests will enable the clinician to actively participate in the care of the patient.

Key Points

- A simple symptom questionnaire (Table 5.1), combined in some cases with a voiding diary (Figure 5.1), provides invaluable information during the initial evaluation of urogynecologic symptoms.

- Examination of pelvic prolapse—including an assessment of each compartment (anterior, posterior, apex)—can be performed in a few minutes, using an ordinary speculum and no high-tech equipment.
- Before initiating medication for women with "overactive bladder" symptoms, the following three conditions should be ruled out: (1) hematuria (simple urinalysis), (2) infection (urine culture), and (3) retention (postvoid residual).
- Cystometry refers to the evaluation of bladder pressure during filling and is one of the most valuable and simple urogynecologic tests. "Eyeball cystometry" allows the primary care provider to perform this test with minimal expense, without high-tech equipment.
- Many women with anal incontinence can improve with simple changes to bowel consistency and habit retraining. Anal incontinence can be evaluated with endoanal ultrasound and several functional tests, if initial therapy fails.

References

1. Burgio K, Matthews KA, Engel BT. Prevalence, incidence and correlates of urinary incontinence in healthy, middle-aged women. *J Urol.* 1991;146:1255–1259.
2. Herzog AR, Fultz NH. Prevalence and incidence of urinary incontinence in community-dwelling populations. *J Am Geriatr Soc.* 1990;38:273–281.
3. Division of Chronic Disease Control and Community Intervention, National Center for Chronic Disease Prevention and Health Promotion, Centers for Disease Control. Urinary incontinence among hospitalized persons aged 65 years and older: United States, 1984–1987. *MMWR Morb Mortal Wkly Rep.* 1991;40:433–436.
4. Day JC. *Population projections of the United States by age, sex, race, and Hispanic origin: 1995–2050.* U.S. Bureau of the Census, Current Population Reports, P25–1130. Washington, D.C.: U.S. Government Printing Office. 1996.
5. Stewart WF, Van Rooyen JB, Cundiff GW et al. Prevalence and burden of overactive bladder in the United States. *World J Urol.* 2003;20:327–336.
6. Sirls LT, Zimmern PE, Leach GE. Role of limited evaluation and aggressive medical management in multiple sclerosis: a review of 113 patients. *J Urol.* 1994;151:946–950.
7. Blaivas JG, Barbalias GA. Detrusor-external sphincter dyssynergia in men with multiple sclerosis: an ominous urologic condition. *J Urol.* 1984;131:91–94.
8. McGuire EJ, Savastano JA. Urodynamic findings and long-term outcome management of patients with multiple sclerosis-induced lower urinary tract dysfunction. *J Urol.* 984;132:713–715.
9. Clemons JL, Aguilar VC, Tillinghast TA, Jackson ND, Myers DL. Risk factors associated with an unsuccessful pessary fitting trial in women with pelvic organ prolapse. *Am J Obstet Gynecol.* 2004; 190:345–350.
10. Jackson SL, Weber AM, Hull TL, Mitchinson AR, Walters MD. Fecal incontinence in women with urinary incontinence and pelvic organ prolapse. *Obstet Gynecol.* 1997;89:423–427.
11. Johanson JF, Lafferty J. Epidemiology of fecal incontinence: the silent affliction. Am J Gastroenterol. 1996;91:33–36.

6
Kegel Exercises, Dietary and Behavioral Modifications: Simple Strategies for Getting Started

Jay-James R. Miller and Peter K. Sand

Introduction

Despite many recent pharmacological and surgical advances in urogynecology, a variety of non-medical, non-operative strategies still represent the best first-line approach for many patients. The most common goal of behavioral treatments is to improve bladder control through systematic changes in patient behavior and environmental conditions. The primary behavioral treatment for stress incontinence, for instance, is pelvic floor muscle training and exercise. For fecal incontinence, the most effective behavioral treatment, in addition to pelvic floor muscle exercise, may include dietary alterations—such as increased dietary fiber—and bowel habit retraining. A number of behavioral treatments are commonly implemented for overactive bladder, including bladder drill and bladder training, pelvic muscle exercises, urge-suppression techniques, self-monitoring, and dietary and fluid alterations.

These treatments offer an effective means of controlling symptoms without the adverse effects that may accompany drug or surgical therapies. Primary care providers can easily administer a number of these strategies. In this chapter, a handful of the most useful strategies will be reviewed, with the primary care provider in mind.

Pelvic Muscle (Kegel) Exercises

In 1951, Arnold Kegel, a gynecologist at the University of Southern California, published a landmark study of the effect of pelvic floor muscle exercises in 500 women with urinary incontinence. He instructed his patients to contract their pelvic muscles against a "perineometer," a cone-shaped balloon inserted into the vagina. They were instructed to alternately contract and relax the pelvic floor muscles—specifically the pubococcygeus muscles—for 20 minutes, three times a day, for a total of 300 contractions (see Figure 6.1). Kegel reported an 84% success rate for stress urinary incontinence.[1]

The purpose of pelvic muscle exercises is to restore tone and function of atrophied pelvic muscles, with the rationale that this helps control involuntary loss of urine during physical activities such as coughing, sneezing, exercising, or laughing. The pubococcygeal muscle acts as a sling extending from the pubic bone in front to the coccyx, or tailbone, encircling the urethra, vagina, and rectum. The location of the pubococcygeal muscle may be identified using the "stop test", which refers to voluntarily stopping the urine stream while voiding. The patient should not, however, practice Kegel exercises repetitively during urination. The stop test should be used only as an infrequent means to check the strength and isolation of the correct muscles, as frequent voluntary interruption of the urinary stream could predispose to voiding dysfunction. Alternatively, a woman may be instructed to squeeze the vagina around an inserted finger, providing a low-tech form of biofeedback. The premise is that, by repeatedly contracting the pubococcygeus, these muscles will become stronger, and stronger muscles will provide more resistance to incontinence.

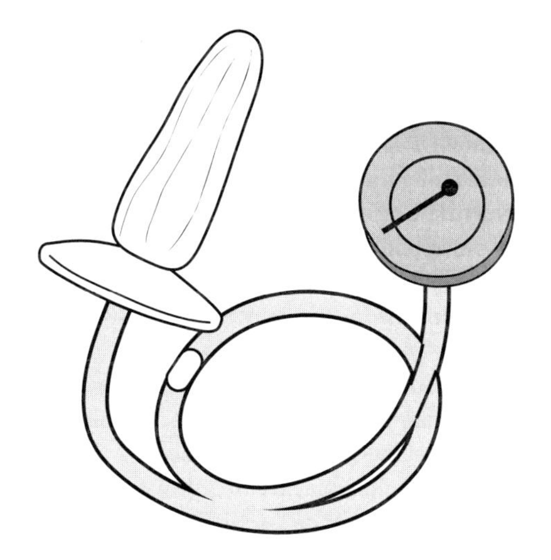

FIGURE 6.1. Perineometer.

It is rarely sufficient to merely ask patients to do "Kegels", because patients frequently use abdominal, leg, or buttock muscles. Contraction of leg and buttock muscles can be seen on examination. Contraction of abdominal muscles is determined by placing a hand on the abdominal wall while the patient is performing these exercises. If the abdominal wall muscles are felt to contract, ask the patient to relax and try again.

Kegel Tips

- Start with the "stop test".
- Avoid leg, buttock contraction.
- Hand on abdomen or thigh.
- Rest between contractions.
- Goal of 10-second contraction.

Once the health care provider is confident that the patient has correctly identified the pubococcygeus muscle, he or she may provide appropriate instruction. In the office, patients are told to empty their bladders before performing pelvic muscle exercises. They are asked to relax completely. These exercises can be done anywhere, anytime, and in any position, but the patient must be relaxed. Pelvic muscle exercises are performed by tightening the pubococcygeus muscle and maintaining the contraction for ten seconds, then relaxing for ten seconds. The patient should feel a sensation of lifting around her vagina or of pulling around her rectum. Some practitioners advise patients to do these exercises for ten-minute sessions and to repeat the exercises three times per day. Others have promoted a much less intensive routine, with only 10 to 20 contractions per day. It remains to be determined which of these approaches is better, with respect to both efficacy and long-term compliance.

Since not all women can hold a ten-second contraction at first, it is important to assess how long a patient can hold a contraction, and this is the amount of time for which a contraction should be held during exercises. It is important that the patient always rest her pubococcygeus for at least as long as she contracts it to avoid fatigue. After two weeks of daily pelvic muscle exercises she may notice some improvement with urinary incontinence. Significant improvement can be expected after twelve weeks of training.

Numerous controlled studies have supported Kegel's findings.[2] In a recently reported 10-year follow-up study, researchers examined questionnaire responses in 52 women who had undergone pelvic muscle exercise training for stress urinary incontinence 10 years earlier. In the 53% of women who had initially responded to pelvic muscle exercises, 66% remained satisfied with their urinary continence status and only 8% had undergone surgery. Of the women who initially failed pelvic floor muscle exercises, 62% had undergone surgery. There was not a significant difference in the levels of satisfaction between the two groups of women.[3] The results of this study reveal the importance of identifying refractory cases that require referral to a urogynecologist or urologist.

In a randomized clinical trial, researchers compared behavioral treatment with drug therapy in a sample of 197 women between 55 and 92 years of age who had urge or mixed incontinence. Subjects were randomly assigned to four sessions of biofeedback-assisted behavioral treatment, which included daily pelvic floor exercises, a drug treatment (oxybutynin chloride), or a placebo drug. Behavioral treatment yielded a mean 81% reduction in incontinence episodes and was significantly more effective than was drug treatment.[4] Pelvic muscle exercises have not been well studied for pelvic organ prolapse, and most practitioners recommend them only for mild cases of prolapse.

Bladder Training

One of the most long-standing forms of behavioral treatment for overactive bladder is timed voiding, or "bladder drill," an intensive intervention that was originally conducted on an inpatient basis as described by Frewen.[5,6] Bladder drill procedures imposed a lengthened interval between voids to establish a normal frequency of urination and were purported to result in normalization of bladder function. Bladder training is a modification of bladder drill that is conducted more gradually on an outpatient basis. Over time, the term "bladder drill" has become synonymous with the term "bladder training."

The rationale for this treatment approach is based on the premise that frequent urination is not only a precursor to, but also a precipitant of, detrusor overactivity. Increased voiding frequency leads to reduced bladder capacity and may eventually result in detrusor instability. By implementing a bladder drill routine, this cycle is broken when patients resist the sensation of urgency to postpone urination and gradually increase the inter-voiding interval.[7]

We usually begin bladder training by asking patients to void at a comfortable starting interval (e.g. every one-to-two hours) while awake, based on a previously recorded bladder diary of when they were urinating and leaking. The initial voiding interval should be selected to ensure initial success. Patients seeking a fairly structured approach are given a stack of "bladder drill cards" with two clocks printed on each one (Figure 6.2).

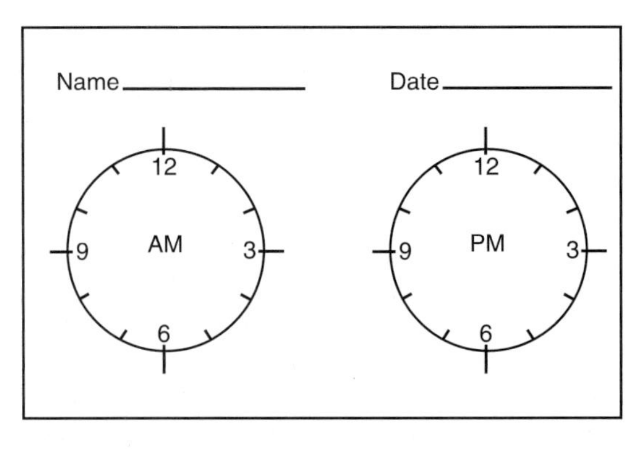

FIGURE 6.2. Bladder card.

The patient is asked to void as soon as she arises and to mark the time on the face of the appropriate clock, usually the one marked "AM". She is then to void only at the specified time interval and to mark the time on the face of the clock. The patient must attempt to empty her bladder completely, even if she does not feel the urge to go. She is only to mark the time on the face of the clock when she actually attempts to empty her bladder.

The patient is asked to ignore all other impulses to void if they occur between the specified times. She is instructed to consciously initiate some other behavior to distract her thoughts from her bladder—for instance, repetitively subtracting three from one hundred to divert her focus (e.g. "100, 97, 94, 91 . . ."). She is also instructed to contract her levator ani and pubococcygeus muscle to activate the vesicoinhibitory reflex—a reflex arc that results in relaxation of the bladder. As a third suppression technique, the patient is instructed to change her position. If she is standing, she should sit down; if she is sitting, then she should lie down, if able to do so. The rule is that she is not allowed to void at any other time than the specified interval.

The last recorded void is at bedtime, and the regimen does not continue through the night. If the patient gets up during the night, she is to mark the number of times she does so on the back of the card, simply as a means to monitor her progress. If nocturia is a problem, the patient is asked to restrict fluids after supper. Any episodes of incontinence are marked on the bladder drill card.

The patient should maintain this routine until her first return visit, usually after two to four weeks. She is instructed to bring all of her bladder drill cards to that appointment so her physician or nurse can review them. Depending on patient progress, a new time interval may be assigned until the next follow-up in two to four weeks. This process continues until the desired interval of every three to four hours is achieved.

Bladder training is widely used for the treatment of urinary complaints in both primary and specialty care, including urge incontinence, urgency, frequency, and nocturia. Bladder training may be started for the mast majority of women on the basis of these symptoms, in a primary care setting. Exceptions would include patients with urinary retention, hematuria, persistent infection, or significant pelvic prolapse, in which case a more formal urogynecologic evaluation is warranted. Bladder training aims to increase the time interval between voids, either by a mandatory or self-adjustable schedule, so that incontinence is avoided and continence ultimately regained.

One randomized clinical trial of bladder training was conducted by Fantl et al.,[8] who demonstrated that older women reduced their episodes of incontinence by a mean of 57% using bladder training, whereas little improvement occurred with a no-treatment control group.

A potential way to improve the efficacy of conservative therapies for overactive bladder is to combine behavioral and drug treatments. Some clinicians combine pharmacotherapy and bladder training with the idea that relaxing the bladder with a pharmacologic agent provides a measure of control that will allow the patient to be better able to learn volitional control of detrusor contraction.

Bladder Diet

Increasing urinary pH by avoiding some foods, drinking plain water, or with bicarbonate of soda, will help reduce urinary symptoms to some degree. It is quite logical that foods that decrease the pH and make the urine more acidic are likely to increase urinary urgency and frequency by irritating inflamed areas of the bladder and urethra or by sensitizing C-fibers. Foods that are high in arylalkylamines (tyrosine, tyramine, tryptophan, aspartate, and phenylalanine) may also irritate the bladder. Partial listings of foods that decrease pH and are high in arylalkylamines are shown in Table 6.1 and Table 6.2, respectively.

TABLE 6.1. Foods That Decrease pH

Alcoholic Beverages	Coffee	Peaches
Apple Juice	Cranberries	Pepper
Apples	Grapes	Pineapple
Ascorbic Acid	Guava	Plums
Cantaloupes	Lemons	Strawberries
Carbonated Beverages	Lemon Juice	Tea
Chili	Lime	Tomatoes
Citrus Fruits	Nectarines	Vinegar
	Oranges	

TABLE 6.2. Foods That Are High in Arylalkamines

Avocados	Cranberries	Prunes
Bananas	Fava Beans	Raisins
Beer	Lima Beans	Rye Bread
Brewer's Yeast	Marmite™	Saccharin
Canned Figs	Mayonnaise	Sour Cream
Champagne	NutraSweet®	Soy Sauce
Cheese	Nuts	Vitamins B & C
Chicken Livers	Onions	Wines
Chocolate	Pickled Herring	Yogurt
Corned Beef	Pineapple	

For patients interested in dietary alterations, we recommend that they try to avoid the acidic foods in Table 1 whenever possible. In addition, foods that are high in arylalkylamines (Table 2) should potentially be avoided. If any symptoms are to be improved by avoiding these foods and substances, patients will begin to feel this improvement within a few weeks. Once patients are feeling better, they may begin to challenge their systems by adding foods back, individually, to see if any specifically irritate them. Alternatively, some patients simply observe which of the foods or beverages in Tables 1 and 2 irritate their bladders. The most common bladder irritants are alcohol, caffeinated beverages, and carbonated beverages.

It is important to be able to offer alternative foods to patients avoiding acidic foods. Apricots, papayas, pears, and watermelons are low-acid fruits that may be substituted for the fruits listed in Tables 1 and 2. Coffee drinkers may substitute Kava or other low-acid instant drinks such as Postum. Tea drinkers can substitute non-citrus herbal or sun-brewed teas that are better tolerated by patients with overactive bladder symptoms.

Drinking plenty of water may help to increase urinary pH and dilute out any of the effects of specific irritants. This can also be used as rescue therapy when dietary indiscretions lead directly to increased symptoms.

The "Bicarbonate Flush"

In situations where bladder symptoms are dramatically increased, it is possible to deliberately increase urinary pH by using a bicarbonate "slush". A dilute solution of bicarbonate of soda may be made by mixing 1 tsp. of baking soda with 8 oz. of water and drinking this, followed immediately by 8 oz. of plain water 3 times an hour for the next 2 to 4 hours. This can be repeated 2 or 3 times a day. Caution is advised in patients who are prone to salt retention or who have high blood pressure.

Some patients find these dietary manipulations useful. They are quite difficult to follow and may be difficult to maintain over a long period of time but, for some women, they provide a degree of benefit. This is not meant as a sole treatment for urinary problems and, in most cases, should be used in conjunction with other therapies.

Caffeine reduction is an accepted treatment strategy for patients with urinary symptoms. A recent prospective randomized trial supported caffeine reduction in order to improve urinary urgency and frequency. The study was conducted among 95 consecutive adult patients with urinary symptoms presenting to two nurse continence advisers. Caffeine intake, frequency, urgency, and leakage episodes were tested one month after enrollment. There were significant reductions in caffeine intake, frequency, and urgency in the experimental group.[9]

Dietary Fiber in Treatment of Fecal Incontinence

Fecal incontinence is a very distressing and common disorder in the general population. It results in work absenteeism, inability to work, self-imposed social isolation, and depression. It affects not only sufferers, but caregivers as well. It is also a frequent cause of admission to nursing homes. Four percent of women over the age of 65 years who live in their own homes report fecal incontinence,[12] and as many as 30% of nursing home residents report fecal incontinence.[13]

Managing fecal incontinence is essential to maintaining the dignity and independence of an individual. If there is a clear cause with an effective cure, such as a rectovaginal fistula or gross disruption of the external anal sphincter, then cure should be the aim. In most cases, however, there is not a clear cause or an effective treatment. Symptom management is indicated in these people. Symptom management of fecal incontinence often includes dietary fiber supplementation. Fiber therapy may precede or accompany pelvic muscle exercises using biofeedback.

Fecal incontinence is exacerbated by liquid stools or diarrhea. Loose and liquid stools are recognized as the primary risk factor for fecal incontinence in acutely ill hospitalized patients.[14] Non-hospitalized patients with chronic diarrhea also experience fecal incontinence when stools are liquid, regardless of stool volume.[15] Therapies that make stool consistency less loose or liquid, or that sequester stool water, are useful in managing fecal incontinence. Dietary fiber supplementation manages fecal incontinence by making stools less loose and liquid.

In addition to advising a patient to take fiber to regulate her fecal incontinence, it is helpful to begin a routine bowel schedule. The optimal time for a bowel movement is in the morning or after a meal. If the patient starts her daily activities with an empty colon, she will be less likely to have fecal incontinence during her daily activities. For this reason, the patient should set aside sufficient time to allow for an undisturbed visit to the bathroom each morning. Also, the urge to have a bowel movement should not be ignored throughout the day. We help patients achieve a consistent habit of predictable bowel emptying by recommending Citrucel®, FiberCon®, or 25 to 30 mg of psyllium dietary fiber supplements at bedtime. Supplementation at this time of day seems to aid morning bowel movements, and the dietary fiber maintains a balanced stool that is easy to pass and more solid.

There are three hypothesized mechanisms that may explain how dietary fiber moderates stool consistency and, thereby, restores fecal continence. First, dietary fiber not fermented by fecal bacteria may trap water in the residual fiber-stool matrix as shown in several in vitro experiments.[16,17] Subsequent research has shown that although this mechanism may hold true for certain types of fiber like psyllium,[18,19] it may not be true of others like xanthan gum.[20] In a prospective randomized trial looking at two different fiber supplements, improvements in fecal incontinence or stool consistency did not appear to occur with unfermented dietary fiber.[21]

Second, bacterial proliferation after fiber fermentation may result in sequestration of stool water in bacterial cells. This mechanism is supported by research that showed increased bacterial mass after ingestion of oat bran and/or gum arabic supplements.[22,23]

Finally, dietary fiber may actually decrease (instead of increase) free stool water and improve continence by fiber fermentation products. These products are short-chain fatty acids that are the preferred energy substrate for colonic cell metabolism and stimulate colonic absorption of water and electrolytes in vitro.[24–26] The effects of these short-chain fatty acids on stool consistency again are dependent on the type of fiber ingested and its fermentation by fecal bacteria.[16,27]

One of the only studies on the use of dietary fiber as a treatment of fecal incontinence is a prospective randomized trial. In this study, 39 subjects with fecal incontinence of loose or liquid stools recorded diet intake and stool consistency, both before and after a 31-day fiber supplementation period. Supplementation with either psyllium or gum arabic was associated with improved stool consistency and fewer incontinent stools when compared to placebo.[21]

Conclusion

A significant limitation of outpatient behavioral treatments is their reliance on the active participation and cooperation of an involved and motivated patient. Improvements are based on the ability to learn and retain skills and on conscious changes in daily behavior. This limits the usefulness of behavioral treatment in patients who have cognitive impairment or those who are not interested in complying with a consistent daily regimen. Their utility has also been limited, in part, by the lack of availability of practitioners trained in these methods.

An obvious advantage of behavioral treatments, in addition to the absence of adverse effects, is that the procedures can be implemented effectively by primary care—and even nonphysician—providers in outpatient office settings. In many cases these simple, cost-effective strategies can vastly improve a woman's quality of life.

Key Points

- Pelvic floor ("Kegel") exercises should be discussed for almost all cases of incontinence. *Stress incontinence* episodes may decrease as muscle tone around the urethra is increased. For *urge incontinent* women, strong pelvic floor muscles will provide a means to "shut off" involuntary bladder contractions and, thereby, suppress the urge to urinate.
- Although Kegel exercises have been shown to improve mild and moderate cases of stress incontinence, "total dryness" will rarely be achieved for more severe symptoms. Regular, long-term patient compliance is the single most important factor in the success of this approach.
- "Bladder drills" refer to behavioral retraining of the bladder by slowly increasing the time interval between voids. Numerous studies have demonstrated the efficacy of this simple, low-tech approach. Bladder drills should be discussed for all cases of overactive bladder.
- Dietary bladder irritants (see "bladder diet") may exacerbate an overactive or, in some cases, painful bladder. Women with irritative lower urinary tract symptoms should receive a listing of foods and beverages to potentially avoid.
- Many cases of fecal incontinence will respond to simple dietary and bchavioral changes. Initial steps include the use of daily bulking agents and timed defecation.

References

1. Kegel AH. Physiologic therapy for urinary stress incontinence. *JAMA.* 1951;146:915–917.
2. Wyman JF, Fantl JA, McClish DK, Bump RC. Comparative efficacy of behavioral interventions in the management of female urinary incontinence. Continence Program for Women Research Group. *Am J Obstet Gynecol.* 1998;179:999–1007.
3. Cammu H, Van Nylen M, Amy JJ. A 10-year follow-up after Kegel pelvic floor muscle exercises for genuine stress incontinence. *BJU Int.* 2000;85:655–658.
4. Burgio KL, Locher JL, Goode PS, et al. Behavioral vs drug treatment for urge urinary incontinence in older women: a randomized controlled trial. *JAMA.* 1998; 280:1995–2000.
5. Frewen WK. Role of bladder training in the treatment of the unstable bladder in the female. *Urol Clin North Am.* 1979;6:273–277.
6. Frewen WK. A reassessment of bladder training in detrusor dysfunction in the female. *Br J Urol.* 1982; 54:372–373.
7. Burgio KL. Influence of behavior modification on overactive bladder. *Urology.* 2002;60:72–77.

8. Fantl JA, Wyman JF, McClish DK, et al. Efficacy of bladder training in older women with urinary incontinence. *JAMA*. 1991;265:609–613.
9. Bryant CM, Dowell CJ, Fairbrother G. Caffeine reduction education to improve urinary symptoms. *Br J Nurs*. 2002;11:560–565.
10. Dallosso HM, McGrother CW, Matthews RJ. The association of diet and other lifestyle factors with overactive bladder and stress incontinence: a longitudinal study in women. *BJU Int*. 2003 Jul;92: 69–77.
11. Dallosso HM, Matthews RJ, McGrother CW. The association of diet and other lifestyle factors with overactive bladder: a longitudinal study in men. *Public Health Nutr*. 2004;7:885–891
12. Edwards NI, Jones D. The prevalence of faecal incontinence in older people living at home. *Age Ageing*. 2001;30:503–507.
13. Peet SM, Castleden CM, McGrother CW. Prevalence of urinary and faecel incontinence in hospitals and residential and nursing homes for older people. *BMJ*. 1995;311:1063–1064.
14. Bliss DZ, Johnson S, Savik K, Clabots CR, Gerding DN. Fecal incontinence in hospitalized patients who are acutely ill. *Nursing Res*. 2000;49: 101–108.
15. Read NW, Harford WV, Schmulen, AC, Read MG, Santa Ana C, Fordtran JS. A clinical study of patients with fecal incontinence and diarrhea. *Gastroenterology*. 1979;76:747–756.
16. McBurney MI, Horvath PJ, Jeraci JL, Van Soest, PJ. Effect of in vitro fermentation using human faecal inoculum on the water-holding capacity of dietary fibre. *Br J of Nutr*. 1985;53:17–24.
17. Stephen AM, Cummings JH. Water holding by dietary fibre in vitro and its relationship to faecal output in man. *Gut*. 1979;20:722–729.
18. Eherer AJ, Santa Ana CA, Porter J, Fordtran JS. Effect of psyllium, calcium polycarbophil, and wheat bran on secretory diarrhea induced by phenolphthalein. *Gastroenterology*. 1993;104:1007–1012.
19. Wenzl HH, Fine KD, Schiller LR, Fordtran JS. Determinants of decreased fecal consistency in patients with diarrhea. *Gastroenterology*. 1995;108: 1729–1738.
20. Daly J, Tomlin J, Read NW. The effect of feeding xanthan gum on colonic function in man: correlation with in vitro determinants of bacterial breakdown. *Br J of Nutr*. 1993;69:897–902.
21. Bliss DZ, Jung H, Savik K, et al. Supplementation with dietary fiber improves fecal incontinence. *Nursing Res*. 2001;50:203–213.
22. Bliss DZ, Stein TP, Schleifer CR, Settle RG. Supplementation with gum arabic fiber increases fecal nitrogen excretion and lowers serum urea nitrogen concentration in chronic renal failure patients consuming a low-protein diet. *Am J Clin Nutr*. 1996; 63:392–398.
23. Chen HL, Haack VS, Janecky CW, Vollendorf NW, Marlett JA. Mechanisms by which wheat bran and oat bran increase stool weight in humans. *Am J Clin Nutr*. 1998;68:711–719.
24. Roediger WE, Moore A. Effect of short-chain fatty acid on sodium absorption in isolated human colon perfused through the vascular bed. *Dig Dis Sci*. 1981;26:100–106.
25. Roediger WE, Rae DA. Trophic effect of short chain fatty acids on mucosal handling of ions by the defunctioned colon. *Br J Surg*. 1982;69:23–25.
26. Ruppin H, Bar-Meir S, Soergel KH, Wood CM, Schmitt MG Jr. Absorption of short-chain fatty acids by the colon. *Gastroenterology*. 1980;78: 1500–1507.
27. Bourquin LD, Titgemeyer EC, Fahey GC Jr. Vegetable fiber fermentation by human fecal bacteria: cell wall polysaccharide disappearance and short-chain fatty acid production during in vitro fermentation and water-holding capacity of unfermented residues. *J Nutr*. 1993;123:860–869.

7
An Overview of Medication for Lower Urinary Tract Dysfunction

Patrick J. Culligan

Introduction

In the last several years, multiple new "bladder medications" have received approval by the Food and Drug Administration. Most of these drugs are designed to treat patients suffering from detrusor overactivity. This chapter will review both old and new pharmacologic treatments for detrusor overactivity and stress urinary incontinence. This chapter *will not* offer a comprehensive review, but instead will focus on the practical advantages and disadvantages of the most commonly used medications. Before using the drugs mentioned in this chapter, practitioners should familiarize themselves in detail with the relevant clinical pharmacology.

Background: Normal Bladder Physiology

No pharmacologic agents offer pure selectivity for the lower urinary tract. Therefore, all medications designed to alleviate lower urinary tract symptoms have side effects caused by their activity in other organ systems. Understanding the normal physiology of bladder activity makes it easy to understand the drugs we use to treat bladder dysfunction.

The bladder is a muscular reservoir that rests in the retropubic space in an extra-peritoneal position. As urine fills the bladder, stretch receptors are activated. These receptors send impulses along pelvic nerve afferent fibers to the spinal cord and on to the sympathetic nucleus, where the hypogastric nerve is activated. The resulting impulse is carried down the hypogastric nerve to the bladder, where beta-adrenergic receptors cause bladder relaxation, and alpha-adrenergic receptors cause increased urethral smooth muscle tone. Urethral skeletal muscle tone is maintained through a different complimentary system that originates in the sacral spinal cord (in Onuf's nucleus). Activity from Onuf's nucleus is conveyed along the pudendal nerve, which releases acetylcholine to stimulate excitatory *nicotinic* receptors and contraction of the striated urethral sphincter.

When the bladder becomes distended to the point at which micturition should occur, activity from the pelvic nerve is carried up to the pontine micturition center, which causes activation of sacral parasympathetic neurons whose axons traverse the pelvic nerve and cause release of acetylcholine to stimulate excitatory *muscarinic* receptors and contraction of the detrusor. Of course, the cerebral cortex comes into play as well, because one should be able to suppress these stimuli if one's social situation does not lend itself to micturition.

Drugs for Stress Incontinence

General Considerations

To date, there are no drugs with an FDA approved indication for the treatment of stress urinary incontinence. The medications listed below all work by increasing either smooth or striated muscle tone within the urethra.

Imipramine Hydrochloride

Imipramine hydrochloride is a tricyclic antidepressant that produces systemic anticholinergic effects as well as direct inhibitory effects on bladder smooth muscle. This drug also has alpha-adrenergic effects in the urethra. Therefore, imipramine hydrochloride decreases bladder contractility and increases outlet resistance. Use of this drug for lower urinary tract symptoms is considered "off-label" by the U.S. FDA, so any practitioner contemplating use of this drug to alleviate bladder symptoms should be thoroughly familiar with potential side effects and relative precautions—some of which are discussed below.

The usual adult dosage is 25 mg to 75 mg once daily. Due to its propensity to cause drowsiness, this drug is taken at bedtime. Usually, patients should be started on 25 mg, and the dosage should be increased by 25 mg increments on a weekly basis (i.e., 25 mg the first week, 50 mg the second week, and 75 mg thereafter). The most common side effects include dry mouth, constipation, CNS effects, postural hypotension, fatigue, and generalized weakness. Patients who want to discontinue this drug due to unpleasant side effects should be weaned slowly (using the reverse of the weekly dosing schedule). Coming off this drug too quickly can produce confusion and disorientation.

Patients with moderate to severe nocturia and mild stress incontinence tend to be the best candidates for imipramine hydrochloride. Significant symptomatic improvements can be expected in approximately 30% of these patients.[1]

Pseudoephedrine

Pseudoephedrine is a common ingredient in over-the-counter cold remedies (e.g., Sudafed) that produces an alpha-adrenergic effect in the urethra. Use of this drug for stress incontinence is considered off-label. Potential side effects include blood pressure elevation, anxiety, insomnia, palpitations, and cardiac dysrhythmias.

The usual dosage is 30 mg to 60 mg QID in patients with mild stress incontinence. Moderate to severe stress incontinence usually does not respond to this medication. Stress incontinent patients who become dry on this medication should be screened for urinary retention via a post-void residual measurement. A recent Cochrane review suggests only weak evidence that alpha-agonists perform better than placebos in the treatment of stress urinary incontinence.[2]

Duloxetine Hydrochloride

A combination norepinephrine and serotonin re-uptake inhibitor, duloxetine hydrochloride produces increased skeletal muscle tone by activating receptors in Onuf's nucleus. This drug is currently available in the U.S. for the treatment of depression; however, it is approved for use in Europe as either an antidepressant or treatment for stress urinary incontinence. After years of clinical trials in the U.S., duloxetine was recently removed from the FDA pipeline by its manufacturer. Therefore, use of this drug for stress incontinence in the U.S. will likely always be considered off-label. Interestingly, the dosage used in clinical trials for stress incontinence was actually higher than currently approved dosages for depression. The dosage for depression is 20 mg to 30 mg BID, and the most likely dosage for stress incontinence would be—if approved—40 mg BID. At that dosage, duloxetine reduced incontinence episode frequency by 59% compared with 40% in a placebo group. In those studies, the most common side effects of this drug seemed to be very much like those of serotonin re-uptake inhibitors—namely, nausea and diarrhea.[3,4,5]

Drugs for Detrusor Overactivity

General Considerations

Once the diagnosis of detrusor overactivity has been established, there are multiple pharmacologic treatment options. In the last few years, several new agents for the treatment of detrusor overactivity have been approved by the FDA. The clinical trials required for FDA approval typically pit the active molecule against a placebo. Unfortunately, there are very few randomized trials comparing these new active drugs to each other. The main outcome measures used in any study involving this class of drugs include incontinence episode frequency, voids per day, and cure or dry rates. Virtually all of the anticholinergic medications mentioned in this section have performed similarly in their respective FDA-approval clinical studies. Common numbers (in placebo-controlled studies) include 60% to 80% reductions of incontinence episode frequency (usually amounting to 2 to 4 fewer leakage episodes per day), 25% to 45% reductions in voids per day (usually amounting to 3–5 fewer voids per day), and cure rates of between 10% and 25%.

When initiating an anticholinergic agent for the treatment of detrusor overactivity, the practitioner should manage patient expectations. None of these drugs have impressive cure rates; therefore, patients should not expect to be "dry" on these medications. Instead, they should be counseled that searching for the proper anticholinergic agent may amount to a trial-and-error process. With each change in dosage or anticholinergic agent, patients should be counseled to weigh the benefits (decreased urgency, frequency and incontinence episodes) against side effects (dry mouth, constipation, etc.). The side-effect profiles for the newer drugs in this class are usually reported within these ranges: severe dry mouth, between 3–7%; *any* dry mouth, between 20% and 35%; discontinuation rates, between 2% and 11%; and CNS side effects, present in 4% to 6%. For the sake of simplicity, only deviations from these ranges will be discussed individually below. In other words, unless specifically stated otherwise, each of the drugs listed below have reported side-effect profiles within these ranges. The average monthly costs of drugs currently approved by the FDA for the treatment of detrusor overactivity are listed in Table 7.1.

All of the FDA-approved agents for detrusor overactivity are relatively safe—in other words, they all have a wide therapeutic index. They are all contraindicated for patients with narrow-angle glaucoma. Caution should be used when prescribing these drugs for patients with urinary outflow problems or poorly contractile bladders. Caution should also be used in patients with intestinal atony or myasthenia gravis. Patients should be warned that any of these drugs can cause drowsiness. Anticholinergics can also produce confusion and short-term memory loss.

Table 7.1. The Average Monthly Cost of FDA-Approved Drugs for Detrusor Overactivity

Drug	Dosage	Average Monthly cost
Oxybutynin IR	2.5–10 mg PO BID – TID	$22.80
Oxybutynin ER	5–30 mg PO QD	$64.20
Oxybutynin Transdermal Patch	1 patch 2x/week (3.9 mg/day)	$88.16
Tolterodine IR	1–2 mg PO BID	$105.60
Trospium chloride	20 mg PO BID	$82.20
Darifenacin	7.5–15 mg PO QD	$99.60
Solifenacin	5 mg PO QD	$100.20

Source: *The Medical Letter*. 2005;47:23–24.

Imipramine Hydrochloride

This drug was covered in the previous section regarding stress urinary incontinence. Briefly, it is most likely to be a good choice for patients with a predominance of nighttime manifestations of detrusor overactivity. Use of this drug to alleviate lower urinary tract symptoms is strictly off-label. The drowsiness that occurs due to imipramine use can actually give some patients a better night's sleep.

Oxybutynin Chloride (Immediate Release)

First approved by the FDA in 1975, oxybutynin chloride is a tertiary amine with relatively nonselective antimuscarinic properties. In clinical studies to date, few agents have performed better than immediate-release oxybutynin in terms of decreasing the symptoms associated with detrusor overactivity. However, this agent undergoes extensive first-pass metabolism, significantly increasing its anticholinergic side-effect profile.[6] In fact, nearly two thirds of patients taking immediate-release oxybutynin experience moderate-to-severe dry mouth symptoms,[7] or other severe side effects that will ultimately result in discontinuation. The severe nature of these unpleasant side effects reported by patients taking immediate-release oxybutynin created the market niche that was later filled by the other drugs mentioned below.

For those few patients who do not experience significant side effects while taking immediate-release oxybutynin, it is clearly the most cost-effective choice. The usual dosage is 5 mg TID, although titration down to 2.5 mg or up to 10 mg TID is sometimes required. However, given the poor side-effect profile of this generic drug, many practitioners only prescribe it for patients who simply cannot afford one of the newer preparations.

Oxybutynin Chloride (Extended Release)

Approved as an extended-release preparation in 1999, this drug (Ditropan XL™) is much better tolerated than its immediate-release counterpart. It uses a unique osmotic drug-delivery system, which releases the drug at a controlled rate over 24 hours. This delivery system should be explained to patients, because the pill is actually just a vessel that passes unchanged in the stool once the drug has been released. A patient unaware of this point may complain that the drug just passes right through them.

The improved side-effect profile of the extended-release version is believed to result from decreased peak serum concentrations as well as a decrease in the number of peaks normally associated with multiple dosing schedules. Another factor in the favorable side-effect profile is the decreased first-pass effect that results from absorption primarily through the distal small intestine. The dosage is 5 mg to 30 mg QD.

Tolterodine Tartrate

First approved in 1998, this agent has selectivity for muscarinic receptors in the bladder over the salivary glands in experimental models.[8] It is available in both immediate release (for BID dosing) and extended release (for QD dosing) versions. Given that the monthly costs of the immediate-release (Detrol) and extended-release (Detrol LA) versions of this medication are very similar, most patients use the QD dosage. However, some patients who mainly experience nighttime symptoms of detrusor overactivity will benefit from a strictly QHS dosing (1 mg to 2 mg) schedule of the immediate release tablets. Doing so can cut the monthly expense of this drug in half. For those patients who only require 1 mg of immediate-release tolterodine at bedtime, further cost savings could be realized by splitting 2 mg tablets in half, because the 1 mg and 2 mg tablets cost roughly the same. The dosage for the extended release capsules (Detrol LA) is 2 mg to 4 mg QD.

Ditropan XL Compared to Detrol LA

There is only one well-designed clinical trial comparing these two drugs.[9] Among nearly 800 patients, the two treatment groups demonstrated similar improvements in incontinence episode frequency (72% for Ditropan XL versus 70% for Detrol LA). Dry mouth was reported less frequently in the Detrol LA group (22% vs 30%, P = 0.02). Total dryness or cure was reported in a higher percentage of the Ditropan XL group (23% vs 17%, P = 0.03). All other outcome measures of interest were similar between the two groups. Unfortunately, this trial left unanswered the question of whether Ditropan XL—which crosses the blood-brain barrier far more readily than Detrol LA—tends to produce more CNS side effects. Although the study patients were asked whether they experienced confusion, etc., no validated outcome measure for CNS side effects was administered.

Oxybutynin Transdermal

This version of oxybutynin chloride (Oxytrol) offers the convenience of a twice-weekly dosing schedule and the decreased side-effect profile associated with avoidance of the first-pass effect in the liver. The transdermal version achieves higher plasma concentrations with a lower dose than oral oxybutynin.[10] The dosage is 3.9 mg/day delivered via a patch that should be changed twice weekly. Steady state conditions are reached within a week (i.e., shortly after placement of the second patch).

Other than the usual anticholinergic side effects, the most common adverse event noted by patients using this medication is localized pruritus, occurring in approximately 14% of patients.

Trospium Chloride

Approved in Europe for the treatment of detrusor overactivity for approximately 20 years, this non-selective antimuscarinic agent is hydrophilic and, therefore, should not cross the blood-brain barrier.[11] It was given FDA approval in 2004 following phase II and phase III trials in which 2975 patients were randomized to trospium chloride (Sanctura, N = 1673), placebo (N = 1056) or other active control medications (N = 246). The dosage is 20 mg BID except for patients with renal insufficiency, who should only receive 20 mg QD. It should be taken on an empty stomach, either 1 hour before or 2 hours after meals. No other strengths of this medication are offered; however, some patients who mainly experience nighttime detrusor overactivity will respond to QHS rather than BID dosing.

Darifenacin

This antimuscarinic agent (Enablex), also approved by the FDA in 2004, is highly selective for the M3 receptors (predominately found in the bladder and GI tract) over M1 receptors (which mediate CNS effects and salivary glands). The dosage is 7.5 mg QD, and this can be increased to 15 mg QD for increased efficacy without significantly worsened side effects.[12] Patients taking the 7.5 mg dose may ask that their prescription be written for the 15 mg tabs, in hopes that they can split the pills in two and thereby save money. However, the coating on these tablets is an important pharmacokinetic factor, so this practice should be strongly discouraged.

Solifenacin Succinate

This antimuscarinic agent (Vesicare), also approved in 2004, has a relatively long half-life and bioavailability of 90%.[13] These properties result in relatively constant plasma concentrations without significant peak levels. The usual dosage is 5 mg QD, but this can be decreased to 5 mg QOD for patients experiencing significant adverse side effects. A 10 mg tablet is also available. Solifenacin tablets are not scored, but splitting a 10 mg tablet to create two 5 mg tablets (again for cost savings) may be possible. Patients desiring to do so should be warned that their dosage may vary from day to day. Otherwise, this practice should be a safe way to save money.

Vesicare Compared to Detrol LA

In a recent well-designed study, solifenacin was compared to tolterodine extended-release. This was a prospective, double-blind, double-dummy, two-arm, parallel-group, 12-week study conducted to compare the efficacy and safety of solifenacin 5 mg or 10 mg and tolterodine extended-release 4 mg QD in patients suffering from detrusor overactivity. After 4 weeks of treatment, patients had the option to request a dose increase but were "dummied" throughout, as approved product labeling only allowed an increase for those on solifenacin.[14] This study demonstrated greater efficacy in the solifenacin group in terms of decreasing urgency episodes, urge incontinence, and pad usage as well as increasing the volume voided per micturition.

Key Points

- All medications designed to alleviate lower urinary tract symptoms have side effects caused by their activity in other organ systems.
- There are no drugs with an FDA-approved indication for the treatment of stress urinary incontinence, although duloxetine hydrochloride has approval for this indication in Europe.
- Virtually all of the anticholinergic medications have performed similarly in their respective FDA-approval clinical studies. Any significant differences between the medications will likely be discovered in future after-market, head-to-head trials.
- The most typical side effects associated with anticholinergic drugs are dry mouth, dizziness, constipation, blurred vision, and confusion.
- Many so-called after-market studies are likely to be published in the next few years as pharmaceutical companies try to differentiate the various anticholinergic medications.

References

1. Urinary Incontinence Guideline Panel. Urinary Incontinence in Adults: Clinical Practice Guideline. AHCPR Pub. No. 920038. Rockville, MD. Agency for Health Care Policy and Research, Public Health Service, U.S. Department of Health and Human Services. March 1992.
2. Clinical Evidence Issue 10. December 2003. BMJ Publishing Group, London.
3. Dmochowski RR, Miklos JR, Norton PA, Zinner NR, Yalcin I, Bump RC. Duloxetine versus placebo for the treatment of North American women with stress urinary incontinence. *J Urol.* 2003;170:1259–1263.
4. van Kerrebroeck P, Abrams P, Lange R, et al. Duloxetine versus placebo in the treatment of European and Canadian women with stress urinary incontinence. *BJOG.* 2004;111:249–257.
5. Norton PA, Zinner NR, Yalcin I, Bump RC. Duloxetine versus placebo in the treatment of stress urinary incontinence. *Am J Obstet Gynecol.* 2002; 187:40–48.
6. Thuroff J, Chartier-Kastler E, Corcus J, et al. Medical treatment and medical side effects in urinary incontinence in the elderly. *World J Urol.* 1998;16:548–561.
7. Davila GW, Daugherty CA, Sanders SW; Transdermal Oxybutynin Study Group. A short-term, multicenter, randomized double-blind dose titration study of the efficacy and anticholinergic side effects of transdermal compared to immediate release oral oxybutynin treatment of patients with urge urinary incontinence. *J Urol.* 2001;166:140–145.
8. Nilvebrant L, Sundquist S, Gillberg PG. Tolterodine is not subtype (m1-m5) selective but exhibits functional bladder selectivity in vivo. *Neurourol Urodyn.* 1996;15:310–311.
9. Diokno AC, Appell RA, Sand PK, et al. Prospective, randomized, double-blind study of the efficacy and tolerability of the extended-release formulation of oxybutynin and tolterodine for overactive bladder: results of the OPERA trial. *Mayo Clin Proc.* 2003; 78:687–695.
10. Appell RA, Chancellor MB, Zohrist RH, Thomas H, Sanders SW. Pharmacokinetics, metabolism and saliva output during transdermal and extended-release oral oxybutynin administration in healthy subjects. *Mayo Clin Proc.* 2003;78:696–702.
11. Zinner N, Gittelman M, Harris R, et al. Trospium chloride improves overactive bladder symptoms: a multicenter phase III trial. *J Urol.* 2004;171:2311–2315.
12. Haab F, Stewart L, Dwyer P. Darifenacin, an M3 selective receptor antagonist, is an effective and well-tolerated once-daily treatment for overactive bladder. *Eur Urol.* 2004;45:420–429.
13. Kuipers ME, Krauwinkel WJ, Mulder H, Visser N. Solifenacin demonstrates high absolute bioavailability in healthy men. *Drugs R D.* 2004;5:73–81.
14. Chapple CR, Martinez-Garcia R, Selvaggi L, et al.: for the STAR study group. A comparison of the efficacy and tolerability of solifenacin succinate and extended release tolterodine at treating overactive bladder syndrome: results of the STAR trial. *Eur Urol.* 2005;48:464–470.

8 Biofeedback and Pelvic Floor Physiotherapy: Introducing Non-Surgical Treatments to Your Office

Charles R. Rardin

Introduction

Among women, the majority of urinary incontinence can be categorized into disorders of urethral support mechanisms (stress incontinence) and disorders of detrusor overactivity (urge incontinence). Disorders of obstruction (e.g., overflow incontinence), anatomy (e.g., urethral diverticula), and extra-urethral incontinence (e.g., urogenital fistulae) should always be considered, but are much less common. Similarly, the beneficial effects of conditioning of the female pelvic floor musculature, as discussed in previous chapters, can also be considered in terms of enhancing urethral support and suppressing detrusor overactivity.

The muscular components of the pelvic floor are collectively known as the levator ani and are affixed to the bony pelvis. In other mammals, these muscle groups are responsible for the balance and locomotion associated with movements of the tail, as can be recognized by their insertion on the distal sacrum and the coccyx. With the advent of erect posture in humans, these muscle groups assumed a new function, namely the support of pelvic organs. In providing support to the pelvic organs, as well as the abdominal contents, these muscles must provide tonic support that is resistant to fatigue. The majority of muscle fibers of the pelvic floor are type II, slow-twitch fibers. In order to counteract the suddenly increased load associated with intra-abdominal pressures, such as a cough or sneeze, a component of fast-twitch muscle fibers provide reflex, or voluntary, extra support to the slow-twitch basal tone. Specifically with regard to urinary incontinence, this system of muscular support, along with its fascial and fibromuscular connections, is believed to act as a hammock or backboard against which the urethra is compressed shut during periods of increased abdominal pressure, in the healthy woman.[1] Although the association of stress incontinence and loss of suburethral support—usually measured with the cotton-swab test[2]—has been long recognized, the contribution of the pelvic muscles to continence is less thoroughly documented. The proportion of fast-twitch fibers in the levator musculature decreases as a woman ages; it has also been noted to be decreased in women with symptoms of stress incontinence.[3] More recent imaging techniques, including ultrasound and MRI, have identified decreases in levator volume and alterations in levator morphology; these have indicated an association with the incidence of prolapse and incontinence.[4–6] One of these studies demonstrated that a program of physiotherapy restored muscle to a degree that patients' muscle thickness was comparable to continent controls.[4]

Many practitioners feel that regular exercises help not only to effect muscle hypertrophy and compensate for the loss of fast-twitch muscle fibers, but also to improve the coordination of the contraction of the involved muscle bundles.[7] Through this variety of mechanisms, urethral support is enhanced. Evidence for this hypothesis can be found in the discovery that pressure-transmission, a measurement of the support of the urethra and the resulting coaptive force, is enhanced after a program of pelvic physiotherapy.[8] In addition, however, to enhancing urethral support, the pelvic floor musculature plays an important role in the regulation of detrusor activity. Functional behavior of the lower urinary tract in both the filling and voiding phases depends on the coordinated reflex pathways that involve the peripheral afferents, sacral and pontine micturition centers, and autonomic and somatic efferent fibers.[9] Evidence for this can be found in the observation that the first step in the process of normal micturition is a decrease in EMG activity of the pelvic floor, and then of urethral pressure; this decreased levator activity is followed by a detrusor contraction. When micturition is not desirable, in the filling phase, activation of pudendal nerve afferent fibers results in reflex inhibition of hypogastric and pelvic splanchnic efferents and, therefore, inhibits detrusor contractility.[10] The sensory apparatus of the pelvic floor is, therefore, felt to play an important role in improving urinary function. While the sensory component of pelvic muscle exercises can be appreciated, this effect is enhanced using physiotherapy modalities that increase the sensory component, such as vaginal weights, manometry or EMG inserts, or electrical stimulation and neuromodulation.

The Role of Physiotherapy in the Treatment of Urogynecologic Disorders

The role of pelvic floor muscle exercises (PFME) has been discussed in previous chapters, and a recent Cochrane Database review concluded that, despite limitations and methodologic heterogeneity, existing data support the superiority of PFME over placebo or no treatment for women with stress or mixed incontinence.[11] Despite this finding, there is no consensus regarding the optimal indication, application, or regimen for their use. Additionally, there is a wide variety of teaching methods to educate patients in their use; and the majority of patients, despite careful and standardized teaching in pelvic floor muscle exercises (PFMEs), are found to perform them incorrectly.[12] Isolation of the target muscle groups— an important principle in muscle strengthening—was found to be difficult; a quarter of women were actually performing maneuvers that could potentially promote incontinence, such as Valsalva maneuvers. Finally, no reliable predictors of successful efforts could be found.

Elia and colleagues performed urodynamic testing on women about to undergo a program of PFMEs and then analyzed these parameters according to clinical response. The authors concluded that PFMEs were much more likely to work in women with mild incontinence and with urodynamic indices that were closer to normal controls[13]; other authors have come to similar conclusions[14]. Another study, investigating predictors of success with a program of electrical stimulation, found that patients with clinical success were more likely to have been compliant with the treatment regimen[15]. As in all practices based on behavioral modification, patient motivation and expectations are important variables to consider.

In the 1940s and 50s, Arnold Kegel, a California gynecologist, published much about the employment of pelvic floor muscle exercises in the treatment of female pelvic floor dysfunction.[16–20] Although he was not the first to describe the physical exercise of regulated contractions of the pelvic musculature, he was its most vocal proponent, and the exercises bear his name. More specifically, however, he did introduce the pelvic manometer, or perineometer, and thus introduced the technique of biofeedback to the domain of pelvic floor dysfunction.

Biofeedback is not a treatment unto itself, but rather a teaching technique in the overall application of behavioral modification and physical therapy. In general terms, biofeedback refers to techniques of converting a physiologic response to a behavior into visual or other cues, in real time. This conversion is usually done through some sort of apparatus or equipment and allows the user to consciously identify, isolate, amplify, and enhance the behavior itself. In terms of pelvic floor therapy, the biofeedback modalities generally convert pelvic muscle activity into visual or auditory stimuli; these senses have much greater sensitivity, acuity, and discrimination than proprioception within the pelvic floor.

Types and Techniques of Biofeedback

Kegel's original perineometer—a version of which remains available for purchase today—consisted of a bulb that, inserted vaginally, reflected the pressure generated within the vaginal canal, presumably by the pubococcygeus muscles. A woman with the device in place could observe, by means of the analog dial, the efficiency and intensity of the pelvic floor contractions. A variety of devices are now available that essentially achieve the same end—conversion of pelvic floor activity into some visible, tactile, or audible cues that provide more accurate feedback than the individual's own proprioception.

An example of such a device is the weighted vaginal cone; adequate pelvic contraction is demonstrated to the individual if the cone is retained vaginally during ambulation. When a woman is able to achieve a certain goal (e.g., 20 minutes), the weight is increased. One advantage of these techniques is that they are readily adaptable to patients' home use.

Vaginal cones represent a variation of perineometric pelvic floor biofeedback; the sensation of the weighted cone slipping out from the vagina informs the user that current tone is inadequate and prompts increased pelvic floor effort. (Figure 8.1) When the first of a series of cones of increasing weight can be successfully retained—usually during ambulatory activity, for a duration of 20 minutes on two or more separate occasions—the weight is increased. This technique does help to isolate the pelvic floor from abdominal muscle activity; components of Valsalva will increase the likelihood of cone expulsion, and the woman will likely learn to adapt her efforts to optimize the exercises.

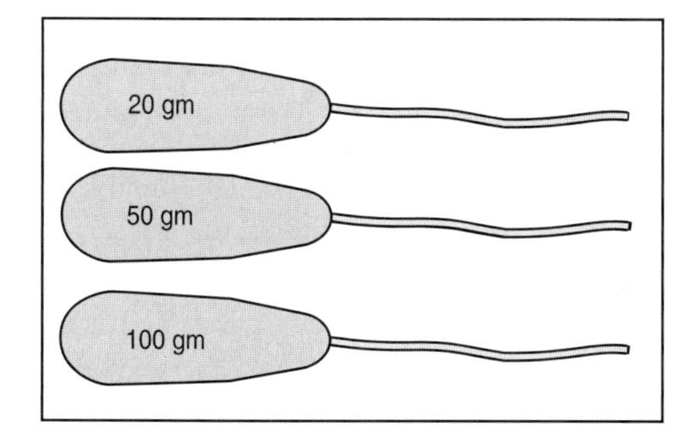

FIGURE 8.1. Weighted vaginal cones.

Studies of the efficacy of vaginal weighted cones Estimate subjective and objective short-term improvement rates of 70% to 90%.[21] Pressure-transmission ratios and maximum urethral closure pressures, urodynamic measures of urethral resistance to leakage, have been shown to be improved after a program of physiotherapy with weighted cones.[8,22] Results are not consistent, however; one series demonstrated a success rate of only 14% to 30%, with successful outcomes found in women with the mildest incontinence,[23] while a randomized trial showed no benefit of cones over a program of supervised PFME.[24] Randomized trials have arrived at conflicting conclusions regarding the superiority of one over the other.[25–26] A subsequent series echoed the finding of benefit for women with only milder forms of incontinence.[27] A Cochrane Database review concluded that there was limited support for cones in the treatment of stress incontinence, with similar results as with PFME and electrical stimulation.[28]

Electromyography (EMG) Biofeedback

Although manometry techniques can offer technical simplicity and ease of home use, there are two limitations. The first is that manometry can provide good information about maximal pelvic muscle contraction strength, but generally provides little information about the relaxation phase. Many women, especially those with pelvic pain or voiding dysfunction, may have chronically elevated tonic levator activity, which is not easily distinguished from ambient pelvic pressure on manometry. Secondly, pelvic manometry does not generally distinguish between pressures generated by the desired levator musculature activity and increased intra-abdominal pressures generated by counterproductive Valsalva maneuvers.

To address this, many modern pelvic biofeedback systems use electromyography to detect the electrical activity of the neuromuscular apparatus of the pelvic floor and of the abdominal musculature. Surface electrodes are mounted on the perineal skin, or on a vaginal or anal insert, and connected to computerized sensing, display, and recording devices. Another channel can be used to detect and register abdominal musculature activity; the patient is then given the information required to isolate the target muscle groups more accurately and to reduce the paradoxical Valsalva. In addition to multi-channel capability, most EMG-type devices can be converted to use for electrical stimulation, which will be discussed later. In addition, advances in electronics have made home-usage devices based on EMG more practical and affordable. The feedback these home units may provide the user can be visual or audible; generally, in addition to real-time biofeedback regarding the performance of pelvic exercises, this information can be stored, reviewed, and downloaded to the clinician for further review and evaluation. (Figure 8.2) (Figure 8.3)

Cystometric, or bladder, biofeedback employs detrusor manometry; a pressure transducer in the bladder converts detrusor activity (as opposed to the voluntary musculature of the pelvic floor) into a visible or, in some cases, audible signal for the patient.[29,30] In addition, the levator and urethral relaxation that accompanies the onset of a detrusor contraction can be identified by the patient, who can respond with voluntary muscular activity and thereby inhibit the detrusor contraction. This provides an additional source of quantifiable information, which may help patients to acquire better control. This may be of particular use among patients whose sensory perception of bladder activity, usually perceived as urgency, may have been altered, either by surgery or by neurologic process or insult. The technique of cystometric biofeedback may be used in conjunction with other biofeedback modalities, although the utility of multiple biofeedback techniques has not been clearly demonstrated.

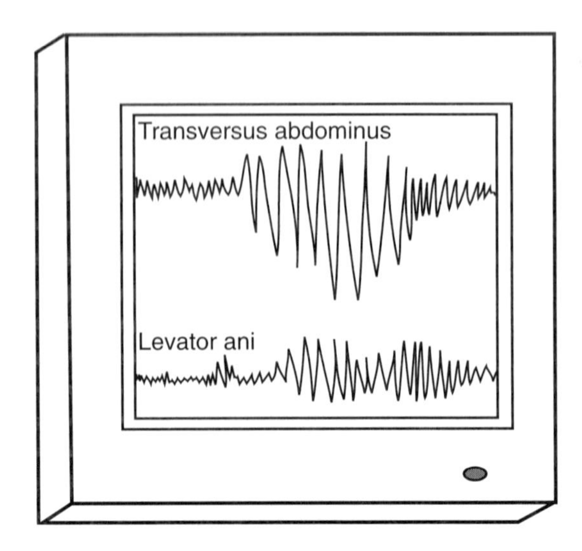

FIGURE 8.3. Biofeedback screen with EMG readings demonstrating failure to isolate levator ani contraction (i.e. Upper EMG line would be flat ideally.)

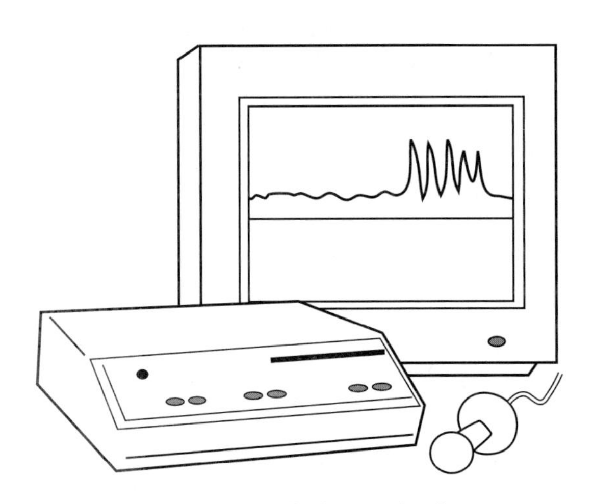

FIGURE 8.2. Biofeedback unit and probes.

The Process of Biofeedback

Bourcier and Burgio describe four main stages of pelvic floor muscle training that include (1) education and awareness of specific musculature, (2) muscle strengthening, (3) reflex, or automatic muscle activity, and (4) the application of these new skills in activities of daily life.[31] The first step involves improved isolation of the muscles of interest; as outlined above, multichannel biofeedback modalities are especially helpful in this step. Muscle strengthening, adapted from sports medicine physical therapy programs includes activation of both fast- and slow-twitch fibers by means of rapid contraction, slow and sustained contraction, and combination patterns. Automatic muscle

TABLE 8.1. Biofeedback for SUI

Author	N	Randomized?	Modality of Biofeedback (Compared to PFME)	Biofeedback significatly better?	Comment
Bo[26]	107	Yes	Cones	No	PFME superior
Arvonen[25]	37	Yes	Cones	Yes	
Castelden[34]	19	No	Perineometry	No	
Shepherd[35]	22		Perineometry	Yes	Maybe due to compliance
Burgio[36]	24	No	Perineometry/cystometry	Yes	
Glavind[37]	40	Yes	Perineometry	Yes	Long-term also better
Berghmans[38]	40	Yes	Perineometry	No	More rapid improvement?
Cammu[24]	60	Yes	Cones vs Observed PFME	No	
Morkved[39]	94	Yes	Perineometry (Home unit)	No	better motivation
Burns[40]	135	Yes	Perineometry	No	Muscle strength better, but not incontinence

contraction describes the subject's ability to use voluntary muscle action in response to, or anticipation of, other events. Examples of this capability include "the knack," the name given to the pre-contraction of the levators in anticipation of a cough or sneeze, which has been shown to reduce stress incontinence,[32,33] as well as to inhibit detrusor activity through pelvic floor activation as described above. The final step involves the application of these skills into activities of daily life.

Clinical Data

The scientific evaluation of the performance of biofeedback techniques is generally comprised of large numbers of small trials comparing PFME combined with biofeedback to PFME alone. The studies that have been published vary in the patient selection, biofeedback modality, frequency and duration of treatment, and duration of follow-up and are of varying methodologic quality. (Table 8.1) (Table 8.2)

Beyond Biofeedback

Electrical Stimulation

The development of physiotherapeutic modalities such as neuromuscular electrical stimulation and neuromodulation arose from the recognition that, in individuals in whom neurologic or muscular disease or injury permanently impairs the pelvic floor contraction mechanism, efficacy of voluntary PFMEs will also be impaired. Electrical

TABLE 8.2. Biofeedback for Mixed or Urge Incontinence

Author	N	Randmized?	Modality of Biofeedback (Compared to PFME)	Outcome	Comment
Cardozo[30]	6	No	No Comparison group	Half of subjects cured	
Burton[41]	27	No	Perineometry/Cystometry	No statistical difference	
Burgio[42]	222	Yes	Perineometry	Outcomes similar	Satisfaction higher among biofeedback group

stimulation of the pelvic floor was introduced in the 1950s;[43,44] and subsequently, a variety of modalities have been described, including transcutaneous, endovaginal, or endoanal delivery of electrical stimulation. This impulse results in depolarization of the peripheral nerve and thereby activates the neuromuscular unit. The action potential generated in the peripheral nerve results in activation of the pelvic floor musculature; in this way, motor units dormant for years following denervation injury can be rehabilitated.

In addition to direct neuromuscular activation through depolarization of somatic efferents, a number of beneficial reflex circuits are triggered by electrical stimulation. Even at voltages insufficient to produce motor unit activation, a reflex arc mediated by the sacral micturition reflex center and the hypogastric sympathetic nerve fibers results in increased tone of the periurethral striated musculature, which reduces the propensity toward stress urinary incontinence.[45,46] There is evidence that this stimulation of the pelvic floor can produce not just muscular hypertrophy, but also a change toward type I, fast-twitch muscle fibers, further enhancing dynamic pelvic and urethral support.[47]

This increased hypogastric sympathetic tone may also serve to inhibit detrusor overactivity, in several ways; first, by increasing urethral tone, funneling of the bladder neck and introduction of urine to the proximal urethra, shown to promote bladder contractions in animal models, is decreased.[48] Secondly, increased sympathetic tone to the bladder served to directly inhibit detrusor activity. Finally, stimulation of the pudendal afferent fibers, by way of another reflex arc mediated by the sacral micturition reflex center, inhibits parasympathetic tone, further decreasing detrusor overactivity[49]. Some investigators have found that the effects of electrical stimulation are more pronounced among patients with urge incontinence than those with stress incontinence.[50,51]

Although many devices are available and marketed in the United States, they generally consist of a battery/control unit and a vaginal or anal insert with metal electrodes. The nature of electrical stimulation is such that tissue penetration is dependent on the impedance of the tissue itself and, therefore, increased current is required to penetrate more deeply. This current may have undesired local effects, such as soreness or pain at the electrode sites. Therefore, electrodes that can be placed in closer proximity to the neural tissue of interest offer the advantage of lower voltage requirements. For this reason, the control unit allows the therapist and user to alter the character of the stimulation, including the current amplitude, pulse width, and frequency, if intermittent stimulation is selected. Techniques of electrical stimulation take advantage of the observation that modifying characteristics of the applied current, including shortening the pulse width and use of biphasic stimulation, can lower the threshold for action potential generation while reducing the likelihood of local chemical changes and tissue injury.[52] The frequency of stimulation plays an important role. In one study using a feline model, a frequency of 5 to10 Hz produced the most robust efferent inhibition of bladder contraction[49]; while in humans, frequencies of 20 to 50 Hz produced the greatest increase in urethral pressure.[53] Electrode location probably plays an important role in achieving the desired effects.[53,54] In addition, a different application of stimulation may affect the different fibers of the pelvic floor; maximal stimulation targets the fast-twitch muscles of the pelvic floor, while low-frequency, low-intensity stimulation may enhance the function of the slow-twitch component.

As with all studies of pelvic physiotherapy, investigations of the performance of electrical stimulation for urinary incontinence employ a variety of techniques, devices, regimens, and treatment durations; generalizability is difficult. Perhaps as a reflection of the multiple pathways through which electrical stimulation can inhibit parasympathetic tone and detrusor activity, a more robust and reproducible benefit has been seen in treating patients with urge or mixed incontinence, rather than pure stress incontinence. A study comparing urethral closure pressures among younger women with SUI showed that voluntary PFMEs resulted in significantly higher urethral pressures than did either of two forms of transvaginal electrical stimulation.[55] Another study showed that, while electrical stimulation improved symptoms of stress incontinence, it was not any more beneficial than a program of physical therapy using vaginal weighted cones.[56] Results of clinical trials are presented in Tables 8.3 and 8.4.

TABLE 8.3. Electrical Stimulation (Estim) for Stress Urinary Incontinence

Author	N	Randomized?	Study Design	Electrical Stimulation Significan Better?	Comment
Olah[56]	54	Yes	Estim vs cones	No	
Parkkinen[57]	33	No	PFME and vaginal weights, with or without Estim	No	
Goode[58]	200	Yes	Behavioral training vs Estim vs self-help book	No	Estim had higher subjective satisfaction than behavioral
Bo[26]	107	Yes	PFME vs Estim vs Cones	No	PFME superior
Wilson[14]	60	Yes (sequentially)	PFME vs Estim	No	
Resplande[59]	30	No (crossover)	Estim (compared to sham, and no electrode)	No	Immediate changes in UDT attributed to probe itself, not Estim
Sand[60]	52	Yes	Estim vs sham	Yes	
Smith[61]	18	Yes	Estim vs PFME	No	

Electrical stimulation has enjoyed greatest clinical success with transvaginal or transanal electrode devices; however, transanal techniques are frequently associated with the development of anal soreness and bowel changes, limiting the clinical utility. For these reasons, many practitioners recommend transvaginal electrical stimulation techniques where feasible. Electrical stimulation, in conjunction with a program of biofeedback, seems most likely to yield benefit among younger patients with less urethral hypermobility, adequate estrogenization, and without intrinsic sphincter deficiency or detrusor instability; another important predictor of success in this study was patient compliance.[67] In addition, the technique requires at least some component of intact, functioning pudendal neuromuscular apparatus; this may explain some of the inconsistency of clinical trial results, particularly in the elderly population. One study evaluated the efficacy of adding electrical stimulation to a program of PFMEs in the elderly; lack of additional benefit, as well as the perceived intensity of the therapy, led the authors to terminate the study early and to discourage the use of the modality in this population.[66]

As with some modalities of biofeedback, electrical stimulation seems to be amenable to use by the patient at home. Home use of electrical stimulation is effective—66% subjectively improved and 55% considered improved by their providers[68]—safe, and feasible, with 79% recommending the therapy to friends.[69] Commercially available products emphasize the utility of home-use electrical stimulation.

Neuromodulation

Sacral Neuromodulation (Figure 8.4)

Neuromodulation differs from the electrical stimulation techniques described above in that electrical impulses are applied not to the pelvic musculature and nerve terminals, but to nerve

TABLE 8.4. Electrical Stimulation for Urge or Mixed Incontinence

Author	N	Study Design	Electrical Stimulation Significantly Better?	Comment
Seo[62]	120	Estim/Biofeedback vs vaginal cone	No	Written in support of new vaginal cone
Barroso[63]	36	Estim vs sham	Yes	1/3 needed retreatment at 6 months
Yamanishi[64]	68	Estim vs sham	Yes	results more durable in active treatment
Brubaker[50]	121	Estim vs sham	Yes (for DI)	SUI symptoms not significantly changed
Fall[51]	40	Estim (no comparison)	Yes (for DI)	SUI not significantly changed
Wang[65]	103	PFME v Biofeedback vs Estim	Yes	Biofeedback still better than PFME
Spruijt[66]	35	PFME with or without Estim	No	Authors denounce its use in the population, study was terminated
Smith[61]	38	PFME vs Estim	No	

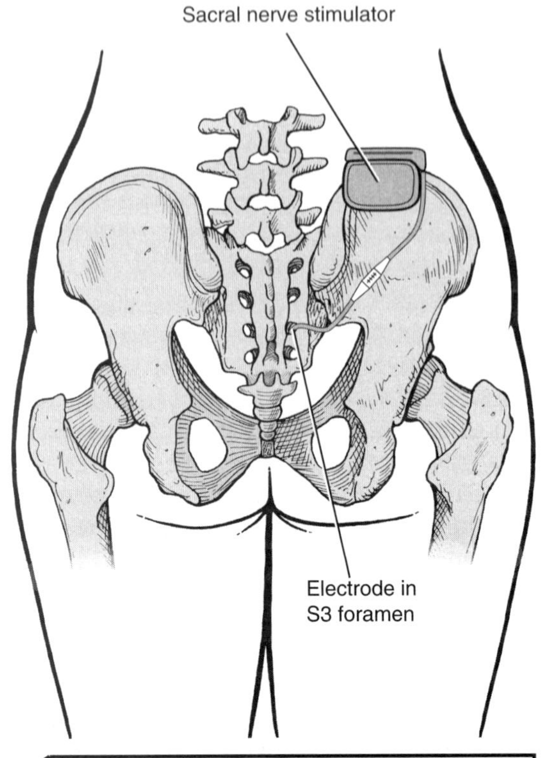

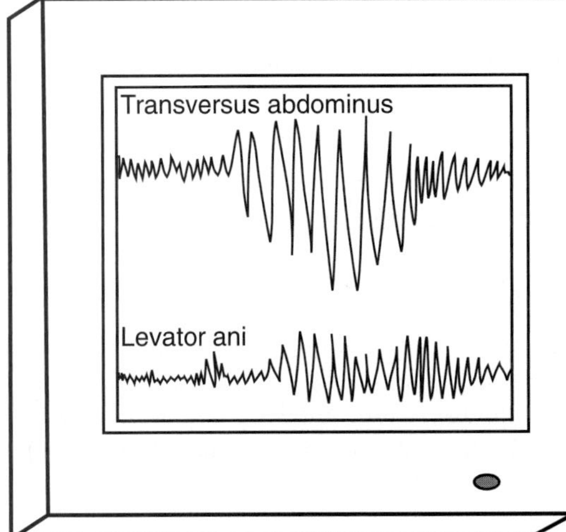

FIGURE 8.4. InterStim device.

roots. Investigations into the utility of neuromodulation for patients with traumatic nerve injuries were reported in the 1970s; more recently, the technique has been applied to patients with chronic lower urinary tract dysfunction. The InterStim sacral neuromodulation device received FDA approval in 1997 for the treatment of urgency, frequency, urge incontinence, and nonobstructive urinary retention. Its original design involved the placement of a percutaneous wire into the S3 foramen, for direct stimulation of the S3 nerve root. For a period of several days, the patient would use the percutaneous lead to apply stimulation from a portable generator; if the indicating symptoms were observed to improve significantly during the test phase, based on voiding diaries, the wire was removed and replaced with a permanent lead, which was then attached to an implanted generator device. Recent modifications to the technique involve the placement of a permanent, but removable, tined lead for the test stimulation; if the test is successful, the implanted generator is connected to the original lead. This increases the technical ease of implantation and also allows for a more accurate test.[70]

The mechanism of action of sacral neuromodulation is not entirely clear; it appears to have both efferent (pelvic floor musculature enhancement) and afferent (reflex inhibition of detrusor activity and stimulation of urethral striated muscle) effects, as seen in other forms of pelvic physiotherapy. In addition, stimulation of and selection for the A-delta myelinated fibers of the sacral nerve roots seems to enhance stability of detrusor activity and to increase the tone of the urethral musculature.

Although the newer modifications of the procedure allow its performance on an outpatient basis and under local anesthesia, the invasiveness and expense relegate it to last-resort status. Although in many ways preferable to the bladder denervation, urinary diversion, or augmentation cystoplasties, it should still be reserved for patients who are unresponsive to or intolerant of more conservative measures.

Peripheral Neuromodulation

Peripheral percutaneous neuromodulation is a non-surgical alternative. This technique takes advantage of the accessibility of the posterior tibial nerve, 3 cm to 4 cm above the level of the medial malleolus. Delivery of current to the afferent fibers of the posterior tibial, and then the sciatic, nerve is hypothesized to result in indirect stimulation of the S3 nerve root, the goals of which are outlined above. In an office-based procedure, a 34-gauge (acupuncture-type) needle is inserted percutaneously, and electrical stimulation is applied for a period of time, typically 30 minutes. The treatments are administered every 7 to 10 days, usually for a course of 12 weeks. The provider adjusts stimulation such that the patient is usually aware of only mild stimulation and little discomfort.

Peripheral neuromodulation has been shown to have an immediate effect on complex cystometric parameters. Bladder capacity, as well as bladder volume at first uninhibited bladder contraction, were significantly improved in patients with detrusor overactivity during the acute application of peripheral posterior tibial nerve stimulation.[71] In a study of patients with detrusor overactivity refractory to medical therapy, a program of percutaneous posterior tibial stimulation produced statistically significant reductions in diurnal and nocturnal urinary frequency as well as a 35% reduction in incontinence episodes.[72] Investigators considered 71% of subjects to be treatment successes, and no significant adverse events related to treatment were described.

Extracorporeal Electromagnetic Neurostimulation

Magnetic fields are generated by the movement of any electrical current; similarly, application of a magnetic field to human tissue will generate a current and voltage differential between points in space. If the differential is sufficient, depolarization of nerves in the exposed tissue occurs, and an action potential is generated. In the mid-1800s, Faraday demonstrated that muscular activity could be induced by the application of a variable magnetic field. The clinical utility of this technique—which differs from electrical stimulation in that the stimulation is applied indirectly and does not require invasive application—has generated interest in the field of pelvic floor dysfunction in recent years. Of particular importance, the nature of magnetic energy is such that its intensity is proportional to the distance from the generating coil and independent of the volume or type of tissue involved. This confers a significant advantage over electrical stimulation, which, due to tissue impedance, requires high voltages to penetrate into tissue, and thus either requires invasive lead placement (such as peripheral or sacral neuromodulation) or is associated with surface tissue injury and discomfort. Refinements to magnetic coils and field generators have allowed for enhanced targeting of tissue and neurologic response, greatly increasing the clinical utility and safety of the modality.[73]

The NeoControl Pelvic Floor Therapy System was introduced, and received FDA approval, for the treatment of female urinary incontinence; other indications are being investigated clinically. The magnetic coils are built into a seat; the patient sits, fully clothed and without the need for invasive probes, and stimulation can be adjusted by the provider to reach maximal effect. Stimulation of the sacral nerve roots results in activation of the pelvic musculature, as demonstrated by increased urethral, rectal, and anal pressures, as well as some activation of toe flexors.[74,75] This stimulation can have immediate effects; bladder contractions elicited by rapid saline infusion are suppressed,[76] and detrusor contraction during normal voiding can be interrupted acutely by the application of magnetic stimulation.[77] Magnetic stimulation has demonstrated therapeutic benefit among patients with detrusor overactivity,[78] as well as hyperreflexia in patients with spinal injuries.[79] mixed incontinence,[80] and pure stress incontinence.[81–83] As with PFMEs and electrical stimulation, there is some suggestion that patients without previous anti-incontinence surgery, and with relatively shorter duration of symptoms, are more likely to benefit from this therapy.[84]

Special Cases and Considerations

Pregnancy

The effects of pregnancy and delivery on the form and function of the pelvic floor are of great interest to obstetric providers. A study investigating pelvic floor function of pregnant nulliparae, in terms of perineometry strength and urogenital diaphragm muscle thickness (measured by ultrasound), found that women with incontinence in pregnancy had thinner and weaker muscles than their continent counterparts[85]; the implication is that pelvic floor conditioning may promote continence among pregnant women. A similar, randomized trial demonstrated that the benefit of PFMEs in pregnancy are carried into the postpartum period, as well.[86] Some practitioners have been concerned that pelvic muscle strength conditioning may, by increasing pelvic diaphragm tone, interfere with vaginal delivery; a randomized study demonstrated that, to the contrary, women assigned to pelvic muscle therapy in pregnancy were less likely to experience protracted second stage labor.[87]

Several studies have indicated that a program of pelvic floor muscle exercises may help to prevent and/or treat postpartum urinary incontinence, both in the immediate postpartum period, and for up to one year afterward.[86,88–91] The addition of physiotherapy techniques to standard PFME programs in the prevention or treatment of postpartum incontinence has shown mixed results. One series investigating postpartum PFMEs with or without the use of vaginal weighted cones determined that the addition of that form of biofeedback enhanced pelvic muscle strength.[92] A recent review of the literature regarding the use of pelvic muscle exercises with some form of biofeedback concluded that, while antepartum treatments were not found to decrease incontinence at three months after delivery, postpartum programs of PFMEs with biofeedback appeared to decrease incontinence and increase pelvic muscle strength.[93] A Cochrane Database review of physical therapies used for prevention of fecal and urinary incontinence in postpartum women revealed that three of seven eligible studies found a benefit of physical therapy over controls, but methodologic heterogeneity precluded quantitative analysis.[94] A randomized, double-blind, sham-control study investigating the use of extracorporeal magnetic stimulation in the postpartum period failed to demonstrate any increased benefit of magnetic stimulation over sham in the restoration of pelvic muscle strength, as measured by perineometry; this study did not evaluate subjective or urodynamic parameters.[95] One study investigated PFMEs with or without anal Estim. Although the intervention of PFMEs appeared to yield lower rates of fecal incontinence among women with third or fourth degree obstetrical lacerations than might be expected, the addition of Estim yielded no discernible benefit. Although this may be attributable to low numbers, the active treatment was abandoned due to anal pain.[96]

Voiding Dysfunction

In the normal condition, bladder emptying is effected by a detrusor contraction; this is usually preceded by relaxation of the pelvic floor musculature and of the urinary sphincter mechanism. In certain conditions, often involving neurologic disease, this sequence is disrupted and the urethra fails to relax, or may actually increase in tone. This condition is known as detrusor-sphincter dyssynergia and is one of the genitourinary hallmarks of central nervous system disorders such as multiple sclerosis, or patients with spinal cord injury. Some authors have demonstrated that, in patients with DSD, visual or audible feedback techniques demonstrating the dysfunctional increase in urethral muscle tone was effective in correcting or improving the condition.[97–99]

Magnetic stimulation has been investigated for the treatment of voiding dysfunction; in an animal model of surgically neurogenic bladder, magnetic stimulation demonstrated improvement in vesical pressures and voiding function[100]; some studies have shown some promise in the treatment of voiding dysfunction among patients with spinal injuries.[101]

Prolapse

Pelvic organ prolapse shares much with urinary incontinence in terms of risk factors and epidemiology; many of the current leading hypotheses of the pathophysiology of incontinence invoke the concept of lack of support, or prolapse, of the bladder outlet mechanisms. It stands to reason, therefore, that the condition and function of pelvic floor musculature is important in the development of prolapse. The role of the levator muscles includes the regulation of the size of the genital hiatus[102]; widening of the genital hiatus, by relaxation or dysfunction of the pubococcygeus muscle, may predispose to prolapse by reducing the support of the levator plate[103] MRI imaging of women with prolapse, like those with urinary incontinence, show significant thinning and presence of gaps of levator musculature, compared with normal controls.[5,6,104,105] However, prolapse clearly involves detachment injury as well as neuromuscular dysfunction; one series of patients undergoing surgery for urethral hypermobility and anterior vaginal wall prolapse found paravaginal detachments in over 85% of cases.[106]

Despite these considerations, few data exist regarding the conservative management of pelvic floor prolapse with pelvic physiotherapy. A recent Cochrane Database review found no eligible studies of treatment of prolapse with PFME or physiotherapy to include in analysis.[107] While the risk involved is exceedingly low with a program of PFME, there is no scientific support as yet for its role in this indication.

Does pelvic floor enhancement protect surgical outcomes? Although this has not been scientifically evaluated, one study demonstrated that reconstructive surgery that resulted in alterations in pudendal nerve terminal motor latency was more likely to fail.[108] Whether or not this neuromuscular pathology can be corrected through pelvic physiotherapy is not clear; however, this finding provides some support for the widely held belief that optimization of the pelvic neuromuscular apparatus is likely to provide some enhancement to surgical prolapse repair.

Anal Incontinence

The role of pelvic muscle exercises in the treatment of fecal incontinence can be readily appreciated with an understanding of the muscular anatomy. The external anal sphincter is intimately associated with the puborectalis component of the levator ani complex, and voluntary contraction of the muscle groups are synchronous and inseparable. The levators play an important role in fecal continence in the healthy subject. The rectoanal angle is created by the sling effect of the puborectalis muscle and is crucial in the continence mechanism and anorectal reflexes central to fecal continence and defecatory function. While the majority of the resting tone of the anal canal is attributed to the action of the smooth muscle of the internal anal sphincter, the puborectalis and the external anal sphincter, which are continuous muscular structures, act together, under both voluntary and spinal reflex control, to increase resistance during episodes of increased intraabdominal pressure.[109] Clearly, neuromuscular integrity and conditioning are important factors in maintaining fecal continence. (Figure 8.5)

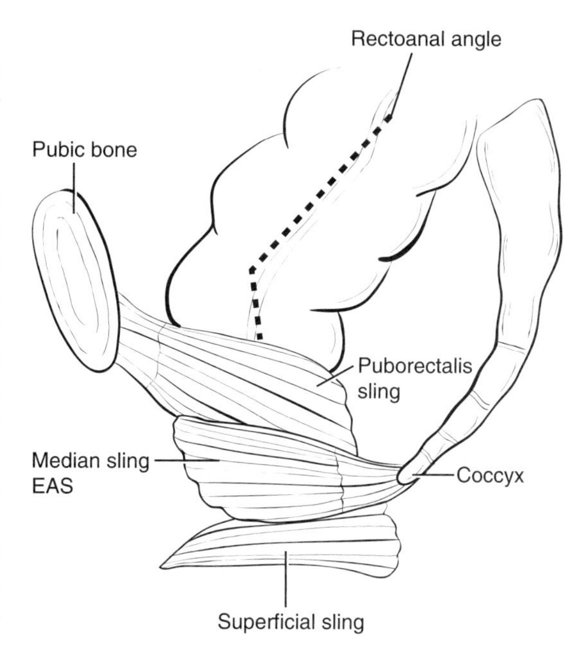

FIGURE 8.5. External anal sphincter.

The addition of physiotherapy techniques to PFME teaching has been investigated in a widely disparate collection of studies, which are limited by small numbers, methodologic flaws, and inconsistencies; the Cochrane Database review was able to identify only five studies meeting inclusion criteria, involving a total of 109 patients. The reviewers determined that there was a suggestion of enhanced benefit in a program of anal biofeedback, electrical stimulation, and exercises over similar programs involving vaginal biofeedback and exercises alone, particularly in the postobstetrical population.[110] Another reviewer reached similar conclusions about trials investigating electrical stimulation alone in the treatment of fecal incontinence.[111]

Conclusion

Pelvic floor physiotherapy plays an important role in the armamentarium against lower urinary tract dysfunction. Scientific studies evaluating the efficacy of these techniques are variable in their support; this likely represents variations in treatment regimens, details of technique, and patient population. Although a great deal of attention is paid to new and expensive pharmacotherapy, scientific data suggests that pelvic floor exercises, behavioral therapy, and pelvic physiotherapy can be equally, or even more, effective than drug therapy; the combination may be more effective still.[112,113] These interventions have a higher success rate among younger women with high motivation, less advanced pelvic floor dysfunction, without previous urogynecologic surgery, and less severe symptomatology. More rigorous trials are needed to come to more definitive conclusions about the comparative efficacy of physiotherapy over other behavioral, surgical, or pharmacologic treatments.

Key Points

- Pelvic floor biofeedback converts muscle activity into visual or auditory stimuli, allowing the patient to identify and amplify her "Kegel squeeze" efforts.
- A simple perineometer represents a "low tech" biofeedback device, whereas more sophisticated machines utilize EMG surface electrodes to enhance muscle isolation.
- Electrical stimulation therapy utilizes vaginal probes, which deliver mild stimulation to the pelvic floor nerves and muscles. Home units are available, allowing women an alternative for both stress and urge incontinence.
- "Neuromodulation" refers to an implantable "pelvic pacemaker" electrode, designed for women with overactive bladder symptoms that fail to respond to non-invasive therapy.

References

1. DeLancey JO. Structural support of the urethra as it relates to stress urinary incontinence: the hammock hypothesis. Am J Obstet Gynecol. 1994; 170:1713–1723.
2. Crystle CD, Charme LS, Copeland WE. Q-tip test in stress urinary incontinence. Obstet Gynecol. 1971;38:313–315.
3. Gilpin SA,Gosling JA, Smith AR, Warrell DW. The pathogenesis of genitourinary prolapse and stress incontinence of urine. A histological and histochemical study. Br J Obstet Gynaecol. 1989;96: 15–23.
4. Bernstein IT. The pelvic floor muscles: muscle thickness in healthy and urinary-incontinent women measured by perineal ultrasonography with reference to the effect of pelvic floor training. Estrogen receptor studies. Neurourol Urodyn. 1997;16:237–275.
5. Hoyte L, Fielding JR, Versi E, Mamisch C, Kolvenbach C, Kikinis R. Variations in levator ani volume and geometry in women: the application of MR based 3D reconstruction in evaluating pelvic floor dysfunction. Arch Esp Urol. 2001;54: 532–539.
6. Hoyte L, Jakab M, Warfield SK, Shott S, Flesh G, Fielding JR. Levator ani thickness variations in symptomatic and asymptomatic women using magnetic resonance-based 3-dimensional color mapping. Am J Obstet Gynecol. 2004;191:856–861.
7. Dougherty MC. Current status of research on pelvic muscle strengthening techniques. J Wound Ostomy Continence Nurs. 1998;25:75–83.
8. Voigt R, Halaska M, Wilke I et. al. Urogynecologic follow-up after conservative therapy of stress incontinence with a vaginal cone (Femcon) [in German]. *Geburtshilfe Frauenheilkd.* 1994;54: 390–393.
9. de Groat WC. Central nervous system control of micturition. In: O'Donnell P. Urinary incontinence. St. Louis: Mosby; 1997 p. 33–47
10. Nygaard I, Dougherty MC. Genuine stress incontinence and pelvic organ prolapse`; Nonsurgical treatment. In: Urogynecology and Reconstructive Pelvic Surgery, Walters MD and Karram MM, Eds. Mosby, St. Louis, 1999, P.150
11. Hay-Smith EJ, Bo Berghmans LC, Hendriks HJ, de Bie RA, van Waalwijk van Doorn ES. Pelvic floor muscle training for urinary incontinence in women. Cochrane Database Syst Rev. 2001; CD001407.
12. Bump RC, Hurt WG, Fantl JA, Wyman JF. Assessment of Kegel pelvic muscle exercise performance after brief verbal instruction. *Am J Obstet Gynecol.* 1991;165:322–329.
13. Elia G, Bergman A. Pelvic muscle exercises: when do they work? *Obstet Gynecol.* 1993;81:283–286.
14. Wilson PD, Al Samarrai T, Deakin M, Kolbe E, Brown AD. An objective assessment of physiotherapy for female genuine stress incontinence. *Br J Obstet Gynaecol.* 1987; 94: 575–582.
15. Miller K, Richardson DA, Siegel SW, Karram MM, Blackwood NB, Sand PK. Pelvic floor electrical stimulation for genuine stress incontinence: who will benefit and when? *Int Urogynecol J Pelvic Floor Dysfunct.* 1998;9:265–270.
16. Kegel AH. The physiologic treatment of poor tone and function of the genital muscles and of urinary

stress incontinence. *West J Surg Obstet Gynecol.* 1949;57:527–535.
17. Kegel AH, Powell TO. The physiologic treatment of urinary stress incontinence. *J Urol*, 1950;63: 808–814.
18. Kegel AH. The physiological treatment of stress incontinence of the urine in women. *Gynecol Prat.* 1960;11:539–560.
19. Kegel AH. Stress incontinence of urine in women; physiologic treatment. *J Int Coll Surg.* 1956;25: 487–499.
20. Kegel AH. Early genital relaxation; new technic of diagnosis and nonsurgical treatment. *Obstet Gynecol.* 1956;8:545–550.
21. Peattie AB, Plevnik S, Stanton SL. Vaginal cones: a conservative method of treating genuine stress incontinence. *Br J Obstet Gynaecol.* 1988;95: 1049–1053.
22. Dellas A, Drewe J. Conservative therapy of female genuine stress incontinence with vaginal cones. *Eur J Obstet Gynecol Reprod Biol.* 1995;62: 213–215.
23. Kondo A, Yamada Y, Niijima R. Treatment of stress incontinence by vaginal cones: short- and long-term results and predictive parameters. *Br J Urol.* 1995;76:464–466.
24. Cammu H,Van Nylen M. Pelvic floor exercises versus vaginal weight cones in genuine stress incontinence. *Eur J Obstet Gynecol Reprod Biol.* 1998;77:89–93.
25. Arvonen T, Fianu-Jonasson A, Tyni-Lenne R. Effectiveness of two conservative modes of physical therapy in women with urinary stress incontinence. *Neurourol Urodyn.* \2001;20:591–599.
26. Bo K, Talseth T, Holme I. Single blind, randomised controlled trial of pelvic floor exercises, electrical stimulation, vaginal cones, and no treatment in management of genuine stress incontinence in women. *BMJ.* 1999;318:487–493.
27. Kato K, Kondo A. Clinical value of vaginal cones for the management of female stress incontinence. *Int Urogynecol J Pelvic Floor Dysfunct.* 1997;8: 314–317.
28. Herbison P, Plevnik S, Mantle J. Weighted vaginal cones for urinary incontinence. *Cochrane Database Syst Rev.* 2000:CD002114.
29. Cardozo LD. Biofeedback in overactive bladder. *Urology.* 2000;55:24–28, 31–32.
30. Cardozo L, Stanton SL, Hafner J, Allan V. Biofeedback in the treatment of detrusor instability. *Br J Urol.* 1978;50:250–254.
31. Bourcier AP, Burgio KL. Biofeedback therapy. In: Bourcier AP, McGuire EJ, Abrams P, eds. *Pelvic Floor Disorders.* Philadelphia: Elsevier Saunders; 2004:301
32. Miller JM, Ashton-Miller JA, DeLancey JO. A pelvic muscle precontraction can reduce cough-related urine loss in selected women with mild SUI. *J Am Geriatr Soc.* 1998;46:870–874.
33. Miller JM, Perucchini D, Carchidi LT, DeLancey JO, Ashton-Miller J. Pelvic floor muscle contraction during a cough and decreased vesical neck mobility. *Obstet Gynecol.* 2001;97:255–260.
34. Castleden CM, Duffin HM, Mitchell EP. The effect of physiotherapy on stress incontinence. *Age Ageing.* 1984;13:235–237.
35. Shepherd AM, Montgomery E, Anderson RS. Treatment of genuine stress incontinence with a new perineometer. *Physiotherapy.* 1983;69:113.
36. Burgio KL, Robinson JC, Engel BT. The role of biofeedback in Kegel exercise training for stress urinary incontinence. *Am J Obstet Gynecol.* 1986; 1541:58–64.
37. Glavind K, Nohr SB, Walter S. Biofeedback and physiotherapy versus physiotherapy alone in the treatment of genuine stress urinary incontinence. *Int Urogynecol J Pelvic Floor Dysfunct.* 1996;7: 339–343.
38. Berghmans LC, Frederiks CM, de Bie RA et al. Efficacy of biofeedback, when included with pelvic floor muscle exercise treatment, for genuine stress incontinence. *Neurourol Urodyn.* 1996;15: 37–52.
39. Morkved S, Bo K, Fjortoft T. Effect of adding biofeedback to pelvic floor muscle training to treat urodynamic stress incontinence. *Obstet Gynecol.* 2002;100:730–739.
40. Burns PA, Pranikoff K, Nochajski TH, Hadley EC, Levy KJ, Ory MG. A comparison of effectiveness of biofeedback and pelvic muscle exercise treatment of stress incontinence in older community-dwelling women. *J Gerontol.* 1993;48:M167–174.
41. Burton JR, Pearce KL, Burgio KL, Engel BT, Whitehead WE. Behavioral training for urinary incontinence in elderly ambulatory patients. *J Am Geriatr Soc.* 1988;36:693–698.
42. Burgio KL, Goode PS, Locher JL. Behavioral training with and without biofeedback in the treatment of urge incontinence in older women: a randomized controlled trial. *JAMA.* 2002;288: 2293–2299.
43. Huffman JW, Osborne SL, Sokol JK. Electrical stimulation in the treatment of intractable stress incontinence; a preliminary report. *Arch Phys Med Rehabil.* 1952;33: 674–676.
44. Bors E. Effect of electric stimulation of the pudendal nerves on the vesical neck; its significance for the function of cord bladders: a preliminary report. *J Urol.* 1952;67:925–935.

45. Godec C, Cass AS, Ayala GF. Electrical stimulation for incontinence. Technique, selection, and results. *Urology*. 1976;7:388–397.
46. Fall M, Erlandson BE, Carlsson CA, Lindstrom S. The effect of intravanginal electrical stimulation on the feline urethra and urinary bladder. Neuronal mechanisms. *Scand J Urol Nephrol Suppl*. 1977; 44:19–30.
47. Brubaker L. Electrical stimulation in overactive bladder. *Urology*. 2000;55:17–23, 31–32.
48. Bourcier AP, Burgio KL. Biofeedback therapy. In: Bourcier AP, McGuire EJ, Abrams P, eds. *Pelvic Floor Disorders*. Philadelphia: Elsevier Saunders. 2004:297–310.
49. Lindstrom S, Fall M, Carlsson CA, Erlandson BE. The neurophysiological basis of bladder inhibition in response to intravaginal electrical stimulation. *J Urol*. 1983;129: 405–410.
50. Brubaker L, Benson JT, Bent A, Clark A, Shott S. Transvaginal electrical stimulation for female urinary incontinence. *Am J Obstet Gynecol*. 1997; 177:536–540.
51. Fall M, Ahlstrom K, Carlsson CA. Contelle: pelvic floor stimulator for female stress-urge incontinence. A multicenter study. *Urology*. 1986;27: 282–287.
52. Benson JT (ed). Pelvic floor disorders: investigation and treatment, urinary incontinence electrical stimulation. In: Benson JT (ed). Pelvic Floor Disorders; Investigation and Treatment. New York: WW Norton and Co, NY, 1992:220.
53. Erlandson BE, Fall M, Sundin T. Intravaginal electrical stimulation. Clinical experiments of urethral closure. *Scand J Urol Nephrol Suppl*. 1977;44: 31–39.
54. Erlandson BE, Fall M, Carlsson CA. The effect of intravaginal electrical stimulation on the feline urethra and urinary bladder. Electrical parameters. *Scand J Urol Nephrol Suppl*. 1977;44: 5–18.
55. Bo K. Talseth T. Change in urethral pressure during voluntary pelvic floor muscle contraction and vaginal electrical stimulation. *Int Urogynecol J Pelvic Floor Dysfunct*. 1997;8:3–7.
56. Olah KS, Bridges N, Denning J, Farrar DJ. The conservative management of patients with symptoms of stress incontinence: a randomized, prospective study comparing weighted vaginal cones and interferential therapy. *Am J Obstet Gynecol*. 1990;162:87–92.
57. Parkkinen A, Karjalainen E, Vartiainen M, Penttinen J. Physiotherapy for female stress urinary incontinence: individual therapy at the outpatient clinic versus home-based pelvic floor training: a 5-year follow-up study. *Neurourol Urodyn*. 2004; 23:643–648.
58. Goode PS, Burgio KL, Locher JL. Effect of behavioral training with or without pelvic floor electrical stimulation on stress incontinence in women: a randomized controlled trial. *JAMA*. 2003;290: 345–352.
59. Resplande J, Gholami S, Bruschini H, Srougi M. Urodynamic changes induced by the intravaginal electrode during pelvic floor electrical stimulation. *Neurourol Urodyn*. 2003;22:24–28.
60. Sand PK, Richardson DA, Staskin DR et. al. Pelvic floor electrical stimulation in the treatment of genuine stress incontinence: a multicenter, placebo-controlled trial. *Am J Obstet Gynecol*. 1995;173:72–79.
61. Smith JJ 3rd. Intravaginal stimulation randomized trial. *J Urol*. 1996;155:127–130.
62. Seo JT, Yoon H, Kim YH. A randomized prospective study comparing new vaginal cone and FES-Biofeedback. *Yonsei Med J*. 2004;45:879–884.
63. Barroso JC, Ramos JG, Martins-Costa S, Sanches PR, Muller AF. Transvaginal electrical stimulation in the treatment of urinary incontinence. *BJU Int*. 2004;93:319–323.
64. Yamanishi T, Yasuda K, Sakakibara R, Hattori T, Suda S. Randomized, double-blind study of electrical stimulation for urinary incontinence due to detrusor overactivity. *Urology*. 2000;55: 353–357.
65. Wang AC, Wang YY, Chen MC. Single-blind, randomized trial of pelvic floor muscle training, biofeedback-assisted pelvic floor muscle training, and electrical stimulation in the management of overactive bladder. *Urology*. 2004;63:61–66.
66. Spruijt J, Vierhout M, Verstraeten R, Janssens J, Burger C. Vaginal electrical stimulation of the pelvic floor: a randomized feasibility study in urinary incontinent elderly women. *Acta Obstet Gynecol Scand*. 2003;82:1043–1048.
67. Susset J, Galea G, Manbeck K, Susset A. A predictive score index for the outcome of associated biofeedback and vaginal electrical stimulation in the treatment of female incontinence. *J Urol*. 1995;153:1461–1466.
68. Indrekvam S, Sandvik H, Hunskaar S. A Norwegian national cohort of 3198 women treated with home-managed electrical stimulation for urinary incontinence–effectiveness and treatment results. *Scand J Urol Nephrol*. 2001;35:32–39.
69. Indrekvam S, Hunskaar S. Side effects, feasibility, and adherence to treatment during home-managed electrical stimulation for urinary incontinence:

a Norwegian national cohort of 3,198 women. *Neurourol Urodyn.* 2002;21:546–552.

70. Kessler TM, Madersbacher H, Kiss G. Prolonged sacral neuromodulation testing using permanent leads: a more reliable patient selection method? *Eur Urol.* 2005;47:660–665.
71. Amarenco G, Ismael SS, Even-Schneider A et al. Urodynamic effect of acute transcutaneous posterior tibial nerve stimulation in overactive bladder. *J Urol.* 2003; 169: 2210–2215.
72. Govier FE, Litwiller S, Nitti V, Kreder KJ Jr, Rosenblatt P. Percutaneous afferent neuromodulation for the refractory overactive bladder: results of a multicenter study. *J Urol.* 2001;165:1193–1198.
73. Jalinous R. Technical and practical aspects of magnetic nerve stimulation. *J Clin Neurophysiol.* 1991;8:10–25.
74. Jost WH, Schimrigk K. Magnetic stimulation of the pudendal nerve. *Dis Colon Rectum.* 1994;37: 697–699.
75. Yamanishi T, Yasuda K, Suda S, Ishikawa N. Effect of functional continuous magnetic stimulation on urethral closure in healthy volunteers. *Urology.* 1999;54:652–655.
76. McFarlane JP, Foley SJ, de Winter P, Shah PJ, Craggs MD. Acute suppression of idiopathic detrusor instability with magnetic stimulation of the sacral nerve roots. *Br J Urol.* 1997;80:734–741.
77. Craggs MD, McFarlane JP, Foley SJ, Wagg AS, Knight SL. Detrusor relaxation following suppression of normal voiding reflexes by magnetic stimulation of the sacral nerves. *J Physiol.* 1997;53: 501P.
78. Yamanishi T, Yasuda K, Suda S, Ishikawa N, Sakakibara R, Hattori T. Effect of functional continuous magnetic stimulation for urinary incontinence. *J Urol.* 2000;163: 456–459.
79. Sheriff MK, Shah PJ, Fowler C, Mundy AR, Craggs MD. Neuromodulation of detrusor hyper-reflexia by functional magnetic stimulation of the sacral roots. *Br J Urol.* 1996;78:39–46.
80. Chandi DD, Groenendijk PM, Venema PL. Functional extracorporeal magnetic stimulation as a treatment for female urinary incontinence: 'the chair'. *BJU Int.* 2004; 93: 539–542.
81. Galloway NT, El-Galley RE, Sand PK, Appell RA, Russell HW, Carlan SJ. Extracorporeal magnetic innervation therapy for stress urinary incontinence. *Urology.* 1999;53:1108–1111.
82. Fujishiro T, Enomoto H, Ugawa Y, Takahashi S, Ueno S, Kitamura T. Magnetic stimulation of the sacral roots for the treatment of stress incontinence: an investigational study and placebo controlled trial. *J Urol.* 2000;164:1277–1279.
83. Yokoyama T, Fujita O, Nishiguchi J et. al. Extracorporeal magnetic innervation treatment for urinary incontinence. *Int J Urol.* 2004;11:602–606.
84. Bourcier AP, Burgio KL. Biofeedback therapy. In: Bourcier AP, McGuire EJ, Abrams P, eds. *Pelvic Floor Disorders.* Philadelphia: Elsevier Saunders; 2004:294.
85. Morkved S, Salvesen KA, Bo K, Eik-Nes S. Pelvic floor muscle strength and thickness in continent and incontinent nulliparous pregnant women. *Int Urogynecol J Pelvic Floor Dysfunct.* 2004;15: 384–390.
86. Morkved S, Bo K, Schei B, Salvesen KA. Pelvic floor muscle training during pregnancy to prevent urinary incontinence: a single-blind randomized controlled trial. *Obstet Gynecol.* 2003;101:313–319.
87. Salvesen KA, Morkved S. Randomised controlled trial of pelvic floor muscle training during pregnancy. *BMJ.* 2004;329:378–380.
88. Glazener CM, Herbison GP, Wilson PD. Conservative management of persistent postnatal urinary and faecal incontinence: randomised controlled trial. *BMJ.* 2001; 323: 593–596.
89. Chiarelli P, Cockburn J. Promoting urinary continence in women after delivery: randomised controlled trial. *BMJ.* 2002;324:1241.
90. Morkved S, Bo K. Effect of postpartum pelvic floor muscle training in prevention and treatment of urinary incontinence: a one-year follow up. *BJOG.* 2000;107:1022–1028.
91. Sampselle CM, Miller JM, Mims BL, Delancey JO, Ashton-Miller JA, Antonakos CL. Effect of pelvic muscle exercise on transient incontinence during pregnancy and after birth. *Obstet Gynecol.* 1998;91: 406–412.
92. Jonasson A, Larsson B, Pschera H. Testing and training of the pelvic floor muscles after childbirth. *Acta Obstet Gynecol Scand.* 1989;68:301–304.
93. Harvey MA. Pelvic floor exercises during and after pregnancy: a systematic review of their role in preventing pelvic floor dysfunction. *J Obstet Gynaecol Can.* 2003;25: 487–498.
94. Hay-Smith J. Herbison P, Morkved S. Physical therapies for prevention of urinary and faecal incontinence in adults. *Cochrane Database Syst Rev.* 2002:CD003191.
95. Culligan PJ, Blackwell L, Murphy M, Ziegler C, Heit MH. A randomized, double-blinded, sham-controlled trial of postpartum extracorporeal magnetic innervation to restore pelvic muscle strength in primiparous patients. *Am J Obstet Gynecol.* 2005;192:1578–1582.

96. Sander P, Bjarnesen J, Mouritsen L, Fuglsang-Frederiksen A. Anal incontinence after obstetric third- /fourth-degree laceration. One-year follow-up after pelvic floor exercises. *Int Urogynecol J Pelvic Floor Dysfunct.* 1999;10:177–181.
97. Maizels M, King LR, Firlit CF. Urodynamic biofeedback: a new approach to treat vesical sphincter dyssynergia. *J Urol.* 1979;122:205–209.
98. Sugar EC, Firlit CF. Urodynamic biofeedback: a new therapeutic approach for childhood incontinence/infection (vesical voluntary sphincter dyssynergia). *J Urol.* 1982;128:1253–1258.
99. Libo LM, Arnold GE, Woodside JR, Borden TA, Hardy TL. EMG biofeedback for functional bladder-sphincter dyssynergia: a case study. *Biofeedback Self Regul.* 1983;8: 243–253.
100. Shafik A. Magnetic stimulation: a novel method for inducing evacuation of the neuropathic rectum and urinary bladder in a canine model. *Urology.* 1999;54:368–372.
101. Lin VW, Wolfe V, Frost FS, Perkash I. Micturition by functional magnetic stimulation. *J Spinal Cord Med.* 1997;20:218–26.
102. Ghetti C, Gregory WT, Edwards SR, Otto LN, Clark AL. Severity of pelvic organ prolapse associated with measurements of pelvic floor function. *Int Urogynecol J Pelvic Floor Dysfunct.* 2005;16: 432–436.
103. Delancey JO, Hurd WW. Size of the urogenital hiatus in the levator ani muscles in normal women and women with pelvic organ prolapse. *Obstet Gynecol.* 1998;91:364–368.
104. Monnerie-Lachaud V, Pages S, Guillot E, Veyret C. Contribution of pelvic floor MRI in the morphological and functional analysis of pre and postoperative levator muscle in patients with genital prolapse [in French]. *J Gynecol Obstet Biol Reprod (Paris).* 2001;30:753–760.
105. Ozasa H, Mori T, Togashi K. Study of uterine prolapse by magnetic resonance imaging: topographical changes involving the levator ani muscle and the vagina. *Gynecol Obstet Invest.* 1992;34:43–48.
106. Delancey JO. Fascial and muscular abnormalities in women with urethral hypermobility and anterior vaginal wall prolapse. *Am J Obstet Gynecol.* 2002;187:93–98.
107. Hagen S, Stark D, Maher C, Adams E. Conservative management of pelvic organ prolapse in women. *Cochrane Database Syst Rev.* 2004: CD003882.
108. Welgoss JA, Vogt VY, McClellan EJ, Benson JT. Relationship between surgically induced neuropathy and outcome of pelvic organ prolapse surgery. *Int Urogynecol J Pelvic Floor Dysfunct.* 1999;10: 11–14.
109. Bourcier AP, Burgio KL. Biofeedback therapy. In: Bourcier AP, McGuire EJ, Abrams P, eds. *Pelvic Floor Disorders.* Philadelphia: Elsevier Saunders; 2004:15.
110. Norton C, Hosker G, Brazzelli M. Biofeedback and/or sphincter exercises for the treatment of faecal incontinence in adults. *Cochrane Database Syst Rev.* 2000:CD002111.
111. Hosker G, Norton C, Brazzelli M. Electrical stimulation for faecal incontinence in adults. *Cochrane Database Syst Rev.* 2000:CD001310.
112. Goode PS. Behavioral and drug therapy for urinary incontinence. *Urology.* 2004;63: 58–64.
113. Burgio KL, Locher JL, Goode PS et. al. Behavioral vs drug treatment for urge urinary incontinence in older women: a randomized controlled trial. *JAMA.* 1998;280:1995–2000.

9
Pessary Devices: A Stepwise Approach to Fitting, Teaching, and Managing

Patrick J. Culligan

Introduction

Although pessaries have been used successfully for thousands of years, they are often overlooked as a first-line treatment option for women with pelvic organ prolapse. When properly fitted, pessaries can provide immediate relief of prolapse symptoms. These devices, which represent the primary non-surgical management option for pelvic organ prolapse, are appropriate for either temporary or long-term use.

Indications for Pessary Placement

Although often considered a treatment option for elderly patients only, pessaries can be appropriate for younger women as well. In fact, *any* patient suffering from pelvic organ prolapse is a potential candidate for pessary placement. Ultimately, the decision about whether a woman will wear a pessary or undergo surgery is hers alone—regardless of her age. That is because surgery to correct prolapse, even if performed via laparoscopic or vaginal techniques, always carries the possibility of a more difficult recuperation than expected. Women undergoing these types of operations are usually asked to restrict their physical activity for twelve weeks while they heal. These restrictions often involve lifting no more than 10 pounds, avoiding significant straining with bowel movements, and refraining from intercourse. Some women who would otherwise undergo surgery choose to use a pessary *temporarily*, because the above-mentioned restrictions do not fit into their immediate plans. Others wear pessaries during their reproductive years and then undergo surgery once they have completed their families. In some cases, pessaries are indicated to provide relief of prolapse symptoms *during* pregnancy.

Pessaries can also be used to *simulate* the benefits of surgery for women whose prolapse symptoms seem worse than their physical findings (i.e., severe symptoms associated with minimal prolapse). If wearing a pessary alleviates the bothersome symptoms in this group of women, then prolapse surgery is likely to be successful as well.

Certain pessaries can also be useful in the management of stress urinary incontinence by providing differential support to the urethra (Figure 9.1). Women who have very predictable stress urinary incontinence during athletic activities such as golf, horseback riding, tennis or soccer sometimes choose this type of pessary, thinking of it as just another "athletic brace."

Still, the most typical pessary wearers are poor surgical candidates age 65 or older,[1] Women with immunosuppressive conditions such as poorly controlled diabetes mellitus or HIV may be subject to serious infections following pelvic reconstructive surgery. Also, any history of pelvic radiation greatly increases the potential for wound breakdown or erosion of graft material. In these situations, the risks of surgery probably outweigh the benefits. For such high-risk patients, surgery should only be considered after pessary management has proven unsuccessful.

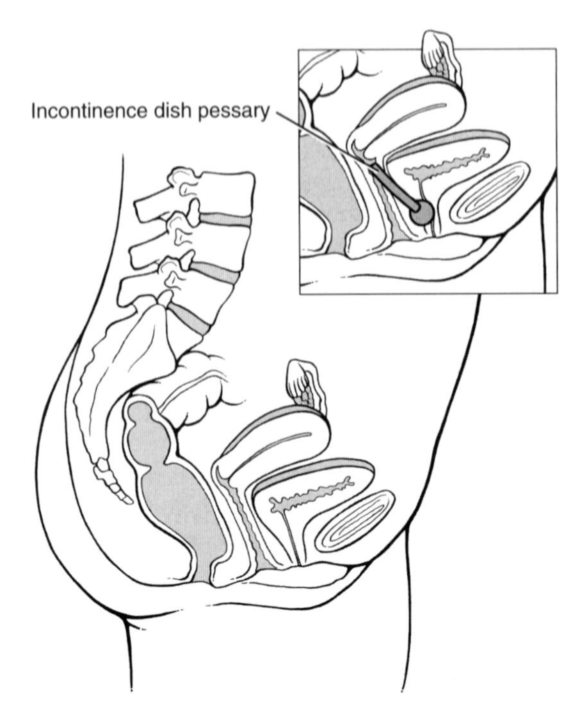

Figure 9.1. The incontinence-dish pessary works to prevent/diminish urinary incontinence because the bulb-like structure compresses the urethra during episodes of increased abdominal pressure.

Choosing the Proper Pessary—the Good, Bad, and Ugly

Even for practitioners with little or no experience, offering pessary management to their patients with pelvic organ prolapse requires only a minimal initial outlay of time and money. In fact, from a "bang for your buck" standpoint, few treatment modalities compare with pessary management. While the wide array of pessary shapes and sizes can be daunting to new users, the vast majority of patients are successfully treated with one of only two basic types—the *ring with support* and the *Gellhorn*. Choosing between these two pessary types is usually quite simple. Figure 9.2 depicts these and other pessaries. All pessaries discussed in this chapter are made of medical grade silicone. They are durable and do not tend to create a foul odor. Older pessaries made of rubber or latex should be considered obsolete.

Regardless of the specific defect present (i.e. cystocele, rectocele, uterine prolapse. etc.), a ring with support will often do the job. When a ring with support works effectively, it is the best choice, because patients can usually be taught to manage these pessaries by themselves. When the ring with support will not work (i.e., when it tends to fall out), the next choice should be a Gellhorn pessary. In most cases, if a Gellhorn pessary does not work, the likelihood of finding a successful pessary device drops precipitously, and the remaining pessary choices carry much higher rates of complications and patient dissatisfaction. Other varieties of pessaries are as follow:

Donut Pessary

This space-filling pessary can be difficult to remove and replace. Patients are almost never able to manage it themselves. It also produces more vaginal discharge than most other pessaries.

Cube Pessary

This pessary should only be used as a last resort for patients who will remove it and replace it themselves on a daily basis. If it is not removed regularly, it will cause serious vaginal ulcerations and a copious vaginal discharge.

Gehrung Pessary

This pessary is technically difficult to place correctly, and it tends to rotate out of the proper position.

Hodge Pessary

This pessary and the other "lever" pessaries (which look very much like this one) work by being wedged behind the pubic bone. While their shape is supposed to allow patients to have intercourse while the pessary is in place, the number of women who actually try to do so is unknown. They are technically difficult to place and tend to cause more pain than either the ring with support or the Gellhorn.

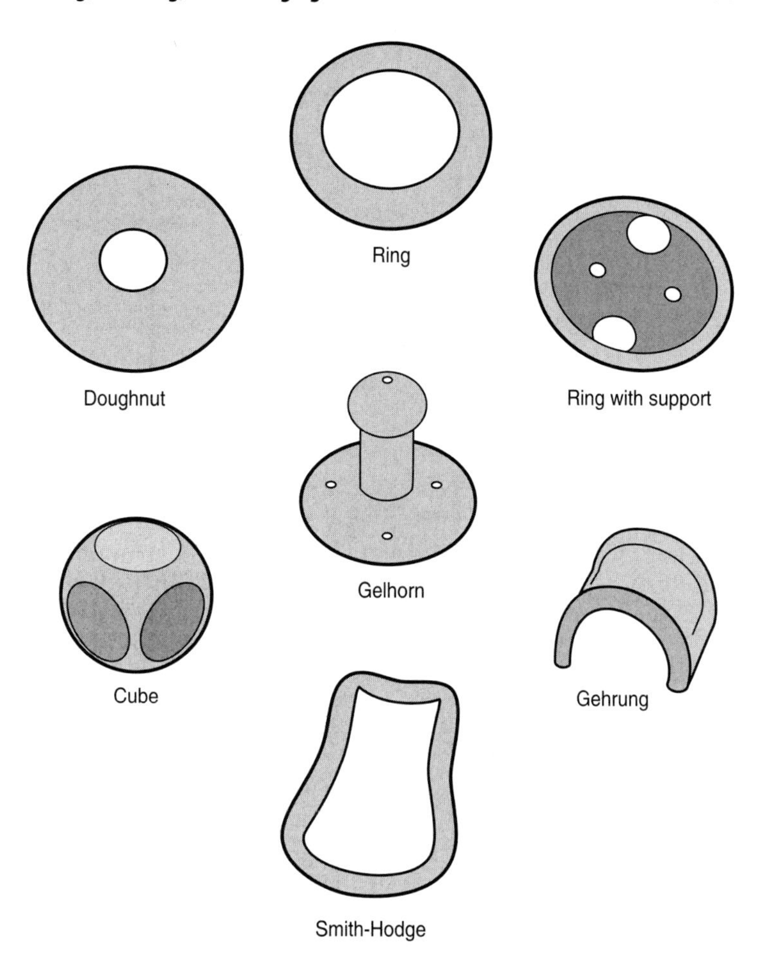

FIGURE 9.2. The various commonly used pessaries. The most useful of these by far are the Gellhorn and ring with support.

Inflatoball Pessary

This pessary is made of latex—NOT silicone. It is in the shape of a donut pessary, but it has a stem through which it can be inflated with air. It is designed to be inflated to a size that matches the patient's defect. The latex material tends to absorb the vaginal discharge, which gives this pessary a foul odor after only short-term use. It also has all of the above-mentioned disadvantages of the donut pessary.

Fitting the Pessary—3 Easy Steps

In a study of nearly 500 women, Swift et al. showed that women do not usually feel prolapse symptoms until their prolapse extends beyond the introitus.[2] Therefore, the goal of pessary placement is to keep the pelvic organs from bulging beyond the opening of the vagina. Regardless of the specific type of pessary, the proper size for a given patient is the smallest one that doesn't fall out. As mentioned above, a ring with support pessary should usually be tried first. Virtually any patient can retain a pessary comfortably as long as one thing is true about her physical exam—the vaginal canal needs to be greater in caliber than the vaginal opening or introitus. That is because the introitus and perineal body tend to hold a pessary in place. As such, women with introitus measurements of less than 4 centimeters are more likely to be the best pessary candidates.

Step 1—Digital Exam

Simply place two fingers inside the vagina as would be done during any bimanual exam. Spread your fingers as wide as you can without causing pain, and remember that width. Keep your fingers at that width while removing them from the vagina. If the introitus and perineal body force you to close your fingers somewhat in order to withdraw them, a pessary will usually work well. If, on the other hand, the vaginal canal is smaller than, or the same size as, the opening, a pessary may tend to fall out. When choosing either a ring with support or Gellhorn pessary, the width of the vaginal canal (determined during your bimanual exam) should be the same as the diameter of the pessary you choose.

Step 2—"How Does It Feel?"

After placing the pessary in the vagina, ask the patient, *"How does that feel?"* The best possible answer is something like, "*How does 'what' feel*?" In other words, a patient will not usually feel the properly fitted pessary. This is usually surprising to the patient. If the pessary is causing any discomfort, it should be immediately removed, because such discomfort always gets worse. If a patient describes a vague sensation of mild irritation but no real discomfort, this feeling could simply be the result of manipulation during the exam. Clinical judgment should be used to determine whether such mild irritation warrants immediate removal of the pessary.

Step 3—The Cough Test

With the patient in the dorsal lithotomy position, immediately after placing the pessary, ask her to cough vigorously. If the pessary is much too small, it may simply fall out. If it doesn't fall out spontaneously, gently tug on the edge of the pessary as the patient coughs again. If it becomes dislodged with only minimal additional pressure, it is too small. If the patient passes both of these tests in the lithotomy position, ask her to stand up and then repeat the process.

The patient herself should perform the final sizing test by herself, in your office bathroom. While sitting on the toilet, she should strain as though she were moving her bowels; you may consider fastening a plastic urometer "hat" to the toilet rim to avoid having the pessary device fall into the toilet itself. If the pessary remains in place, there is little chance that it will become dislodged during the patient's day-to-day life.

If the pessary falls out during any of these tests, repeat the process with a slightly larger, or perhaps a different type of, pessary.

Pessary Management

Once the proper pessary has been chosen, the patient should attempt to answer one simple question: *Is her quality of life better while wearing the pessary?* We usually ask patients to leave the pessary in place continuously and return to the office in 1 to 2 weeks. When the patient returns to the office, she is simply asked whether she wants to continue using the pessary. If her answer is "*yes*", we then attempt to teach her to insert and remove it herself. For those patients unable or unwilling to do this, an office management schedule is set up. For most of these patients, office visits are scheduled every 2 to 3 months. During those visits, the pessary is removed, cleaned, and replaced. The vagina is irrigated and inspected for abrasions and ulcerations.

Complications Associated with Pessary Use

True pessary complications are rare and are almost always associated with non-compliance to the management plan described above. Other common problems that fall short of complication status include (1) a tendency toward urinary incontinence, (2) vaginal discharge. (3) minor vaginal spotting, or (4) spontaneous expulsion.

The most common *true* complication of pessary use is vaginal ulceration or abrasion. Such lesions are easily treated by leaving the pessary out for 2 to 3 weeks while the patient uses vaginal estrogen cream each night. For persistent lesions, discontinuation of pessary use—and even biopsy—may be necessary. If a pessary is left in place continuously, with no intervening office management visits, it can even become incarcerated or migrate into adjacent viscera.

Key Points

- Although pessaries have been used successfully for thousands of years, they are often overlooked as a first-line treatment option for women with pelvic organ prolapse. In fact, any patient suffering from pelvic organ prolapse is a potential candidate for pessary placement.
- The goal of pessary placement is to simply keep the pelvic organs from bulging beyond the opening of the vagina.
- Virtually any patient can retain a pessary comfortably as long as one thing is true about her physical exam—the vaginal canal needs to be greater in caliber than the vaginal opening or introitus.
- The most useful pessaries are the ring with support and the Gellhorn. They should be tried in that order, with patients who cannot retain the ring with support subsequently receiving a trial of the Gellhorn.

Other Information—Pessary Pearls

- Not all pessary wearers require treatment with vaginal estrogen. Use of vaginal estrogen can be limited to those patients with urogenital atrophy or a proven tendency toward vaginal ulceration.
- A thorough vaginal inspection *prior* to pessary fitting is the only way to determine whether a vaginal lesion was caused by the pessary itself.
- Many patients will only have a tendency toward pessary expulsion during bowel movements. If these patients are willing to simply hold the pessary in place with their fingers during a bowel movement, many of them will continue pessary use rather than choose surgery.
- A pessary will sometimes cause otherwise normal Pap smears to be read as atypical. Knowledge of this phenomenon can aid practitioners as they decide whether to perform colposcopy and biopsy as follow-up to such Pap smears.
- Posterior defects (rectocele or perineocele) are the most difficult to treat with a pessary.

Antibiotic gels are usually only useful for patients with a copious foul-smelling vaginal discharge. For instance, metronidazole may be helpful for bacterial vaginosis that presents as a homogeneous, copious grey discharge.

References

1. Clemons JL, Aguilar VC, Tillinghast TA, Jackson ND, Myers DL. Risk factors associated with an unsuccessful pessary fitting trial in women with pelvic organ prolapse. *Am J Obstet Gynecol.* 2004;190: 345–350.
2. Swift SE, Tate SB, Nicholas J. Correlation of symptoms with degree of pelvic organ support in a general population of women: what is pelvic organ prolapse? *Am J Obstet Gynecol.* 2003;189: 372–377.

10
Surgery for Incontinence and Pelvic Dysfunction: Overview for the PCP

Miles Murphy and Vincent R. Lucente

Introduction

Although nonsurgical treatments outlined in the preceding chapters are invaluable to countless women, it is an unavoidable fact that at least 11% of women ultimately elect to undergo surgery to correct vaginal prolapse or incontinence.[1] When behavioral and pharmacological modalities fail to provide adequate symptom relief, surgery is often the only option available to improve a patient's quality of life.

The female pelvis presents a number of unique challenges that, until recently, rendered traditional surgical procedures susceptible to high rates of failure or limited long-term success. However, numerous recent innovations in surgical technique and materials are addressing many of these shortcomings. As a result, women today enjoy higher rates of long-term surgical cure than those of the previous generation, most often with a shorter hospital stay and recovery time when compared with the surgical alternatives of years past.

It is important for primary care providers to understand the latest options available to patients pursuing surgery so that accurate advice can be provided. In this chapter we will review the most common operations performed for urinary incontinence, pelvic organ prolapse, anal incontinence, and defecatory dysfunction, including new and emerging techniques. Moreover, we will review what patients and their primary care providers can expect in terms of post-operative recovery, physical activity limitations, and a return to their daily routine.

Surgery for Urinary Incontinence

Urinary incontinence can be divided, as previous chapters have discussed, into two basic categories—stress and urge. The vast majority of surgeries performed for incontinence are done to treat stress urinary incontinence (SUI). Approximately 135,000 women per year have inpatient surgery for the treatment of SUI, and many more may have outpatient surgery.[2] Stress urinary incontinence has generally been considered to be a result of either poor anatomical support of the urethra and bladder neck (urethrovesical junction hypermobility) or a weakness of the urethral sphincter muscles themselves (intrinsic urethral sphincter deficiency). The various types of operations used to treat this condition reflect these two theoretical etiologies.

Surgery for Stress Urinary Incontinence

Traditional Vaginal Surgeries

One long-standing theory used to explain the pathophysiology of stress urinary incontinence is that of the hypermobile urethrovesical angle. Many continence operations have been designed to correct this anatomical defect by reinforcing the "shelf" of vaginal support upon which the bladder neck and urethra normally rest. In the early part of the twentieth century two surgeons popularized a vaginal approach to re-supporting the bladder neck. This procedure—known as the

Kelly-Kennedy plication—is often referred to in layman's terms as a "bladder tack." It is performed through a midline vertical incision in the anterior vaginal wall. The pubocervical fascia layer beneath the vaginal epithelium is then plicated across the midline, creating a shelf under the urethra and stabilizing it during rises in intra-abdominal pressure.

One of the virtues of this procedure is that it, like other vaginal operations, is minimally invasive. But its use over the last few decades has declined. Cure rates in studies investigating this procedure vary greatly; but in our opinion, the Kelly-Kennedy plication should no longer be considered a primary treatment for stress incontinence.

A vaginal procedure related to the Kelly plication is the *bladder neck needle suspension.* Sutures are looped through the periurethral tissue on either side of the bladder neck and passed from the vagina to the anterior abdominal wall, using long needles. The goal, again, is to elevate, support, and stabilize the urethrovesical junction during rises in intra-abdominal pressure. Three of the most common names associated with needle suspensions are *Pereyra*, *Raz*, and *Stamey*.

Although these procedures represented an important step in the evolution of incontinence surgery, a recent systematic Cochrane review[3] concluded that they do not provide satisfactory results compared with other, newer options.

Retropubic Urethropexies

As mentioned in Chapter 2, the retropubic space, also known as the space of Retzius, is a potential space that exists between the posterior surface of the pubic bone and the bladder. A *retropubic urethropexy* (or *colposuspension*) is performed by entering this space and suspending the bladder neck to a fixed anchoring point. In the case of an "*MMK*"—named for Drs. Marshall, Marchetti and Krantz[4]—this point is the periosteum of the pubic bone. For a *Burch procedure*,[5,6] it is the pectineal (Cooper's) ligament.

A number of modifications to the Burch procedure have been described since this original publication, but the core surgery remains the same. The purpose, anatomically speaking, is to correct hypermobility of the urethrovesical angle thus reestablishing continence. When grouped together, these two procedures have a great deal of medical evidence to support their use. A review of 33 trials involving over 2400 women showed a range of overall cure rates from 69% to 88% for the Burch procedure,[5] with a moderate drop to 70% cure at five years. Further reviews have shown no clear difference in cure rates between these procedures when performed from either an open or laparoscopic approach.[7] With these data and decades of experience establishing its safety profile, the retropubic urethropexy remains an important surgical treatment of stress urinary incontinence in women.

As the next section will demonstrate, however, an argument can be made that a new generation of suburethral slings—beginning with the "TVT", and followed by numerous second generation products in recent years—has fast replaced the urethropexy as a new gold standard in the first line treatment of stress incontinence.

Suburethral Slings

Suburethral sling procedures can be divided into two basic categories: *traditional pubovaginal slings* and *minimally invasive midurethral slings.* In traditional sling procedures a strip of material, be it biological (i.e., autologous or cadaveric fascia) or synthetic (i.e., Mersilene or polytetrafluoroethylene), is tunneled underneath the proximal urethra and secured to the rectus muscles, pubic bone, or iliopectineal (Cooper's) ligaments. This sling stabilizes and may even provide a kinking mechanism during rises in intra-abdominal pressure, such as a cough or sneeze, which prevents incontinence.

The first suburethral slings were performed via a combined abdominal and vaginal approach. When autologous material is used for the sling, this must be harvested first (usually rectus fascia or fascia lata). An abdominal incision is used to gain access to the retropubic space. A vaginal incision is then made under the urethra. The sling is then generally passed from the retropubic space down into the vaginal incision at the bladder neck and then back up into the retropubic space on the contralateral side. As mentioned above, various materials and points of securement can be used during for sling procedures. Many of these various techniques and materials are effective; however, the fixed nature of these slings can result in significant voiding dysfunction and/or urinary retention in a certain percentage of patients.

In an attempt to avoid these adverse outcomes while maintaining the excellent continence rates seen with traditional suburethral slings, a move has been made in the last ten years towards developing less invasive slings. In 1996 a procedure was described in which a synthetic sling was placed as an ambulatory procedure under local anesthesia and sedation; this came to be known as tension-free vaginal tape (TVT).[8]

Unlike traditional slings, the TVT sling is placed at the mid-urethra, not the urethrovesical junction; and rather than attaching the sling to a fixed structure, it is placed in a "tension-free" manner. Only minimal vaginal and periurethral dissection is performed, and the ends of the sling are attached to narrow trocars that allow passage of the sling behind the pubic bone and upwards to two small suprapubic skin incisions. Figure 10.1 depicts the differences between the Burch procedure, the traditional sling, and the TVT-type mid-urethral sling. Once the TVT gained worldwide popularity, other surgical device companies

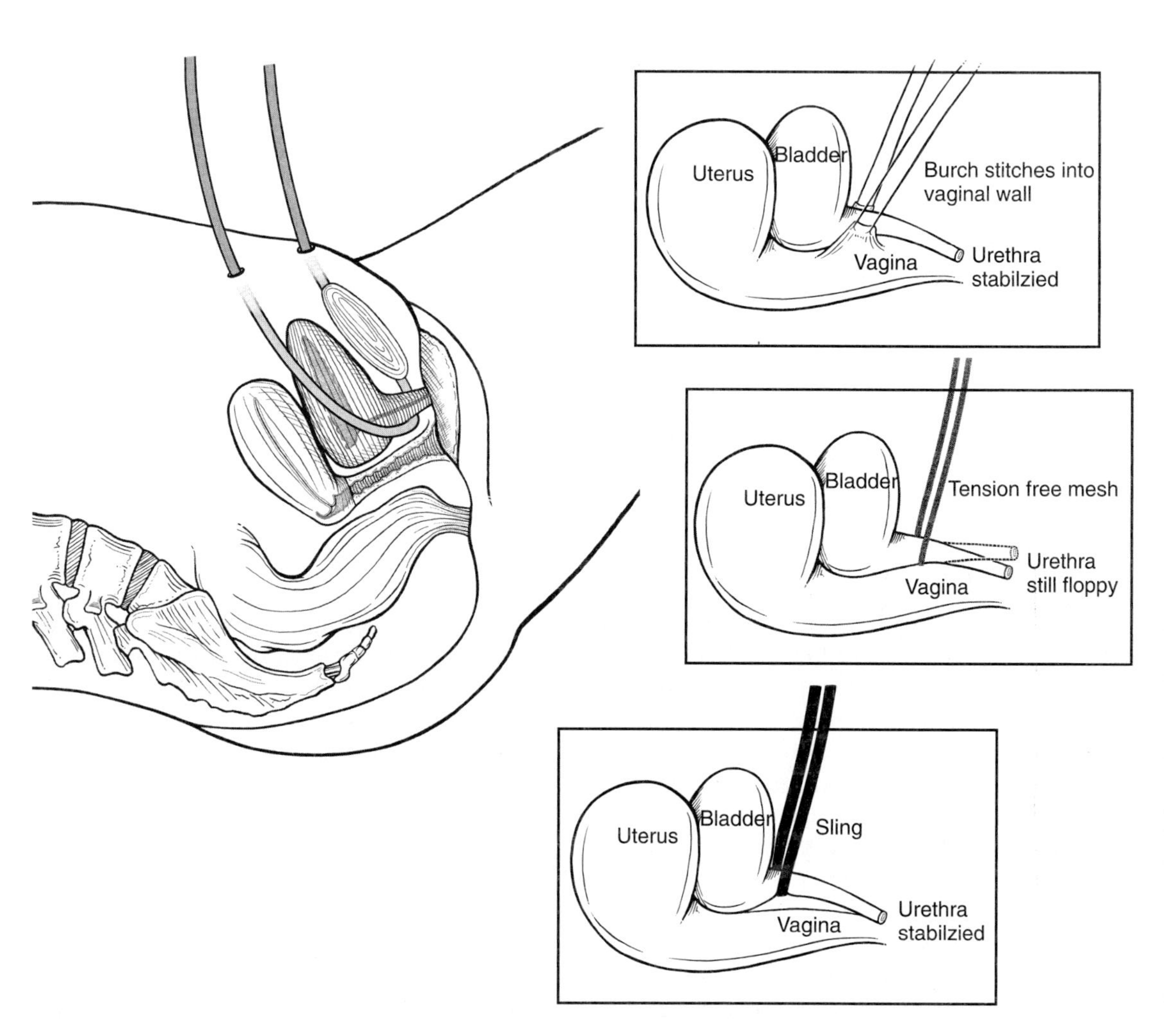

FIGURE 10.1. The Burch procedure creates a "hammock" of vagina tissue to support the urethra—by suspending vaginal tissue to Cooper's ligament. Mid-urethral slings are much looser and allow the urethral mobility to engage the sling itself. Traditional slings compress and elevate the proximal urethra to decrease urethral mobility.

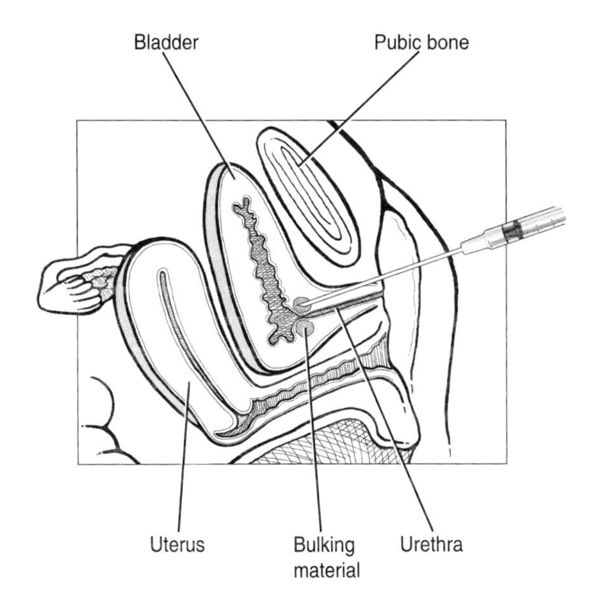

FIGURE 10.2. Periurethral bulking agents compress or "squish" the urethra closed during episodes of intra-abdominal pressure.

began to bring modified versions to the market. These include various shapes of passing devices and different sling materials, both synthetic and biologic. The majority of current mid-urethral sling products utilize a polypropylene mesh "tape" measuring 1 cm wide. In the last few years a number of device companies have also developed minimally invasive slings that are placed through the obturator foramen rather than the retropubic space. Figure 10.2 depicts the difference between transobturator and retropubic slings. At least part of the rationale for developing the transobturator technique is that, in theory, the obturator sling should have a greater safety profile than the retropubic version. With the obturator approach, bladder perforation should be less likely and, more importantly, it is virtually impossible to enter the intraperitoneal cavity with this technique. This negates the rare, but potentially devastating, risk of bowel perforation sometimes seen with the retropubic approach.

To date, there are no randomized trials comparing traditional slings to any of the newer, minimally invasive mid-urethral slings. However, two-year data from a prospective, multicenter randomized trial comparing TVT and colposuspension (open Burch) in 344 women has recently been published.[9] This study showed that the TVT procedure was at least as effective as colposuspension. In a related analysis, TVT was found to also be more cost effective, at least in short-term follow-up, than colposuspension.[10] Similar analyses have projected continued cost effectiveness within five years after surgery.[11] Another randomized trial comparing TVT to *laparoscopic* Burch colposuspension showed greater objective (at one year) and subjective (at one and two years) cure rates with TVT.[12]

There are still many unanswered questions regarding this new generation of minimally invasive mid-urethral slings, but they are certain to play a very large role in the surgical management of stress urinary incontinence in the foreseeable future.

Periurethral Bulking Agents

Injection of periurethral bulking agents represents another minimally invasive treatment alternative for female SUI, and one that can be performed as an office procedure (Figure 10.3).

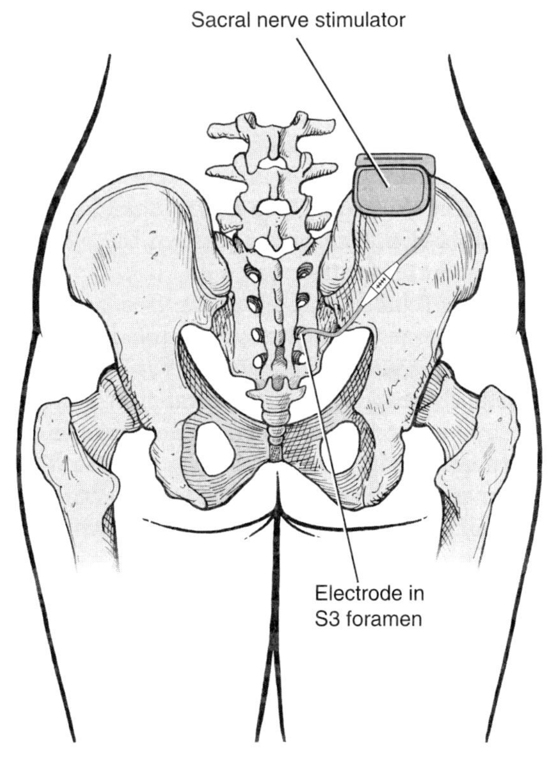

FIGURE 10.3. The InterStim sacral neuromodulation device.

Injection is performed under cystourethroscopic guidance, with the bulking agent injected behind the epithelial lining of the proximal urethra until this tissue bulges into the lumen of the urethra. This procedure is then repeated on the contralateral side until complete closure of the urethral lumen is seen.

The use of periurethral bulking agents appears to be best suited to patients without urethrovesical junction hypermobility (sometimes referred to as a "fixed" or "drainpipe" urethra). Over the years, many materials have been studied as potential bulking agents. But until recently, only glutaraldehyde cross-linked (GAX) collagen has been consistently used by practitioners in the United States. Use of collagen requires a skin test weeks in advance of periurethral use, but it is generally quite well tolerated by the majority of patients. Serious complications are exceedingly rare, but there is a time-related decline in cure rates with collagen.[13]

In 1999 the use of carbon-coated zirconium oxide microbeads (Durasphere) was approved for use a periurethral bulking agent, and a randomized trial found it to be equally effective as collagen.[14] In 2005 a third material was approved for periurethral injection. It is a solution of ethylene vinyl alcohol copolymer in a dimethyl sulfoxide carrier (Tegress) that forms a hydrophilic implant that helps prevent involuntary loss of urine through the urethra.

A recent review involving periurethral bulking agents showed equivalence between these three materials at 12 months.[15] The only trial comparing periurethral bulking agents to surgical management showed a significantly better objective outcome in the surgical group.[16] An acceptable outcome with periurethral bulking agents often requires multiple injections over a number of months.

The advent of mid-urethral slings, which can be placed under local analgesia with IV sedation, has reduced the need for periurethral bulking agents. Nevertheless, the technique still provides an excellent option for certain patients with intrinsic sphincter deficiency, particularly for elderly or medically complicated patients when an office-based technique is preferred.

Surgery for Urge Urinary Incontinence

Sacral Neuromodulation

In the past there were no surgical treatments for overactive bladder and urge urinary incontinence, save highly invasive procedures such as bladder augmentation or urinary diversion. In the past decade two new minimally invasive therapies have emerged which provide a surgical option for patients with severe disease who have failed traditional pharmacologic therapy.

The first of these is sacral neuromodulation. As far back as the 1970s, animal models were used to evaluate the effect of sacral nerve stimulation on bladder function. But it was not until 1997 that the FDA approved the first permanent, implantable device for the treatment of refractory urge urinary incontinence, urgency–frequency syndrome, and non-obstructive urinary retention in humans. This device, known as InterStim (Figure 10.4)), can now be inserted under local analgesia with IV sedation.

Sacral neuromodulation is a two-stage procedure that can be accomplished during two outpatient surgeries scheduled a few weeks apart. Prior to the first stage of the procedure, the patient

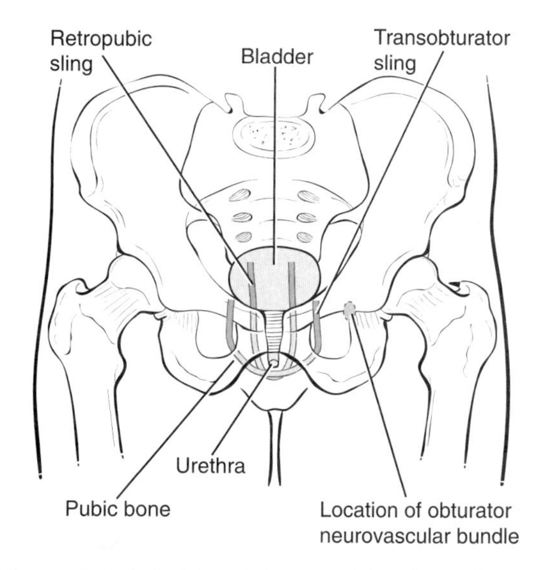

FIGURE 10.4. A depiction of the retropubic and transobturator approach to suburethral slings.

keeps a record of all her voids and incontinent episodes for at least five days. During the Stage I procedure, a permanent lead is implanted percutaneously through the S3 foramen. This lead is connected to an extension wire that exits through the patient's skin along the lower back and is plugged into an external stimulator that the patient clips to her clothes as she would a pager or cell phone. With mild pulsatile stimulation delivered to the sacral nerve roots from this external device, the patient completes a series of voiding diaries over the next several days (i.e., the "test period"). If she reports greater than 50% improvement in her symptoms, she is considered an appropriate candidate to proceed to Stage II. The Stage II procedure, which takes approximately 15 to 30 minutes to perform under local anesthesia, involves reconnecting the lead to an implantable pulse generator (IPG) that is placed between the buttock and iliac crest. The battery life of the IPG is approximately 7 years.

In a multi-center, randomized controlled clinical trial of 51 patients, those who underwent treatment with sacral neuromodulation had a significant decrease in the number of voids daily and their degree of urgency, as well as an increase in the volume voided when compared to the controls.[17] This, and another study with longer follow-up,[18] also showed significantly improved quality of life following sacral neuromodulation. Figure 10.4 depicts the InterStim device in place.

Surgery for Pelvic Organ Prolapse

Prolapse is caused by defects in the connective tissue supporting the vagina and uterus as well as neuromuscular damage to the levator ani muscles that form the pelvic floor.

In recent years practitioners have come to appreciate that, more often than not, women with POP suffer from some combination of defects in the anterior, posterior, and apical compartments of the vagina. One trend receiving much attention is the use of graft materials to augment traditional surgical repairs. Much research is now being conducted to determine their efficacy and safety in pelvic reconstructive surgery.

Anterior and Posterior Vaginal Wall Repair

Traditional Anterior and Posterior Repair

Vaginal hysterectomy with *anterior and posterior colporrhaphy ("A & P repair")* has long been the mainstay for surgical treatment of utero-vaginal prolapse. Anterior and posterior repairs can also be performed independently with uterine preservation or in a patient who has had a prior hysterectomy.

Prolapse of the anterior vaginal wall is commonly referred to as a cystocele, often described as a "dropped bladder." It is important to emphasize that cystocele bulges result from defects in support of the vagina, not an inherent flaw of the bladder itself.

The technique of an *anterior colporrhaphy* ("anterior repair") is the traditional repair for a cystocele. It involves a midline vertical incision through the anterior vaginal wall, followed by dissection of the vaginal epithelium from the underlying pubocervical fascia. The fascia is then plicated across the midline with delayed absorbable or permanent suture. Excess vaginal epithelium is trimmed away, and the incision is closed.

Posterior colporrhaphy ("posterior repair") is the traditional repair for a rectocele, employing a similar surgical technique. A midline vertical incision is made through the posterior vaginal epithelium, which is then dissected off the underlying rectovaginal fascia until the medial edges of the levator ani muscles are reached. The redundant rectovaginal fascia is then plicated in the midline using absorbable suture. Repair of a relaxed vaginal outlet *(perineorrhaphy)* is often performed concomitantly, with sutures placed to re-approximate damaged bulbocavernosus and transverse perineal musculature. Excess vaginal epithelium is trimmed away, and the incision is closed.

Paravaginal Repair

The paravaginal defect repair was initially described as an open abdominal procedure in which the retropubic space is entered and breaks in the attachments of the vagina to the pelvic sidewalls are identified. Permanent sutures, placed through the lateral aspects of the anterior vaginal wall, reattach the vaginal fornices to their normal site of fixation: the arcus tendineus fascia pelvis (ATFP). The ATFP is a condensation of fascia that lies on the obturator internus muscle and spans from the ischial spine to the pubic ramus. Approximately 3 to 5 interrupted sutures are used on each side, to close a paravaginal defect. This repair has also been described as a vaginal and laparoscopic procedure.

Severe or Recurrent Defects

If the support defects are extensive enough, the integrity of the anterior or posterior vaginal fascia is severely compromised; or if the patient has had a previously failed reconstructive surgery, many of the above repairs can be augmented by the use of surgical grafts. These grafts can be autologous (such as fascia lata), xenografts (porcine dermis) or synthetic (such as polypropylene).

Very recently, several surgical device companies have developed "prolapse kits" which include synthetic mesh and specially shaped needles designed to pass arms of the mesh through the obturator membrane (much like the transobturator slings depicted above). These devices (such as the Gynecare Prolift® by Ethicon, Inc., Somerville, NJ) are all placed through a vaginal route and show great promise as minimally invasive solutions to correct prolapse.

Vaginal Apical Suspensions

Sacrospinous Ligament Suspension

Numerous procedures have been described to reestablish adequate support in women with apical prolapse. One common procedure used to resuspend the vaginal apex is the sacrospinous ligament suspension (SSLS). The sacrospinous ligaments are retroperitoneal structures spanning from the ischial spines to the lateral, lower aspect of the sacrum and coccyx. They are among the firmer points of attachment for reconstructive pelvic surgery, and access is usually obtained through a midline posterior vaginal incision. The sacrospinous sutures are then placed through the vaginal apex, thus resuspending the apex when tied down.

Potential complications of this procedure are hemorrhage, buttock pain, nerve injury, rectal injury, and recurrent anterior vaginal wall prolapse. Cure rates vary from 60% to 90%. One recent observational study over a 16-year period demonstrated few serious complications and few failures for support of the vaginal apex.[19]

Uterosacral Vault Suspension

The uterosacral ligaments are the primary suspensory structures in normal female pelvic anatomy. The uterosacral vault suspension (USVS) is predicated on the belief that normal anatomical support can be recreated by suturing the vaginal apex to portions of these ligaments.

Two landmark studies describing this technique, published in 2000, demonstrated an optimal anatomic outcome in approximately 90% of subjects.[20,21] This procedure can be performed at the time of hysterectomy or in a patient who has previously undergone hysterectomy and presents with vaginal vault prolapse. While access to these ligaments can be gained through a retro- or extra-peritoneal approach, it is most frequently performed intraperitoneally. In the case of hysterectomy, the sutures are placed through the vaginal cuff prior to cuff closure. In the case of post-hysterectomy prolapse, the ligaments are reached after opening the enterocele hernia sac at the apex of the vagina.

Two to three non-absorbable sutures are placed through the proximal aspect of each uterosacral ligament. Care should be taken to identify and avoid the ureters when placing these sutures. In one series of vaginal USVS, ureteral occlusion was noted in 5 of 46 cases, with two of these women requiring ureteral reimplantation[21]; thus, cystoscopic evidence of ureteral patency should be confirmed before leaving the operative suite. One end of each suture is then brought through the fascia of the anterior and posterior vaginal walls. By tying down these sutures the anterior and posterior fascia are brought together, correcting or preventing any future enterocele and also resuspending the vaginal apex. One cadaveric study comparing the vaginal and laparoscopic approach demonstrated comparable tensile strength in suturing between the two techniques.[22]

Abdominal Sacral Colpopexy

The abdominal sacral colpopexy (ASC) is a vaginal suspension procedure performed abdominally, which allows a more diffuse distribution of tension over the vagina by attaching surgical graft material to the anterior and posterior vaginal walls and then attaching this graft up to the sacrum. Like the USVS, ASC can be performed at the time of hysterectomy or in patients with prior hysterectomy.

The technique involves an incision in the posterior peritoneum running from the sacral promontory to the vagina, carried anteriorly into the vesicovaginal space and posteriorly into the rectovaginal space. Permanent suture is then used to attach synthetic mesh, or a biological graft, to the undersurface of the anterior and posterior vaginal walls. The tail of mesh attached to the anterior and posterior grafts is then sutured to the anterior longitudinal ligament of the sacrum. The peritoneum is then reapproximated over the grafts to prevent contact between the graft and bowel so as to minimize the risk of bowel obstruction.

While the ASC can be performed laparoscopically, it is usually performed through an open abdominal incision. As such, it is more invasive than the previously described reconstructive surgeries, but it is a very durable procedure and is considered by many to be the "gold standard" for vaginal vault prolapse—especially for recurrent defects. Another benefit of the ASC is that, if the dissection is extensive enough and the graft is placed far enough down the walls of the vagina, this procedure often corrects other defects such as cystoceles and rectoceles.

A recent comprehensive review of close to 100 studies investigating ASC found a success rate ranging from 78% to 100%, for correcting apical prolapse.[23] The median re-operation rate for prolapse was 4.4%, and the overall rate of graft erosion into the vagina was 3.4%. The authors concluded—and we agree—that ASC "is a reliable procedure that effectively and consistently resolves vaginal vault prolapse."

Obliterative Surgery

The objective of the above reconstructive surgeries is not only to relieve the patient of her symptoms of prolapse, but also to create a functional vagina with satisfactory coital ability. If future coital activity is not planned or desired and/or a patient does not feel like she will be psychologically impaired without a functional vagina, an obliterative procedure is an option for women with complete apical prolapse. The ultimate result of a successful obliterative procedure is that of normal appearing external genitalia, but an obliterated vaginal canal.

In patients with complete post-hysterectomy vaginal vault prolapse the procedure is called a *total colpectomy*. The vaginal epithelium is completely excised from the prolapse bulge, leaving just the fibromuscular tube of the vagina. Through a series of transverse rows or purse-string sutures starting at the leading edge of the prolapse, the apex of the vagina is inverted. This process is repeated until the prolapse bulge is reduced above the introitus. The perineum and levator ani musculature are then closed in the midline prior to reducing the introital size.[24,25]

Patients with uterovaginal prolapse can undergo a *LeFort colpocleisis*. As with a colpectomy, after removal of vaginal skin a series of transverse rows of sutures are placed, and the cervix and vagina are inverted and the sutures tied such that the anterior wall of the vagina is in direct opposition to the posterior wall. Unlike total colpectomy, however, tunnels of vaginal epithelium are left intact to allow drainage of any potential future cervical mucous or blood.

These surgeries are best suited for elderly, medically frail patients who understand the consequences of the surgery. The benefits of obliterative procedures are that they can be performed relatively quickly under regional or even local anesthesia with minimal blood loss. The peritoneal cavity is usually not entered, so there is quick return of bowel function and little risk of damage to the bowels.

Surgery for Anal Incontinence and Defecatory Dysfunction

As embarrassing as it is for patients to talk about their urinary incontinence, it is even harder for them to talk about anal incontinence (AI). For this reason, AI is a grossly underreported condition that is nonetheless devastating for women. AI can refer to the loss of gas, liquid stool, and/or solid stool. Flatal incontinence is the most common of these three and the hardest to treat. We do not recommend surgical repair for flatal incontinence by itself, as the risks of the procedure in the face of a low success rate do not justify the risks associated with the procedure. But in the case of a woman who is incontinent of solid stool on a regular basis and has failed conservative management, surgery is often the only option.

Reconstructive Surgery

In women who have a definable defect in the external anal sphincter, such as is often seen with obstetrical trauma, *overlapping sphincteroplasty* is the most common procedure of choice. For this repair, a semilunar incision is made parallel to the cephalad edge of the sphincter. Dissection is then performed from medial to lateral, until the two ends of the disrupted sphincter are identified and isolated. The muscle edges are then pulled into an overlapping position. A series of delayed absorbable or permanent mattress sutures are placed through the two overlapping ends, and the skin is then closed Failure rates generally range from 20% to 30%.[26]

A number of other reconstructive surgeries can be used in the treatment of AI. Most of these are performed at a limited number of medical centers and are usually reserved for recurrent cases. In-depth discussion of these is beyond the scope of this chapter but they include: postanal pelvic floor repair, gracilis and gluteus maximus muscle transposition, artificial anal sphincter, and colostomy or ileostomy.

Sacral Neuromodulation

Two new minimally invasive techniques that have recently been described in the treatment of AI are the Secca procedure, which involves radiofrequency energy delivery to the sphincter, inducing tissue contraction,[27] and a bulking procedure which involves injection of silicone biomaterial into the internal anal sphincter.[28] Experience with these techniques is limited.

Treatment of AI with sacral neuromodulation—a technology more commonly used for urinary incontinence, as discussed in Chapter 8—is generally reserved for patients with an intact external sphincter. The technique of sacral neuromodulation for these patients is the same as that performed for urinary incontinence. In a recent review of over 100 relevant reports, 56% of patients went on to the second stage of permanent implantation of the nerve stimulator,[29] 41% to 75% achieved complete fecal continence, and over 75% experienced reduced incontinence episodes.

Operative Experience

Before Surgery

Patient preparation will vary from procedure to procedure and from patient to patient. As with most surgeries, if a patient has ongoing medical conditions such as diabetes or heart disease, preoperative medical clearance is an essential step. Patients may be asked to discontinue medications and supplements that can increase the risk of bleeding, such as nonsteroidal anti-inflammatory medications (i.e., ibuprofen), aspirin products, Coumadin, clopidogrel (Plavix), and some herbal medications. Post-menopausal women with vaginal atrophy who are going to have reconstructive surgery may be instructed by their surgeon to apply estrogen creams or tablets locally, into the vagina, to improve the quality and vascularity of the vaginal skin and thereby help with healing.

Finally, most patients will be asked to not take anything by mouth after midnight the night before surgery and may be asked to perform a bowel preparation, particularly before abdominal, and especially laparoscopic, surgery.

Just before surgery, most patients receive single-dose intravenous antibiotics. Procedure times may vary from 30 to 300 minutes, depending on the complexity of the reconstruction. The anesthesia used can also vary from simple local and intravenous sedation, in the case of a mid-urethral sling or sacral neuromodulation, to regional anesthesia (i.e., epidural or spinal) for some vaginal reconstructive procedures, to general anesthesia for open and laparoscopic abdominal surgeries. During surgeries where general anesthesia is not being used, the patient will be sedated to the point of sleep in most cases. However, in the case of a mid-urethral sling for stress urinary incontinence, after the sling has been placed, the patient's sedation may be lightened and she may be asked to cough repetitively. This allows precise adjustment of the tightness of the sling to the point where leakage is no longer seen coming from the urethra and has been shown to result in greater improvements in post-operative continence.[30]

After Surgery

An increasing number of urogynecology procedures can be performed on an outpatient basis; currently, the mid-urethral sling for SUI represents the most common example. However, most other reconstructive surgeries require an overnight stay. Patients who have vaginal or laparoscopic procedures may be ready for discharge home one to two days after surgery. If an open abdominal incision is made, hospital stays are usually a bit longer due to a slower return of bowel function.

Anti-incontinence procedures may make complete bladder emptying difficult in the immediate post-operative period. While some patients may be able to void prior to leaving the hospital, others may need to go home with an indwelling Foley or suprapubic catheter, to be removed in the physician's office after discharge. Most patients will be sent home with prescriptions for pain medication and a stool softener such as docusate sodium (Colace). This is to prevent the need to strain during defecation, which can lead to disruption of the surgical repair.

Patients are usually asked to refrain from lifting objects heavier than eight pounds (roughly the weight of one gallon of milk) for 6 to 12 weeks. They are also encouraged not to place anything in the vagina, nor have coitus, for a similar period of time to allow for proper healing and scarring of the reconstructive surgery. However, in most other respects, patients are encouraged to be active. Walking can be initiated immediately in most cases, including the use of stairs, and most patients will be able to begin driving within 1–2 weeks. After a simple procedure such as an outpatient mid-urethral sling, patients may return to low-impact jobs as soon as 72 hours after surgery. The more complex reconstructive surgeries generally require longer convalescent periods (2 to 6 weeks), especially when performed under general anesthesia.

Conclusion

Within the field of female pelvic medicine, invasive surgeries that were commonplace ten years ago are rapidly being replaced by less invasive, more durable procedures. While further research is surely needed, it is important for women and their primary care providers to understand that many options are available to patients who suffer from these debilitating conditions and that these options are vastly different than what was available for their mothers' generation. In this day and age, superior outcomes are being achieved with less invasiveness than ever before.

Key Points

- In the last 5 to 10 years, new technology and surgical techniques have improved the results of surgery to correct pelvic floor disorders, while at the same time becoming less invasive than older techniques.
- The Kelly-Kennedy plication and "needle suspension" surgeries such as the *Pereyra*, *Raz*, and *Stamey* procedures have been replaced by mid-urethral slings such as the TVT.
- Sacral neuromodulation can be very effective for relieving urinary frequency, urge incontinence episodes, and urinary retention for patients unresponsive to other non-surgical treatments.
- There are two basic ways to correct pelvic organ prolapse with surgery: (1) the reconstructive procedures that seek to restore normal anatomy all around and (2) the obliterative techniques that seek to alleviate symptoms by closing the space through which organs can prolapse.
- The advantages of the reconstructive operations are obvious.
- The obliterative operations are very useful for non-sexually active patients who are poor

surgical candidates in need of a fast, reliable, minimally invasive operation.

- Surgical techniques to correct anal incontinence are generally not as successful as those designed to correct urinary incontinence and should usually be reserved for patients with incontinence to solid stool. If a patient is already continent to solid stool, every effort should be made to change her diet and or medications in such a manner that minimal loose or liquid stools result.

References

1. Olsen AL, Smith VJ, Bergstrom JO, Colling JC, Clark AL. Epidemiology of surgically managed pelvic organ prolapse and urinary incontinence. *Obstet Gynecol.* 1997;89:501–506.
2. Waetjen LE, Subak LL, Shen H, et. al. Stress urinary incontinence surgery in the United States. *Obstet Gynecol.* 2003;101:671–676.
3. Glazener CM, Cooper K. Bladder neck needle suspension for urinary incontinence in women. *Cochrane Database of Syst Rev.* 2004:CD003636.
4. Marshall VF, Marchetti AA, Krantz KE. The correction of stress urinary incontinence by simple vesicourethral suspension. *Surg Gynecol Obstet.* 1949;88:509–18.
5. Lapitan MC, Cody DJ, Grant AM. Open retropubic colposuspension for urinary incontinence in women. *Cochrane Database of Syst Rev.* 2003: CD002912.
6. Burch JC. Urethrovaginal fixation to Cooper's ligament for correction of stress incontinence, cystocele, and prolapse. *Am J Obstet Gynecol.* 1961;81: 281.
7. Moehrer B, Carey M, Wilson D. Laparoscopic colposuspension: a systematic review. *BJOG.* 2003;110: 230–235.
8. Ulmsten U, Henriksson L, Johnson P, Varhos G. An ambulatory surgical procedure under local anesthesia for treatment of female urinary incontinence. *Int Urogynecol J Pelvic Floor Dysfunct.* 1996;7:81–86.
9. Ward KL, Hilton P, UK and Ireland TVT Trial Group. A prospective multicenter randomized trial of tension-free vaginal tape and colposuspension for primary urodynamic stress incontinence: two-year follow-up. *Am J Obstet Gynecol.* 2004;190:324–331.
10. Manca A, Sculpher MD, Ward K, Hilton P. A cost-utility analysis of tension-free vaginal tape versus colposuspension for primary urodynamic stress incontinence. *BJOG.* 2003;110:255–262.
11. Kilonzo M, Vale L, Stearns SC et al. Cost effectiveness of tension-free vaginal tape for the surgical management of female stress incontinence. *Int J Technol Assess Health Care.* 2004;20(4):455–463.
12. Paraiso MF, Walters MD, Karram MM, Barber MD. Laparoscopic Burch colposuspension versus tension-free vaginal tape: a randomized trial. *Obstet Gynecol.* 2004;104:1249–1258.
13. Herrmann V, Arya LA, Myers DL, Jackson ND. GAX collagen for female stress urinary incontinence—where are we now? *J Pelvic Surg.* 2001;7: 83–89.
14. Lightner D, Calvosa C, Andersen R, et al. A new injectable bulking agent for treatment of stress urinary incontinence: results of a multicenter, randomized, controlled, double-blind study of Durasphere. *Urology.* 2001;58:12–15.
15. Pickard R, Reaper J, Wyness L, Cody DJ, McClinton S, N'Dow J. Periurethral injection therapy for urinary incontinence in women. *Cochrane Database Syst Rev.* 2003:CD003881.
16. Corcos J, Collet JP, Shapiro S, et al. Surgery vs. collagen for the treatment of female stress urinary incontinence (SUI): results of a multicentric randomized trial. *J Urol.* 2001;165:198.
17. Hassouna MM, Siegel SW, Nyeholt LA, et al. Sacral neuromodulation in the treatment of urgency-frequency symptoms: a multicenter study on efficacy and safety. *J Urol.* 2000;163:1849–1854.
18. Cappellano F, Bertapelle P, Spinelle M, et al. Quality of life assessment in patients who undergo sacral neuromodulation implantation for urge incontinence: an additional tool for evaluating outcome. *J Urol.* 2001;166:2277–2280.
19. Cruikshank SH, Muniz M. Outcomes study: A comparison of cure rates in 695 patients undergoing sacrospinous ligament fixation alone and with other site-specific procedures-a 16-year study. *Am J Obstet Gynecol.* 2003;188:1509–1512.
20. Shull BL, Bachofen C, Coates KW, Kuehl TJ. A transvaginal approach to repair of apical and other associated sites of pelvic organ prolapse with uterosacral ligaments. *Am J Obstet Gynecol.* 2000;183: 1365–1373.
21. Barber MD, Visco AG, Weidner AC, Amundsen CL, Bump RC. Bilateral uterosacral ligament vaginal vault suspension with site-specific endopelvic fascia defect repair for treatment of pelvic organ prolapse. *Am J Obstet Gynecol.* 2000;183:1402–1410.
22. Culligan PJ, Miklos JR, Murphy M, et al. The tensile strength of uterosacral ligament sutures: a comparison of vaginal and laparoscopic techniques. *Obstet Gynecol.* 2003;101:500–503.

23. Nygaard IE, McCreery R, Brubaker L, et al. Abdominal sacrocolpopexy: a comprehensive review. *Obstet Gynecol.* 2004;104:805–823.
24. von Pechmann WS, Mutone M, Fyffe J, Hale DS. Total colpocleisis with high levator plication for the treatment of advanced pelvic organ prolapse. *Am J Obstet Gynecol.* 2003;189(1):121–126.
25. Hoffman MS, Cardosi RJ, Lockhart J, Hall DC, Murphy SJ. Vaginectomy with pelvic herniorrhaphy for prolapse. *Am J Obstet Gynecol.* 2003;189: 364–70.
26. Jorge JM, Wexner SD. Etiology and management of fecal incontinence. *Dis Colon Rectum.* 1993;36:77–97.
27. Takahashi T, Garcia-Osogobio S, Valdovinos MA, Belmonte C, Barreto C, Velasco L. Extended two-year results of radio-frequency energy delivery for the treatment of fecal incontinence (the Secca procedure). *Dis Colon Rectum.* 2003;46:711–715.
28. Kenefick NJ, Vaizey CJ, Malouf AJ, Norton CS, Marshall M, Kamm MA. Injectable silicone biomaterial for faecal incontinence due to internal anal sphincter dysfunction. *Gut.* 2002;51:225–228.
29. Jarrett ME, Mowatt G, Glazener CM et al. Systematic review of sacral nerve stimulation for faecal incontinence and constipation. *Brit J Surg.* 2004;91: 1559–1569.
30. Murphy M, Culligan PJ, Arce MA, Graham CA, Blackwell L, Heit MH. Is the cough-stress test necessary when placing the tension-free vaginal tape? *Obstet Gynecol.* 2005;105:319–324.

11
Female Sexual Dysfunction: Effective Treatment Strategies for All Ages

Laura A.C. Berman and Kerrie A. Grow McLean

Introduction

Sexuality is one of the most important quality-of-life issues; therefore, female sexual dysfunction is an important primary care issue. The potential for every woman to live an active, healthy, and fulfilling sexual life is possible, regardless of age. While there may be many different factors that contribute to sexual issues throughout the lifespan, it is essential to understand that a woman's sexual response is influenced by emotional, relational, and medical factors. It is the combination of these factors that create a unique sexual identity for every woman and which must be taken into consideration when assessing and treating women with sexual function complaints.

Throughout a woman's lifespan, expressions of her need for intimacy constantly change and, as a result, affect all areas of her life. The female sexual response involves a unique and complex set of factors that are different from those of males; therefore the template that is used to address female patients and their sexual function should remain separate from the approach taken for males. A woman's sexual response is influenced by a variety of psychological, relational, and physical factors (see Figure 11.1),[1] which are not mutually exclusive, meaning that each factor can and likely will have an impact on the other. For many women, their physiologic response to sexual stimuli is frequently less of a factor to a meaningful sexual encounter than is their emotional response.[2] Possible physiological barriers to a healthy and satisfying sexual life, however, should be considered for every woman. A comprehensive approach, addressing the physiological, psychological, and relational factors, is instrumental to the evaluation and treatment of female patients with sexual complaints.

Sexual dysfunction has been shown to affect individual mental health, relationship satisfaction, quality of life, and family functioning.[3,4] (More specifically, sexual function complaints can affect a woman's ability to establish and maintain intimate relationships and has been related to low self-esteem, depression, anxiety, and overall psychological distress[5]) With approximately 43 percent of American women experiencing sexual dysfunction,[3] it is clear that sexuality is an important women's health issue that affects the quality of life of many female patients. Clinicians at the primary care level can play a key role in the recognition of female sexual dysfunction and initiate a wide array of initial treatment strategies.

Female Sexual Response Cycle

In order to understand the etiologies and treatments for female sexual dysfunction, it is important to consider the sexual response cycle. The successive phases of sexual response include arousal (otherwise considered excitement and plateau phases), orgasm, and resolution.[6] The component of "desire" as preceding and inciting the entire sexual response cycle was first proposed by Helen Singer Kaplan.[7] Kaplan's three-phase model of desire, orgasm, and resolution is the basis for the DSM IV definitions of female sexual dysfunction, as well as the recent re-classification

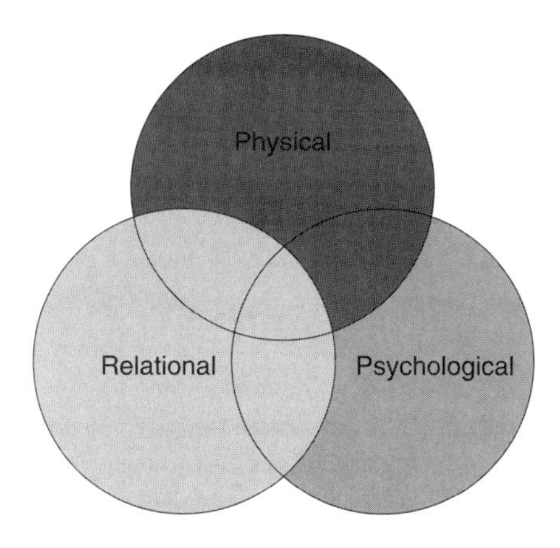

FIGURE 11.1. Factors influencing female sexual function.

system made by the American Foundation of Urologic Disease (AFUD) Consensus Panel in October of 1998.[8] Recently, Basson proposed a five-phase model focusing on intimacy. In this model, the desire to enhance intimacy is seen as the driving force of the female sexual response cycle. The cycle begins with the basic needs for intimacy, which include mutuality, respect, and communication. When these needs are met, a woman will seek out and will be more receptive to sexual stimuli. A woman's intimacy is enhanced and the cycle strengthened if there is an overall positive emotional and physical interaction.[9]

Classification and Definition of Female Sexual Dysfunction

In 1998, the American Foundation of Urologic Disease (AFUD) Consensus Panel classified female sexual dysfunction into four areas: desire, arousal, orgasmic, and sexual pain disorders.[8]

The objective of the panel was to evaluate and revise existing definitions and classifications of female sexual dysfunction so that they would cross disciplines. Specifically, medical risk factors and etiologies for female sexual dysfunction were incorporated with the pre-existing psychologically based definitions. Most importantly, in order for a woman to be diagnosed with FSD, she must be experiencing significant personal distress. The etiology of any of these disorders may be multifactorial, and oftentimes the disorders overlap.[8]

Hypoactive Sexual Desire Disorder (HSDD)

HSDD is defined as the persistent or recurring deficiency (or absence) of sexual fantasies thoughts, and/or receptivity to sexual activity that causes personal distress (see Figure 11.2 for Assessment and Treatment Model for HSDD). Sometimes the lack of receptivity takes on a phobic quality that is known as Sexual Aversion Disorder. Hypoactive sexual desire disorder may have physiologic roots, such as hormone deficiencies, and medical or surgical interventions. Any disruption of the female hormonal balance caused by natural menopause, surgically or medically induced menopause, or endocrine disorders, can result in inhibited sexual desire (see etiologies below). Furthermore, the lack of desire may actually be secondary to poor arousal, response, or pain.

HSDD is sometimes a psychologically or emotionally based problem that has its roots in a variety of reasons beyond history of abuse or trauma. For instance, depression and the treatment of depression are common intrapsychic problems in patients with low sexual desire.[10] The depression can be caused by general life events, or it can be secondary to sexual conflicts in the relationship. Substance abuse—particularly drug and alcohol abuse—can result in problems of dependency, depression, and lack of self-esteem. Additionally, there is an abundance of research supporting that how a woman feels about her body can have a negative impact on her sexual health and functioning.[11–14] Furthermore, a woman's genital image—how she feels about the size, shape, odor, and function of her genitals[15]—has been found to specifically affect a woman's sexual desire and level of sexual distress.

From the standpoint of the impact of HSDD on the woman's life, when there is uneven desire in a relationship, conflicts often arise. If one partner contains feelings of anger, resentment, fear, hostility, or disappointment, the result can be a withdrawal from the intimate relationship. A chronically conflicted relationship with a struggle for control may result in a further voluntary blocking of sexual appetite perpetuated by the partner who feels less valued or less powerful.

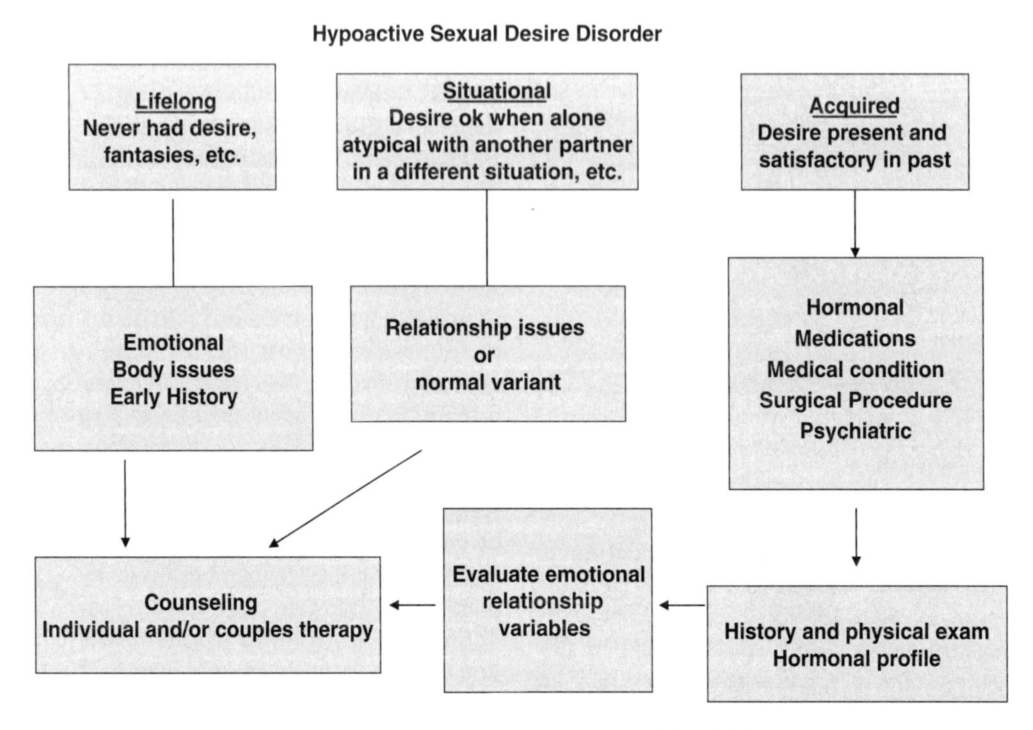

Figure 11.2. Assessment and treatment model for HSDD.

Female Sexual Arousal Disorder (FSAD)

FSAD is the persistent or recurring inability to attain or maintain adequate sexual excitement, causing personal distress. It may be experienced as a lack of subjective excitement or a lack of genital (lubrication/swelling) or other somatic responses (see Figure 11.3 for Assessment and Treatment Model for FSAD). Disorders of arousal include, but are not limited to, lack of or diminished vaginal lubrication, decreased clitoral and labial sensation, decreased clitoral and labial engorgement, or lack of vaginal smooth muscle relaxation. There are medical/physiologic factors such as diminished vaginal/clitoral blood flow, prior pelvic trauma, hormonal decline, pelvic surgery, or medications (see medical etiologies below) that contribute to FSAD.

These conditions may occur secondary to psychological factors as well. If a woman is struggling with body-image issues, low self-esteem, depression, or anxiety, her general emotional state may preclude her from relaxing into the arousal process. If a woman is not feeling good enough about herself, her body, and the person she is with, or of she is distracted by something to do with work or home life, it may be difficult for her to focus on the sexual scenario and reach arousal.[1] This is actually quite different from male sexual response. In the research done on Sildenafil in men, it was found that only about 10% of male erectile dysfunction is psychogenic, and that psychogenic erectile dysfunction is resolved with Viagra in over 80% of cases. In other words, with the added advantage of increased blood flow, men could focus on the sexual scenario and move past the psychogenic factors. The same has not been found to be true with women.[1,16] Yet, similar to erectile dysfunction, a woman's lack of arousal may, in some cases, be connected to performance anxiety. If she is unable to respond sexually, regardless of situational or circumstantial reasons, her future response may become even more inhibited due to her fear of this happening again. Anxiety itself may, in theory, become a cause of vasoconstriction leading to dryness and lack of arousal.

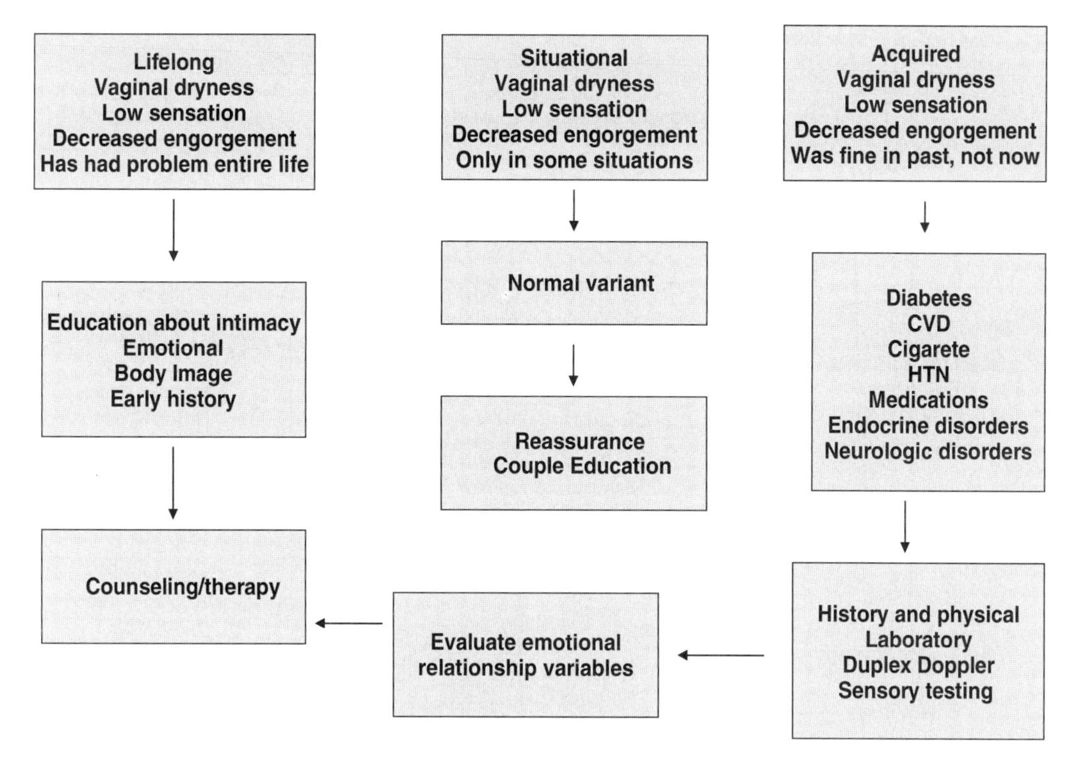

FIGURE 11.3. Assessment and treatment model for FSAD.

Female Orgasmic Disorder (FOD)

FOD is the persistent or recurrent difficulty, delay in, or absence of attaining orgasm, following sufficient sexual stimulation and arousal, that causes personal distress. FOD may be a primary (never achieved orgasm) or a secondary condition (was able to achieve orgasm at one point in time, but now no longer able). (See Figure 11.4 for Assessment and Treatment Model for FOD). FOD can even be situational, referring to the woman who can experience orgasm in some circumstances (e.g., masturbation), but cannot in other situations. Secondary FOD is often a result of surgery, trauma, or hormone deficiencies (see medical etiologies below). Primary FOD is typically secondary to emotional trauma or sexual abuse, and Situational FOD, while often also associated with a trauma history, is also commonly related to emotional stressors and relationship conflicts. However, in both of these cases medical/physical factors, as well as medications (i.e., selective serotonin re-uptake inhibitors), can contribute to or exacerbate the problem (see medical etiologies below).

Another kind of anorgasmia commonly experienced by women is Coital FOD, or the inability to achieve orgasm from coital thrusting without added sexual stimulation. Only 30% of women experience orgasm regularly from sexual intercourse, 30% never reach orgasm during intercourse, and 40% have difficulty achieving orgasm from coital thrusting alone.[17] In the primary care setting, many women describing themselves as anorgasmic are, in fact, experiencing coital anorgasmia. The majority of heterosexual women and their partners believe that they should be able to obtain orgasm through sexual intercourse. When this belief, held by either the man or the woman, is incompatible with the woman's actual stimulation needs, failure to achieve this goal can result in sexual dissatisfaction, relationship conflict, and a lack of sexual confidence.

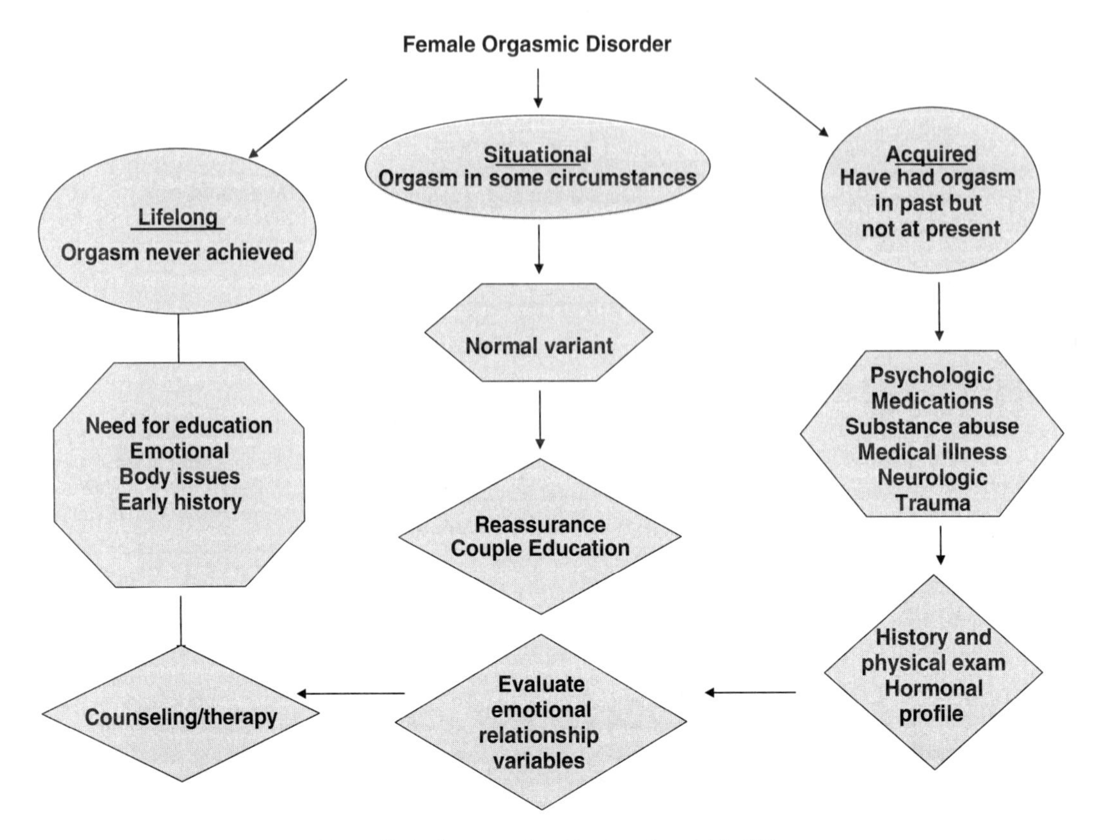

FIGURE 11.4. Assessment and treatment model for FOD.

The effect of anorgasmia on women is unpredictable. Some women can "accommodate" intercourse with minimal levels of arousal, no discomfort, and no apparent psychological effect. Women who achieve high levels of sexual arousal but are unable to complete their sexual response into resolution phase often experience emotional frustration and may experience pelvic pain indicative of chronic pelvic congestion. As with the etiology of other sexual complaints, the etiology of orgasmic disorder can be categorized into physical factors, intrapsychic factors, and interpersonal factors. The factors alone or together can play a role in the evolution of this problem.

Sexual Pain Disorders

Vulvodynia

In 1985, the International Society for the Study of Vulvar Disease (ISSVD) recommended the term vulvodynia to describe any vulvar pain, regardless of the etiology (see Figure 11.5 for Assessment and Treatment Model for Sexual Pain Disorders). Vulvodynia is often accompanied by both physical and psychological disabilities. The prevalence of vulvodynia is estimated to be as high as 15% in the general population.[18] The precise etiology for vulvodynia is unclear. At present there is no definitive evidence favoring autoimmune, infectious, inflammatory or structural etiology.[19]

Several subsets of vulvodynia have been identified. For instance, one is cyclic vulvovaginitis (CVV), where the pain usually worsens just before or during menses. The etiology of CVV is thought to be multifactorial, including hypersensitivity to Candida antigen, cyclic changes in pH, and selective IgA (immunoglobulin, class A) deficiency. Another category is vulvar vestibulitis syndrome (VVS), involving inflammation of the Bartholin's glands and/or the minor vestibular glands at the base of the hymen. Symptoms include vulvar

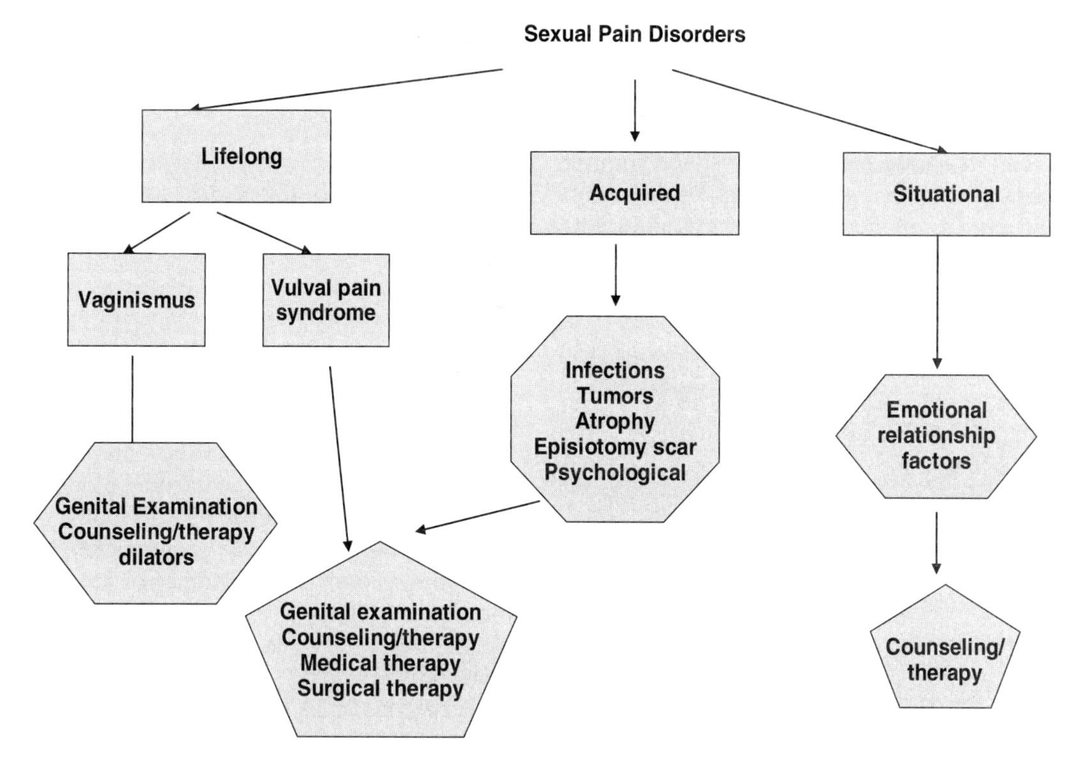

FIGURE 11.5. Assessment and treatment model for sexual pain disorders.

stinging, burning, irritation, and excoriation. Etiology for this syndrome is also multifactorial, including recurrent yeast vaginitis, use of chemicals or other irritants, previous treatment with carbon dioxide laser or cryotherapy, and allergic drug reactions. Vulvar burning has also been associated with higher levels of urinary calcium oxalate and can coexist with other pain disorders, such as interstitial cystitis and fibromyalgia. Dysesthetic vulvodynia is known as essential or idiopathic vulvodynia and refers to altered cutaneous perception or nerve sensory damage. Pudendal neuralgia and reflex sympathetic dystrophy have been implicated in causing vulvar dysesthesia. Vulvar dermatosis can produce a noncyclic, acute or chronic vulvar pruritus or burning pain and patients are typically perimenopausal or postmenopausal. Inflammatory dermatosis is often seen in patients with topical steroid overuse or intolerance. Contact dermatosis should be considered in patients who use feminine hygiene products, such as deodorant sprays, or scented douches, soaps or lubricants.[19,20]

Other etiologic explanations in these cases include previous obstetric or gynecologic trauma to the vagina; menopausal or radiation atrophy; inflammation of the urinary tract, rectum, or vagina; or pelvic adhesive disease.

Symptoms are often not only physiologically based, but may be psychologically based or some combination of the two.[21,22] Intrapsychic issues are, in fact, the main contributing factor in up to 43% of patients presenting with dyspareunia. Elements of fear, anxiety, and intimacy problems are often identified. Interpersonal conflict is the primary contributing factor in 27% of cases of dyspareunia, often characterized by poor communication, with special difficulty in talking about sex and emotions. Psychologic pressure to "perform" sexually can be present, especially when sexual intercourse is the primary or sole source of sexual pleasure and coital orgasm is a measure of intimacy for one or both partners.[21,22]

In an otherwise healthy woman, pain may be due to a change in the physiologic sexual response (arousal phase) that promotes comfortable intercourse. The three elements necessary for comfortable intercourse include vaginal lubrication, vaginal expansion, and relaxation of the pelvic floor muscles. In patients with pain due to these factors, basic education, over-the-counter lubricants, and pelvic floor relaxation may help, but in many cases, further evaluation and treatment is needed.

Vaginismus

Vaginismus involves the recurrent or persistent involuntary spasms of the musculature of the outer third of the vagina that interferes with vaginal penetration and which causes personal distress. Vaginismus usually develops as a conditioned response to painful penetration, or secondary to psychological/emotional factors. Vaginismus can be diagnosed by careful history and digital examination.

Primary vaginismus is often related to some past psychosexual or physical trauma. Psychosexual trauma based on misinformation, sexual interference, or religious proscription can result in phobic reactions to inserting anything in the vagina. On occasion, this problem can be produced iatrogenically by an unskilled or insensitive physician.

In the past, the problem of vaginismus has been badly managed by physicians. Patients are still treated surgically for this problem with hymenotomy, or Fenton's procedure. Because this is primarily a problem of muscle contraction or spasm, enlarging the introitus is not helpful. Some well-meaning physicians attempt to teach the patient "stretching exercises," which again are not helpful. This approach conceptually encourages the patient to force the dilator into the vagina with the hope of enlarging the space. This suggestion reinforces the spasm and increases the pain. For vaginismus, a combination of brief office psychotherapy and gynecological physical therapy can be useful in promoting understanding and muscle relaxation.

Other Sexual Pain Disorders

Other pain disorders involve recurrent and persistent genital pain induced by noncoital sexual stimulation. This includes anatomic and inflammatory conditions, including infections (i.e., HSV), vestibulitis, prior genital mutilation or trauma, and endometriosis.

General Etiologies of Female Sexual Dysfunction

Vasculogenic

Sexual dysfunction in women and impotence in men have been associated with high blood pressure, high cholesterol levels, smoking, and heart disease. The recently named clitoral and vaginal vascular insufficiency syndromes are, in fact, directly related to diminished genital blood flow, secondary to atherosclerosis of the iliohypogastric/pudendal arterial bed.[23] Diminished pelvic blood flow secondary to aortoiliac or atherosclerotic disease leads to vaginal wall and clitoral smooth muscle fibrosis, ultimately resulting in vaginal dryness and dyspareunia. While the precise mechanism is unknown, it is possible that the atherosclerotic changes that occur in clitoral vascular and trabecular smooth muscle interfere with normal relaxation and dilation responses to sexual simulation.

Aside from atherosclerotic disease, alterations in circulating estrogen levels associated with menopause contribute to the age-associated changes in clitoral and vaginal smooth muscle. Vaginal atrophy and vaginal dryness are common factors contributing to genital pain issues in menopausal women. Additionally, any traumatic injury to the iliohypogastric/pudendal arterial bed from pelvic fractures, blunt trauma, surgical disruption, or chronic perineal pressure from bicycle riding, for instance, can result in diminished vaginal and clitoral blood flow and complaints of sexual dysfunction.

Musculogenic

The muscles of the pelvic floor are invested in female sexual responsiveness as well as in sexual function. A duo of small superficial muscles (bulbocavernosus and ischiocavernosus) encircles the vagina and is responsible for the involuntary rhythmic contractions during orgasm. When exercised regularly, they can intensify and contribute to arousal and orgasm. In addition, the muscles of the deep pelvic floor (pubococcygeus or PC) also modulate motor responses vaginal receptivity during orgasm. Hypertonicity within these two groups can lead to sexual dysfunction and pain disorders.

Pregnancy and childbirth carry a high risk of muscular and neurological injury to the pelvic floor, as detailed in Chapter 3. Particularly after vaginal birth, neuromuscular trauma may predispose to sexual pain, and/or loss of responsiveness.

Neurogenic

The same neurogenic etiologies that cause erectile dysfunction in men can also cause sexual dysfunction in women. These include (1) spinal cord injury or disease of the central or peripheral nervous system, including diabetes, and (2) complete upper motor neuron injuries affecting sacral spinal segments. Women with incomplete injuries may retain that capacity for psychogenic arousal and vaginal lubrication.[16] With regard to orgasm, women with spinal cord injury have significantly more difficulty achieving orgasm than normal controls.[24] The effects of specific spinal cord injuries on female sexual response as well as the role for vasoactive pharmacotherapy in this population are being investigated.

Hormonal/Endocrine

Dysfunction of the hypothalamic/pituitary axis, hypopituitarism, Addison's disease, corticosteroid therapy, ovarian failure or oophorectomy, menopause, oral estrogen replacement therapy or oral contraceptive use, and surgical or medical castration are the most common causes of hormonally based female sexual dysfunction. The most common complaints associated with decreased estrogen and/or testosterone levels are decreased libido, vaginal dryness, and lack of sexual arousal.

Although estrogen replacement therapy comes with its own host of risks, we know that estrogen improves the integrity of vaginal mucosal tissue and has beneficial effects on vaginal sensation, vasocongestion, and secretions, which all leads to enhanced arousal. Estrogen deprivation causes a significant decrease in clitoral intracavernosal blood flow and vaginal and urethral blood flow. Histologically, it causes diffuse clitoral fibrosis, thinned vaginal epithelial layers, and decreased vaginal submucosal vasculature. Thus, a decline in circulating estrogen levels can produce significant adverse effects on structure and function of the vagina and clitoris, ultimately affecting sexual function. Protocols for replacing testosterone will be addressed in the treatment section.

Psychogenic

It is important to emphasize that in women, independent of physical factors, emotional and relationship issues significantly affect sexual function and response. In every woman with a sexual function complaint, there are relationship, emotional, and medical factors happening simultaneously and interacting with one another in a nonlinear fashion. From the relationship standpoint, partner sexual dysfunction, uneven levels of desire, lack of communication, relationship conflict, lack of information about sexual stimulation, and how each defines sexual satisfaction/gratification can all impact on a woman's sexual response.

The same is true for the emotional part of the equation. For the woman herself, issues such as self-esteem and body image, a history of sexual trauma or emotional abuse, drug and/or alcohol abuse, and sexual addiction can affect her sexual response. An inability to respond is often connected to performance anxiety. If she is unable to respond sexually regardless of situational or circumstantial reasons, due to her fear and anxiety of this happening again, her response may be inhibited.

Other mood disorders and psychological stressors like depression, anxiety, chronic stress and fatigue are all associated with female sexual function complaints. In addition, the medications commonly used to treat depression can significantly affect the female sexual response. The most frequently used medications for uncomplicated depression are the selective serotonin re-uptake inhibitors (SSRIs). Women receiving these medications often complain of decreased desire, arousal, genital sensation, and difficulty achieving orgasm.

Assessment of Female Sexual Dysfunction

Every woman is at risk for sexual dysfunction, and the more open the physician is to hearing about these complaints, the more likely the patient will bring them up. It is crucial that the clinician provide appropriate cues that he or she is open to discussion of sexual concerns, and this can be achieved in many ways. The primary care clinician may give patients a sexual function questionnaire along with their paper work, or just include a question like, *"Do you have any questions or concerns about your sexual response or interest,"* in the history. It is also helpful to place flyers or booklets about sexual function in the waiting and exam rooms to let your patients know you are receptive to hearing their concerns.

The few studies that have addressed the treatment of sexual complaints in a medical setting have found that family physicians are more likely to be consulted for a sexual problem than anyone else.[25,26] One web-based survey asked 4000 women with sexual dysfunction about their experiences seeking help from their health care professionals,[27] and found that 54% reported that they would like to but didn't, for reasons including embarrassment and a belief that the physician would not be able to help.

Psychosexual Exam

Ideally, assessment of female sexual function complaints should include a psychosexual exam. One interesting study compared the effectiveness of three simple questions applied routinely to patients admitted to a gynecologic service with a more detailed interview conducted by an experienced sex therapist.[28] Patients reported sexual problems to a receptive physician who displayed a willingness to discuss the subject. Ease with the subject matter was proven less important than had been estimated previously. Three simple questions applied by an inexperienced interviewer yielded the same results as a more detailed interview conducted by an experienced interviewer. This should be encouraging to inexperienced physicians, who may feel relatively lacking in their comfort and skill regarding patients' sexual concerns.

A simple screen for sexual dysfunction can include two or three nonintrusive questions related to *desire, discomfort,* and *satisfaction.* These simple questions benefit the relationship between the physician and patient, even if the patient declines to respond to the questions, for two reasons: (1) the patient is informed that he or she can discuss these issues with the physician when he or she is ready; and (2) the mere asking of the questions create an expectation of continued clinical interest in the patient's sexual function.

In assessing a specific sexual concern raised by the patient, a more detailed history is appropriate (see Table 11.1). Elements conducive to eliciting a sexual problem in detail include sufficient time to explore the complaint, a setting that ensures privacy, listening while the patient explains her concern in detail, a comfortable attitude on the part of the physician, and the use of language that is common to and understood by both the physician and the patient.

A problem-solving approach to the patient's sexual complaint is recommended and will enlist relevant questions to clarify whether the complaint relates to desire, arousal, orgasm, or pain. Specific questions can assess the presence of a

TABLE 11.1. Sexual Dysfunction Clinical Assessment Questioning

1) Clarification of the sexual problem. (e.g. "Can you tell me more about it?" What are all the sexual symptoms? Which symptom came first?)
2) How long has the problem been occurring? (Primary = lifelong or Secondary = following a period of "normal" sexual functioning)
3) Is the problem present in all situations? (global; e.g., with all partners, different locations, positions) or only in certain situations (situational; e.g., no symptoms with self-stimulation or when on vacations)
4) Is there anything that makes the situation better? (e.g., going away to a hotel for the weekend, positioning) Is there anything that makes it worse? (e.g., menstrual cycle; partner or self expectations)
5) How is it affecting her relationship with her partner? (e.g., current intimate relationship? partner's reaction to problem)
6) What is the motivation for evaluation and treatment? (e.g. dissolving of marriage/partnership, reached a "breaking point")
7) Does the partner have any sexual problems (e.g., low libido, erectile dysfunction, early ejaculation)
8) Any prior assessment or treatment for problem? What was the outcome?
9) What are the patient's thoughts regarding possible causes for the problem?
10) What is the patient's medical, surgical and psychological history?

dysphoric disorder and a history of medication ingestion. Intrapsychic factors of particular importance include stress, fatigue, depression, and substance abuse. Questions about the patient's early sex life may reveal a life-long inhibited sexual desire, sexual avoidance, or revulsion suggestive of childhood sexual trauma or abuse. If trauma or abuse history is discovered, it is crucial to send the patient for further support and evaluation by a trained therapist (discussed further below).

Relationship factors should be assessed for their relevant impact on the presenting complaint. Issues of grief, power, intimacy, and communication each require assessment to clarify whether the sexual concern is recent or a product of more serious longstanding conflicts. The importance of listening skills cannot be overemphasized. If the patient is allowed to talk, she will likely narrow the list of possible explanations of the problem to one or two in a very short discussion. The physician's comfort in exploring these issues is most important. A relaxed physician in a comfortable atmosphere will encourage full disclosure by the patient. Staccato questions that run through a list of issues will likely yield little information and much frustration. If time is a factor, the assessment can be done over several visits. These complaints are rarely an emergency and may be better dealt with over more than one visit, as long as the second visit is not long after the first. Understanding the myriad of factors that contribute to sexual dysfunction and employing a mind-body approach to assessing and treating women's sexual health will allow for greatest successes in improving sexual function for women. Knowing when and how to refer a patient to a trained therapist for further evaluation and treatment will be discussed below.

Medical Testing

To understand what role physiologic factors may play in a woman's ability to respond sexually, the physician should conduct a full medical and surgical history with the patient. Birth control pills, chronic stress, depression, and childbirth can all contribute to response, as well as, desire problems. Medications or medical conditions that adversely affect libido or sexual function should be noted (see Table 11.2 for a complete list of medications that may affect sexual function).

Table 11.2. Medications that Affect Sexual Function

Anti-androgen drugs:	Lupron, spironolactone, ketoconazole, cytotoxic chemotherapeutic agents
Psychoactive drugs	
Antidepressants:	SSRIs, Tricyclics
Cardiac drugs:	Hydrochlorothiazide, beta blockers, calcium channel blockers
Drugs that bind with testosterone or increase SHBG levels:	Tamoxifen, contraceptive drugs, etc.

The internal and external genitalia should be examined for signs of phlogosis, which can lead to vulvar pain in younger women as well as vaginal atrophy, pain, and arousal disorders in older menopausal women. The muscular tone and strength of the pelvic floor as well as bulbocavernosus reflex should also be determined. Assessment of the genital and perineal sensation should be performed. If abnormalities are noted, further neurologic evaluation may be warranted.

It is important in some circumstances to also assess physiologic changes that occur during the sexual response. Measurements of genital vibratory perception thresholds and genital hemodynamics can be recorded post-sexual stimulation in the clinical setting. Blood-flow assessment—especially clitoral, labial, urethral, vaginal, and uterine arteries—is recorded, and an assessment of blood velocity and venous pooling can be made. In many patients, observations show that despite complaints of sexual dysfunction, sexual stimulation does, in fact, result in significant increases in genital blood flow.[29] Currently, normative data is being gathered to determine normal physiologic responses.

Treatments for Female Sexual Dysfunction

Hormone Therapy

Estrogen

In light of the recent findings of the Women's Health Initiative, it has become clear that the use of oral estrogens—whether bio-identical or traditional HRT—must be considered only after a careful discussion of potential risks and benefits. Estrogen may relieve hot flashes, improve clitoral sensitivity, increase libido, and decrease pain and burning during intercourse. Local or topical estrogen application relieves symptoms of vaginal dryness, burning, and urinary frequency/urgency. In perimenopausal, menopausal, or oophorectomized women, complaints of vaginal irritation, pain, or dryness may be relieved locally with low-dose topical estrogen cream, vaginal estradiol rings, or vaginal estradiol pellets, which may help to minimize the systemic absorption of estrogen, and thereby minimize its risks.

Testosterone

The only FDA approved testosterone replacement available to women is methyltestosterone, indicated for menopausal women, used in combination with estrogen (Estratest), for symptoms of inhibited desire, dyspareunia, or lack of vaginal lubrication, as well as for its vaso-protective effects. A testosterone patch is presently being tested, and early trials indicate the patch may improve sexual activity as well as help create an overall sense of well-being.[30] According to the Princeton Consensus Panel on Female Androgen Insufficiency, if a woman exhibits symptoms of low testosterone (e.g., low libido, decreased energy and well-being), it is important to first determine an alternative explanation for these symptoms. This means ruling out major depression, chronic fatigue symptoms, as well as the range of other emotional and relationship conflicts that may impact on a patient's desire and happiness. The next step is to determine if the patient is in an adequate estrogen state and, if not, consider the pros and cons of replacement.[31]

At the primary care level, measurement of testosterone levels is not common, but can be included in a first-line evaluation. This does, however, require at least 2 to 3 measures of total and free testosterone. Normal value ranges are for total testosterone, 30 to120 ng/dL, and for free testosterone, 3.0 to 8.5 pg/mL for premenopausal women and 3.0 to 6.7 pg/mL for postmenopausal women. If the patient has a treatable cause for the androgen deficiency (e.g., oral estrogens or contraceptive use) treat the specific causes by changing medications. If not, a trial of androgen replacement therapy may be considered. There are conflicting reports regarding the "best" way to administer testosterone, particularly in premenopausal women. All premenopausal woman treated with testosterone must be on some form of reliable birth control and understand the risks. Topical vaginal testosterone is often used in premenopausal women as a first step in the treatment of sexual dysfunction and vaginal lichen planus. Topical testosterone preparations can be compounded in 1% to 2% formulations and should be applied up to 3 times per week. The suggested dose of oral testosterone (pill, sublingual spray, or lozenge) for premenopausal and postmenopausal women ranges from .25 to 1.25 mg/day. The dose can be adjusted according to symptoms, free testosterone levels, cholesterol levels, triglyceride levels, HDL levels, and liver function test. The potential side-effects of testosterone include weight gain, clitoral enlargement, increased facial hair, and hypercholesterolemia. Testosterone can also be converted into estrogen, with attendant risks that should be taken into account when counseling patients. Increased clitoral sensitivity, decreased vaginal dryness, and increased libido have been reported with the use of a 2% testosterone cream. The potential hazards of long-term testosterone administration, both known and unknown, should not be minimized.

Pharmacological Therapy

Aside from hormone replacement therapy, all medications listed below, while used in the treatment of male erectile dysfunction, are still in the experimental phases for use in women. Currently, we have limited information regarding the exact neurotransmitters that modulate vaginal and clitoral smooth muscle tone. Nitric oxide (NO) and Phosphodiesterase Type 5 (PDE5), the enzyme responsible for both the degradation of cGMP and NO production, have been identified in clitoral and vaginal smooth muscle.[26] In addition, organ bath studies of rabbit clitoral-cavernosal muscle strips demonstrate enhanced relaxation in response to the nitric oxide donors, sodium nitroprusside, L-Arginine, and Sildenafil.

Sildenafil

Functioning as a selective type 5 (cGMP specific) phosphodiesterase inhibitor, this medication decreases the catabolism of cGMP, the second messenger in nitric oxide mediated relaxation of clitoral and vaginal smooth muscle. Sildenafil may prove useful alone, or possibly in combination with other vasoactive substances, for treatment of female sexual arousal disorder. Two recent placebo-controlled studies demonstrated that sildenafil is successful in treating female sexual arousal disorder in hormonally replete women without psychosexual causal factors.[32,33] However, Phase II clinical trials were halted. The company conducting the research reported that they were not finding a difference in effectiveness between sildenafil and placebo, but this was most likely due to difficulties recruiting appropriate candidates. It proved difficult to identify women who did not have emotional or relationship causal factors influencing their sexual functioning, much less women who were hormonally replete with both estrogen and testosterone. Other studies have found that sildenafil helps to alleviate arousal problems associated with aging, menopause, and arousal problems experienced secondary to selective serotonin re-uptake inhibitors (SSRI) use.[34]

Sildenafil and other vasodilators will likely have their place as part of a multi-disciplinary treatment plan with a certain kind of candidate. These are most likely women who are hormonally replete and were satisfied with their sexual response at one point in time and now, for medical reasons (hysterectomy, menopause, pelvic injury, etc.) are no longer able to respond as they once could.

L-Arginine

This amino acid functions as a precursor to the formation of nitric oxide, which mediates the relaxation of vascular and nonvascular smooth muscle. L-Arginine has not yet been used in clinical trials in women. However, preliminary studies in men appear promising. A combination of L-Arginine and yohimbine (an alpha 2 blocker) is currently under investigation in women.

Yohimbine

Yohimbine is an alkaloid agent that blocks presynaptic alpha-2 adrenoreceptors. This medication affects the peripheral autonomic nervous system, resulting in a relative decrease in adrenergic activity and an increase in parasympathetic tone. There have been mixed reports of its efficacy for inducing penile erections in men, and no formal clinical studies have been performed in women to date, nor have potential side effects been effectively determined.

Prostaglandin E_1 (MUSE)

An intra-urethral application, absorbed via mucosa (MUSE), is now available for male patients. A similar application of Prostaglandin E_1 delivered intravaginally is currently under investigation for use in women. Clinical studies are necessary to determine the efficacy of this medication in the treatment of female sexual dysfunction.

Phentolamine

Currently available in an oral preparation, this drug functions as a nonspecific alpha-adrenergic blocker, and causes vascular smooth muscle relaxation. This drug has been studied in male patients for the treatment of erectile dysfunction. A pilot study in menopausal women with sexual dysfunction demonstrated enhanced vaginal blood flow and subjective arousal with the medication.[35]

Apomorphine

This short-acting dopamine agonist facilitates erectile responses in both normal males and males with psychogenic erectile dysfunction or organic impotence. Data suggests that dopamine is involved in the mediation of sexual desire and arousal. The physiologic effects of this drug are currently being tested in women with sexual dysfunction.

Nitroglycerin

Nitroglycerin (glyceryl trinitrate) has been used for over a century to relieve anginal symptoms associated with coronary artery disease. It has been administered to humans via oral, sublingual,

TABLE 11.3. Pharmacological Treatments for Female Sexual Dysfunction

Drug/Product	Maker	Key Ingredient	Use/Potential Use	Status
Androsorb	Novavax	Testosterone	HSDD	Phase II
Alista	Vivus	Prostaglandin E1	FSAD	Phase II
EROS	Urometrics	Clitoral therapy device	FDA Approved	With Rx
Estrace Cream	Warner Chilcott	Estrogen	HRT vaginal dryness & discomfort	With Rx
Estratest (pill)	Solvay Pharmaceuticals	Estrogen-testosterone combination	HRT to treat hot flashes. Heightens desire in some women	With Rx
Evista	Eli Lilly	SERM	Osteoporosis, HRT, thickens vaginal walls	With Rx
Femprox (cream)	NexMed	PGE1	FSAD	Phase II
Livial (pill)	Organon	SERM	Osteoporosis, libido & arousal txmt	Phase III
Nitroglycerin (glyceryl trinitrate)	Off label Rx			
NM1-870 (pill)	NitroMed	African tree bark w/nitric oxide	FSAD in postmenopausal women	Phase II
Premarin (pill, cream, or injection), Prempro (pill), Premphase (pill)	Wyeth	Estrogen	Osteoporosis, menopausal sxs, FSAD, & dyspareunia	With Rx
Testosterone Creams	Off-label from compounding pharmacies	Testosterone	T hormone replacement therapy	Not FDA approved for use in women
Testosterone patch	P & G	Testosterone	In 6th month study women reported increased sexual activity & pleasure	FDA denied, approval pending further research
Tostrelle (gel)	Cellegy	Testosterone	Controlled delivery system for testosterone	Phase II/III
Vasofem (tablet)	Zonagen	Blood vessel dilator	Increases blood flow to clitoris	Phase II
Viagra	Pfizer	Blood vessel dilator	Male Erectile dysfunction	Off-label Rx
VIP (cream)	Senetek PLC	Synthetic version of brain chemical	Vaginal dryness & discomfort associated w/menopause	Phase II

intravenous, and transdermal routes. Nitroglycerin has been found to relax most smooth muscle, including bronchial, gastrointestinal tract, urethral, and uterine muscle. It also produces dilation of both arterial and venous vascular beds. Metabolism of nitroglycerin leads to the formation of the reactive free radical nitric oxide. Recent evidence suggests that application of nitroglycerin to painful areas, including the genitals, may provide analgesia to the affected areas.[19,36] More work needs to be done in this area, but many experts are finding this an effective treatment for helping women manage vulvar pain, especially when in combination with topical estrogen and testosterone creams and gynecological physical therapy.

Herbal remedies

Many women are interested in and have been exploring herbal treatments for female sexual dysfunction. However, only two herbal products have had placebo-controlled trials. Zestra, a massage oil formulated to enhance sexual arousal[37] and ArginMax, an herbal remedy that is used to increase sexual desire in women. In the study on ArginMax, 77 women who reported symptoms of sexual dysfunction were surveyed using the Female Sexual Function Index (FSFI). Results showed that after using ArginMax, 71% of the women reported improved sexual desire.[37]

Both of these studies demonstrate the potential role that herbal supplements can play in enhancing sexual functioning. Further placebo-controlled studies are needed (see Table 11.3 for a complete list of pharmacological treatments currently being tested for female sexual dysfunction).

Medical Devices

Eros Therapy

Eros Therapy is the first FDA-approved treatment on the market for arousal and orgasmic disorders in women. It is a small, handheld, medical device with a soft cup, which is placed over the clitoris. When activated, a gentle vacuum is created, thereby increasing blood flow to the clitoris and surrounding tissue. Initial clinical trials showed improvement in premenopausal and postmenopausal women with female sexual arousal disorder or female orgasmic disorder.[39,40]

Sexual Aids and Devices

The quality and accessibility of vibrators, silicone toys, and other sensual accessories has improved dramatically. Unfortunately, adequate information and scholarly research on the subject of masturbation—especially the use of erotic aids to enhance sexuality—still remains difficult to find.[41] Recently, however, a study examined vibrator use, perceptions, and sexual function of a random national sample of 1656 women. Results indicated that vibrator use was significantly correlated with higher levels of sexual function. Specifically, women who used vibrators reported higher levels of sexual desire, arousal, and less pain during and following intercourse.[42]

While taboo in the past, vibrators have become more mainstream; with improved products and accessibility, women no longer have to go into a dark erotica shop in a rough part of town to find a sexual device to improve their sexual response and satisfaction. Although more accessible, it may not yet be common for a physician to recommend a vibrator for improved sexual functioning. There is likely significant anxiety, hesitation at overstepping one's bounds, and the possibility of offending the patient. Physicians, therapists, and other treatment providers must be open to learning about sexual devices and help to normalize their use as a treatment for their patients.

Gynecological Physical Therapy

Chronic sexual pain disorders can effectively be treated with the use of gynecological physical therapy. With the use of manual therapies (internal or external), electrical therapy, exercise, and pelvic floor retraining, normal muscle balance—as well as bowel and bladder function—can be restored, all of which results in improved sexual function.

Yoga

To supplement gynecological physical therapy, yoga can also be used to strengthen and maintain the pelvic floor muscles that are central to sexual function. Yoga exercises are used to focus on the abdomen and pelvic floor for increased flexibility, blood flow, and strength for improved sexual function.

Psychosocial Interventions & Referral to a Trained Sex Therapist

As previously mentioned, female sexual dysfunction is, in most cases, a product of both psychological and relationship factors. Even if the primary etiologic domain is physical, there are emotional and relationship outgrowths to the problem which cannot be ignored (see Figure 11.6). Similarly, not all women are candidates for medical intervention and are better suited to other psychological or couples therapies.[39,40] Usually the best treatment is a combination of medical interventions and psychotherapy. It should be noted here that beginning psychotherapy without evaluating the potential medical causes for female sexual dysfunction is not recommended. Extensive psychotherapy with a woman with undiagnosed medical issues can be a very frustrating experience for both the patient and caregiver.

The ideal way to determine candidates for medical intervention in a clinical setting is to collaborate with a trained sex therapist. The key to making a therapy referral is in helping the patient understand where psychotherapy fits into the treatment equation. It may need to be clarified that, while you do not think her problems are "all in her head," she would benefit from psychotherapy as well as medical treatment. If the physician refers to and supports the role of the psychotherapy and helps the patient understand how psychotherapy will be incorporated into her treatment plan, she will feel validated and encouraged, knowing that her symptoms will be addressed, rather than minimized.

There are a number of specific instances when patients should be referred to specialists. These include patients with longstanding dysfunction or

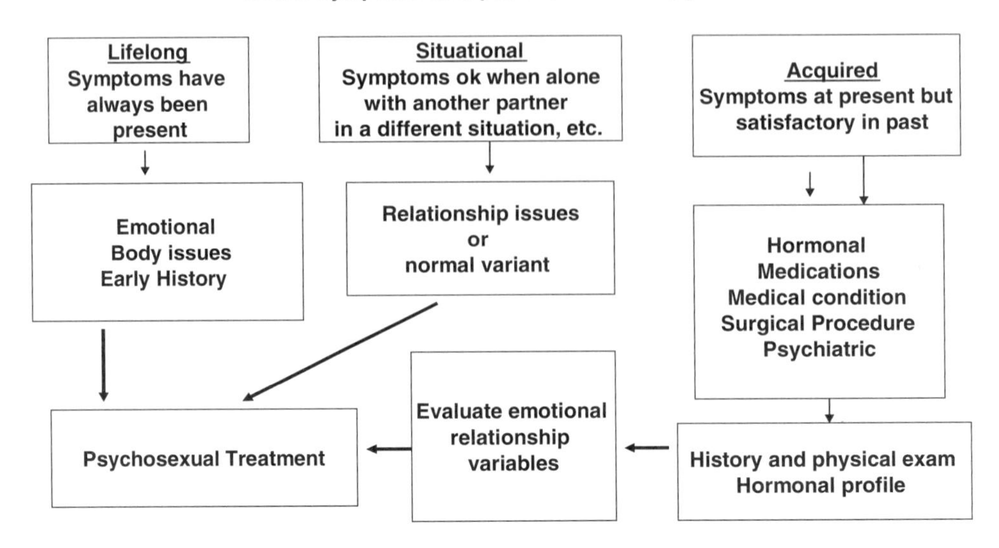

Figure 11.6. Sexual symptoms.

with multiple dysfunctions; patients who have suffered current or past abuse, have a psychiatric history, current depression, stress or anxiety; or if there are any relationship conflicts, including the partner having sexual dysfunction. Additionally, patients whose problems have no known etiology, and patients who do not respond to any type of therapy, will likely benefit from a referral for further assessment and treatment (see Table 11.5).

Many qualified therapists who work with sexual issues can be located through the American Association of Sex Educators, Counselors, and Therapists (AASECT, online at www.assect.org.)

Table 11.4. Red Flags for Further Psychosexual Assessment*

The couple is experiencing relationship conflicts (e.g., lack of intimacy, conflict, etc.).
The symptoms are life-long, not acquired.
The symptoms are situational (e.g., do not exist when stress removed or when with another partner).
The patient has a history of sexual abuse or trauma.
The patient has a psychiatric history.
The patient has a history of or is presently experiencing depression, anxiety and/or stress.
The partner has a sexual dysfunction.

*None of these factors guarantee the problem is psychosexually based, suggest a need for a referral to a trained sex therapist.

Conclusion

Using a comprehensive and holistic approach to women's sexual health is essential in effectively evaluating and treating sexual dysfunction.

Table 11.5. Sexual Challenges at Significant Life Stages

Early sexual experiences/development
Sexual inexperience/lack of education
Body Image issues
Sexual Inhibitions
Sexual culture within family of origin (sexual messages)
Friends influence/Peer Pressure
Performance Anxiety
Sexual Identity
Pregnancy
Body image issues
Shifting sexual identity
Pelvic floor issues often lead to pain, prolapse, and incontinence
Post-partum hormonal issues
Relationship challenges
Perimenopause/Menopause
Diminishing hormones
Incontinence/pelvic floor prolapse
Vaginal Atrophy, dryness
Diminishing genital sensitivity, arousal
Decreased sexual desire
Empty nest challenges to self-esteem, and relationship
Mood/sleep changes affecting relationship dynamics

Regardless of age or stage of life, women face various sexual challenges that can be affected by physical, emotional, and relational health (Table 11.5). Understanding women's sexual health and satisfaction is complex and multifaceted. Primary care providers can have a significant impact on their patients' physical and mental health as well as their overall quality of life. Asking about a woman's sexual functioning in the context of a routine evaluation will help to communicate the openness in which sexuality can be discussed. Learning how to discuss sexual concerns in an appropriate, matter-of-fact way, understanding how to address various areas of a woman's life, and knowing when and how to refer a patient for further assessment are all keys to successfully being a women's health care provider.

Key Points

- FSD is highly prevalent, and its causes are multifactorial. These causes include vascular, neurologic, hormonal, and psychogenic disorders.
- Taking a mind/body approach to FSD is the most effective way of understanding and treating it.
- Women typically experience sexuality and sexual response in a more complicated context than men.
- Part of your medical history and assessment should include consideration of medications the patient is presently taking that may be contributing to symptoms.
- Female Sexual Dysfunction can be categorized into four different disorders that may coexist.
  - Hypoactive Sexual Desire Disorder
  - Female Sexual Arousal Disorder
  - Female Orgasmic Disorder
  - Sexual Pain Disorders
- Treatments for FSD may include hormone therapy, pharmacological therapy, medical devices, gynecological physical therapy, psychosocial interventions or some combination thereof.
- Women who use sexual aids and devices have better sexual functioning than those who do not.
- All physicians treating FSD should have access to a sex therapist in their community and be able to identify psychosexual red flags for referral.
- Effective framing of psychosexual referral is crucial for the patient's willingness to follow through. Make sure you explain to the patient what psychosexual treatment entails and how it will play a role in the larger treatment plan you are managing.

References

1. Berman L, Berman J. Viagra and beyond: Where sex educators and therapists fit in from a multidisciplinary perspective. *J Sex Educ Ther.* 2000;25: 17–25.
2. Berman L, Berman J. *Secrets of the Sexually Satisfied Woman: Ten Keys to Unlocking Ultimate Pleasure.* New York, Hyperion, 2005.
3. Derogatis L, Meyer J, King K. Psychopathology in individuals with sexual dysfunction. *American Journal of Psychiatry* 1981;138:757–763.
4. Laumann EO, Paik A, Rosen RC. Sexual dysfunction in the United States prevalence and predictors. *JAMA.* 1999;281:537–544.
5. Morokoff P, Gillilland R. Stress, sexual functioning, and marital satisfaction. *J Sex Res.* 1993;30:43–53.
6. Masters EH, Johnson VE. *Human Sexual Response.* Boston: Little Brown; 1966.
7. Kaplan HS. *The New Sex Therapy.* London: Bailliere Tindall; 1974,1966.
8. Basson R, Berman J, Burnett A et. al. Report of the international consensus development conference on female sexual dysfunction: definitions and classifications. *J Urol.* 2000;183:888–893.
9. Basson R. Using a different model for female sexual response to address women's problematic low sexual desire. *J Sex Marital Ther.* 2001;5:395–403.
10. Segraves RT. Sex and the depressed patient. *Current Canadian Psychiatry Neurology.* 1995.
11. Faith M., Schare, M. The role of body image in sexually avoidant behavior. *Arch Sex Behav.* 1993;22: 345–346.
12. Ackard D, Kearney-Cooke A, Peterson C. Effect of body image and self-image on women's sexual behaviors. *Int J Ea Disord.* 2000;28:422–429.
13. Liss-Levinson N. Disorders of desire: women, sex, and food. *Women Ther.* 1988;7:121–129.

14. Wiederman MW, Pryor T. Body dissatisfaction and sexuality among women with bulimia nervosa. *Int J Eat Disord.* 1997;21:361–365.
15. Berman L, Berman J, Miles M, Pollets D, Powell JA. Genital self-image as a component of sexual health: relationship between genital self-image, female sexual function, and quality of life measures. *J Sex Marital Ther.* 2003;29:11–21.
16. Goldstein I, Lue TF, Padma-Nathan H, Rosen RC, Steers WD, Wicker PA. Oral sildenafil in the treatment of erectile dysfunction. *N Engl J Med.* 1998; 338:1397–1404.
17. Lamont JA. Vaginismus: A reflex response out of control. *Contemporary Obstetric Gynecology* 1994; 30.
18. Lamont JA. Anorgasmia. *Contemporary Obstetric Gynecology* 1994;30.
18. Goetsch MF. Vulvar vestibulitis: prevalence and historic features in a general gynecologic practice populations. *Am J Obstet Gynecol.* 1991;164:1609–1614.
19. Walsh KE, Berman JR, Berman LA, Vierregger K. Safety and efficacy of topical nitroglycerin for treatment of vulvar pain in women with vulvodynia: A pilot study. *J Gend Specif Med.* 2002;5: 21–27.
20. McKay M. Subsets of vulvodynia. *J Reprod Med.* 1988;33:695–698.
21. Lamont JA. Female dyspareunia. *Am J Obstet Gynecol.* 1980;136:282–285.
22. Lamont JA. Dyspareunia and vaginismus. In: Droegemueller W, Sciarra JJ (eds): *Gynecology and Obstetrics*, p 1. Philadelphia, JB Lippincott, 1990.
23. Tarcan T, Park K, Goldstein I et al., Histomorphometric analysis of age-related structural changes in human clitoral cavernosal tissue. *J Urol.* 1999;161: 940–944.
24. Sipski ML, Alexander CJ, Rosen RC. Orgasm in women with spinal cord injuries: a laboratory-based assessment. *Arch Phys Med. Rehabil.* 1995;5:1097–1102.
25. Houge D. Sex problems in family practice. *Faily Pct Re J.* 1988;7:135–140.
26. Nease DE Jr., Liese BS. Perceptions and treatment of sexual problems. *Fam Med.* 1987;11: 468–470.
27. Berman L, Berman J, Felder S et al. Seeking help for sexual function complaints: what gynecologists need to know about the female patient's experience. *Fertil Steril.* 2003;79:572–576.
28. Plouffe L Jr. Screening for sexual problems through a simple questionnaire. *Am J Obstet Gynecol.* 1985;151:166–169.
29. Berman JR, Berman L, Goldstein I. Female sexual dysfunction: incidence, pathophysiology, evaluation and treatment options. *Urology.* 1999; 54(3):385–391.
30. Shifren JL, Braunstein GD, Simon JA et al. Transdermal testosterone treatment in women with impaired sexual function after oophorectomy. *N Engl J Med.* 2000;343(10):682–688.
31. Bachmann G, Bancroft J, Braunstein G, et al. Female androgen insufficiency: the Princeton consensus statement on definition, classification, and assessment. *Fertil Steril* 2002;77(4):660–665.
32. Caruso S, Intelisano G, Lupo L, Agnello C. Premenopausal women affected by sexual arousal disorder treated with sildenafil: a double-blind, cross-over, placebo-controlled study. *BJO G.* 2001; 108:623–628.
33. Berman JR, Berman LA, Toler SM, Gill J, Haughie S; Sildenafil Study Group. Safety and efficacy of sildenafil citrate for the treatment of female sexual arousal disorder: a double-blind, placebo controlled study. *J Urol* 2003;170:2333–2338.
34. Min K, Kim NN, McAuley I, Stankowicz M, Goldstein I, Traish AM. Sildenafil augments pelvic nerve-mediated female genital sexual arousal in the anesthetized rabbit. *Int J Impot Res.* 2001;12:S32–S39.
35. Rosen RC, Phillips NA, Gendrano NC 3rd, Ferguson DM. Oral phentolamine and female sexual arousal disorder: a pilot study. *J Sex Marital Ther.* 1999;25:137–144.
36. Berrazueta JR, Losada A, Poveda J et al. Successful treatment of shoulder pain syndrome due to supraspinatus tendonitis with transdermal nitroglycerin: A double blind study. *Pain.* 1996;66: 63–67.
37. Ferguson DM, Steidle CP, Singh GS, Alexander JS, Weihmiller MK, Crosby MG. Randomized, placebo-controlled, double-blind, crossover desire trial of the efficacy and safety of Zestra for Women in women with and without female sexual arousal disorder. *J SexMarital Ther.* 2003;29: 33–44.
38. Ito TY, Trant AS, Polan, ML. A Double-blind placebo-controlled study of ArginMax, a nutritional supplement for enhancement of female sexual function. *J Sex Marital Ther.* 2001;27:541–549.
39. Billups KL, Berman L, Berman J, Metz ME, Glennon ME, Goldstein I. A new non-pharmacological vacuum therapy for female sexual dysfunction. *J Sex Marital Ther.* 2001;27:435–441.

40. Berman J, Berman L. For Women Only: A Revolutionary Guide to Reclaiming Your Sex Life. New York: Henry Holt and Company; 2001.
41. Hall D. Good vibrations: Eros and instrumental knowledge. *Journal of Popular Culture* 2000;34:1–7.
42. Berman L. A Survey of Vibrator Use: Prevalence, Perceptions and Relationship to Sexual Function and Quality of Life Measures. Presented at the Women's Sexual Health State of the Art Series, September 11–12. 2004; Chicago, IL.

12
Urinary Tract Infections: Managing Acute, Chronic and Difficult Cases

Christine A. LaSala

Introduction

Urinary tract infection (UTI) is a common diagnosis seen by primary care providers. The majority of UTIs occur in young, otherwise healthy women and respond to antimicrobial therapy. The pathogenesis and management of UTIs is generally straightforward. However, in populations with complicated UTIs, urosepsis may occur and treatment may be more difficult in those with inadequate host defenses or genitourinary abnormalities.

The impact of urinary tract infections on patients and on the healthcare system is substantial; thus, it is imperative that primary care physicians understand the approaches in diagnosing and treating this common condition.

Epidemiology

Urinary tract infection is one of the most common bacterial infections. It accounts for more than 7 million physician visits and 1 million hospital admissions annually in the United States.[1,2] The cost of treating uncomplicated UTIs approximates 1 billion dollars annually.[3] Up to 50% of women will experience a UTI at sometime in their life, with 20% to 50% of these developing a recurrent UTI.[4,5]

The highest incidence is in young, sexually active women aged 20 to 40 years of age and in postmenopausal women. Recurrent UTIs increase in frequency with sexual intercourse and advancing age.[6,7]

In premenopausal women, estrogen encourages normal colonization of Lactobacillus in the vagina. This bacterium produces lactic acid and hydrogen peroxide, which help maintain the acidic pH of the vagina and inhibit growth of uropathogens. With estrogen deficiency and the reduction of lactobacilli, the rise in vaginal pH facilitates colonization of the vagina and periurethral tissue with uropathogenic gram-negative bacteria, particularly E. coli.[12]

Except in neonates, the prevalence and incidence of UTIs is greater in females by a ratio of 30:1. In neonates and infants, UTI is more common in males and is usually associated with congenital anomalies. In early childhood, bacteriuria is more common in girls, is often asymptomatic, but when symptomatic may be associated with vesicoureteral reflux.[8] UTIs are among the most common causes of bacterial infection among febrile pediatric patients, with a prevalence of 4% to 7% in both boys and girls.

The majority of UTIs present as symptoms of acute, uncomplicated bacterial cystitis or pyelonephritis in otherwise healthy women. These patients are at low risk for genitourinary abnormalities and predictably respond to antibiotics.

Other populations have complicating conditions that increase the risk for acquiring infection or failing therapy. Complicated UTIs may occur in men, children, pregnant women, and elderly or immunocompromised patients. Infections in these groups may be mild or lead to life-threatening urosepsis and may be more difficult to treat if there is a structural or functional genitourinary tract abnormality. Resistant organisms or inadequate host defenses may also complicate treatment.

Urinary tract infection is the most common infectious complication in pregnancy. Bacteriuria in pregnant, as compared to non-pregnant, women has a greater risk of progressing to pyelonephritis (28% vs. 1.4%) and is also associated with premature labor and delivery.[10,11]

While acute, uncomplicated UTI is considered a benign condition, the impact on quality of life is significant. A study by Ellis et. al. compared quality of life scores using the SF-36 index in healthy, community-dwelling women with and without acute UTI. Those with UTI had significantly lower quality-of-life scores, including emotional health, vitality, social functioning, pain, and role limitation.[9]

Pathophysiology of Urinary Tract Infection

The lower urinary tract is equipped with a variety of host defense mechanisms that prevent infection. However, there are certain host susceptibility factors, as well as bacterial virulence factors, that increase the risk of infection.

Host defense mechanisms include the acidic pH of the vagina, which inhibits the growth of enterobacteria and promotes the growth of lactobacilli. Immunoglobulins and high urea concentrations in the urine block bacterial adherence. The Tamm-Horsfall protein produced in the ascending loop of Henle inhibits bacterial adherence.

The normal genitourinary tract is sterile except for the distal urethra. The periurethral area in women is colonized with intestinal flora, some of which are uropathogens. Urination flushes bacteria from the urethral orifice, but occasionally the periurethral organisms ascend and cause infection.

Women are at higher risk for UTI because of shorter urethral length, as well as the proximity of the urethral to the perianal area. The shorter the distance between the anus and urethra, the higher the risk for UTI.[13] Men are usually protected due to the length of urethra and scrotum providing a barrier to the perianal area.

Efficient bladder emptying is needed to prevent stagnation. Bladder emptying may be affected in the presence of pelvic organ prolapse (i.e., cystocele, uterine, or vaginal vault prolapse.)

Urinary tract infection occurs through two primary mechanisms—ascending route, which is the most common, and hematogenous spread, which is uncommon. Bacteria enter the genitourinary tract from the fecal reservoir. Bacteria colonize the periurethral area and ascend through the urethra into the bladder, then up to the kidney, in the case of pyelonephritis. Reflux of urine is not required for ascending infection, although edema associated with cystitis may cause changes at the ureterovesical junction, which results in reflux. Ascent is increased if the bacteria have virulence factors (P-fimbriae of E. coli) that allow increased adhesion.

Host defense mechanisms are important in determining the outcome of vaginal colonization. Susceptibility to UTIs is associated with changes in the adhesive characteristics of epithelial cells.[14] Increased receptivity of epithelial cells for bacteria may have a role in the increased frequency of vaginal colonization observed in UTI-susceptible patients. This increased receptivity may result in increased bacterial adherence. In these cases, UTIs may recur despite spontaneous or pharmacologically induced remissions.

Mucosal epithelial cell-surfaces may be genetically altered, resulting in enhanced bacterial adherence. Women with blood group phenotype Lewis antigen non-secretors, Le(a–b–) and Le(a+b–), have a significantly higher rate of recurrent UTI as compared to Lewis-type secretors. Lewis antigen secretors may be protected as a result of fucosylated structures on the cell surface that reduce the number of receptors for E. coli.[15]

Other risk factors for developing uncomplicated UTI in women include sexual activity and contraceptive use.[16,18] Spermicide use alters vaginal flora, resulting in loss of normal lactobacilli. Diaphragm use independently increases the risk of UTI through a potential obstructive process at the urethra. Increased frequency and recency of sexual intercourse increases risk of UTI.[17] Other identified risk factors for recurrent UTI in young women include having had a first UTI at an age younger than 15 years, as well as a history of UTI in the mother.[18]

Risk factors for uncomplicated UTI in the postmenopausal woman differ. Increased post-void residual volume (as may be seen in women with pelvic organ prolapse), history of previous genitourinary surgery, and estrogen deficiency are all risk factors in this population.

Other behavioral factors such as direction of wiping after voiding, use of baths, frequency of voiding, type of menstrual protection, douching practices, and type of undergarments worn are not risk factors for developing UTI. The practice of voiding soon after intercourse to prevent urinary tract infections is debatable.[7,30]

Cranberry juice to prevent UTIs reduces bacteriuria and pyuria in postmenopausal women and inhibits the adherence of E. coli to uroepithelial cells.[31] Cranberry juice has not been studied in the prevention or treatment of UTIs in younger women.

Bacterial Virulence Factors:
Infection of the urinary tract is related to the ability of bacteria to adhere and colonize in the gut, perineum, urethra, bladder, renal calyces and renal interstitium. Bacterial adherence depends on various factors. Uropathogens, especially enterobacteria, are electronegatively charged and too small to overcome repulsion by the negatively charged urothelial cells. Bacterial attachment relies on fimbriae or other surface adhesion systems, which are hydrophobic and favor adhesion to cell membranes.

The presence of adhesions on bacterial fimbria (pili) and on the bacteria's surface determines its virulence, or ability to cause UTI. Type 1 pili facilitate adherence to vaginal, periurethral, and bladder epithelial cells. P-fimbriae adhere to blood group antigens located on erythrocytes and uroepithelial cells.

Bacterial virulence increases as drug resistance increases. Drug resistance occurs via a plasmid-mediated transfer in uropathogens. Plasmid-mediated resistance has been found for beta-lactams, trimethoprim, sulfonamides and aminoglycosides, but not yet to fluoroquinolones.

Definitions

Urinary tract infection: Infection anywhere along the urinary tract from the urethral meatus to the kidney. Significant quantities of bacteria are present in the urine associated with typical signs and symptoms. Significant bacteriuria, implying infection, is traditionally defined as a urine culture containing greater than 10(5) colony-forming units (CFU) of an organism per milliliter. However, a lower count such as 10(2) may be applied in pregnant women, men, or young women with significant symptoms of dysuria. Urinary tract infections may be defined as those occurring in the lower urinary tract (i.e., urethritis or cystitis) or upper tract (ureteritis, pyelonephritis).

Bacteriuria: Presence of bacteria in the urine, not necessarily implying infection. Bacteriuria is preceded by colonization of the vaginal mucosa and/or periurethral mucosa with the organism responsible for the infection. Cultures obtained from patients between their episodes of bacteriuria showed a higher incidence and a greater density of vaginal colonization with urinary pathogens when compared with similar cultures from women who never had an infection.

Pyuria: Presence of WBC in urine, indicating an inflammatory response to bacteriuria, such as occurs during an infection (symptomatic or asymptomatic), or due to fastidious organisms that do not grow on typical urine culture agar plates. One must also consider contamination from a different source, such as the vagina.

Hematuria: Presence of RBC in urine. Hematuria is common with UTI but not with urethritis or vaginitis. Hematuria does not imply a complicated infection unless it persists after the infection has been cleared.

Urethritis: Inflammation of the urethra, which may or may not be bacterial in origin. The primary symptom is dysuria, but not typically urinary frequency. Urethritis is often associated with sexually transmitted diseases such as gonorrhea, chlamydia, and trichomonas.

Cystitis: Inflammation of the bladder that may be due to infection (bacterial or viral) vs. nonbacterial (chemical, radiation, or interstitial cystitis). Clinical symptoms include urinary urgency, frequency, suprapubic pressure, and dysuria.

Pyelonephritis: Inflammation of the kidney, usually caused by bacterial infection. Clinical symptoms include fever, chills, and flank pain accompanied by bacteriuria and pyuria. Acute nonobstructed pyelonephritis occurs in the same population of women who experience acute uncomplicated cystitis. The bacterial organisms are similar, but may be more virulent.

Uncomplicated UTI: Occurs in patients with intact host defenses and a functionally and structurally normal genitourinary tract.

Complicated UTI: Occurs in patients with congenital or surgically anatomic anomalies, stones, or indwelling catheters. Persons with diabetes; pregnant women; men; those exposed to nosocomial pathogens or who have recently taken antibiotics; those with neurogenic bladders, vesicoureteral reflux, medullary sponge or polycystic kidney; renal transplant patients; those with sickle cell anemia; and those who are chronically immunosuppressed are all at risk for complicated UTI. The prevalence of UTI in HIV-infected patients is 8% to 50%. Low CD-4 counts (less than 200), IV drug use, and antineoplastic and antiretroviral therapy are additional risk factors. Diabetic patients may develop renal and perinephric abscesses, emphysematous cystitis or pyelonephritis, fungal infections, xanthogranulomatous pyelonephritis, and renal papillary necrosis. In diabetes, poor glycemic control, per se, is not a risk factor for recurrent UTIs, but duration of the disease is.

The inability to effectively eradicate bacteria from the urinary tract and the inability for antimicrobials to penetrate or concentrate at the site of bacterial presence are two risk factors for complicated UTI.

Presence of an indwelling transurethral catheter is a risk for complicated UTI. Most are asymptomatic, but bacteremia and septic shock may occur. For short-term use, there is a 5% incidence of infection per day, despite the use of prophylactic antibiotics. Within one month of having an indwelling catheter, all patients will have bacteriuria.[19]

Differentiating between complicated and uncomplicated UTI is important in considering potential morbidity, as well as the type and extent of treatment and evaluation required in the diagnosis. Patients with complicated UTI are more likely to be infected with a broader spectrum of uropathogens and experience higher clinical failure rates when treated with antimicrobial therapy for less than 7 days. Tables 12.1 and 12.2 list the types of microbes associated with uncomplicated and complicated UTIs.

Table 12.1. Microbiology of Uncomplicated Urinary Tract Infections

Most common
Escherichia coli (gram-negative) accounts for 90%
Staphylococcus Saprophyticus (gram positive) accounts for 10–20% in young, sexually active women
Less common (other gram-negative Enterobacteriaceae) account for 5–10%
Klebsiella, Proteus, Enterobacter, Providencia, Morganella, Serratia
Gram positive bacteria: staphylococcus aureus, group B streptococcus, enterococcus

Recurrent UTI: Defined as 3 or more infections over a 1-year period, or 2 occurring within 6 months.

Reinfection represents approximately 95% of recurrent UTIs and refers to a new infection from a point outside the urinary tract following initial successful eradication and sterilization of the urine. The majority of recurrent UTIs are due to reinfection with a new strain or by the same strain from a past infection. Colonic flora is the likely reservoir for reinfecting strains.

Bacterial persistence occurs when a later infection arises from a persistent site within the urinary tract with an identical, previously diagnosed, organism. This may be caused by a structural or anatomic abnormality (i.e., renal calculi), inadequate drug dosage or length of therapy, or bacterial resistance.

Recurrent UTIs are common in those with underlying genitourinary tract abnormalities.

Table 12.2. Microbiology of Complicated Infections *These strains are more resistant to antimicrobial therapy*

Enterobacteriaceae
E. coli (accounts for 20%), Klebsiella, Enterobacter, Proteus, Providencia, Morganella
Other gram-negative organisms
Pseudomonas, Acinetobacter
Gram-positive organisms
Staphylococcus aureus (often hematogenous spread), coagulase-negative staphylococcus (other than Staphylococcus saprophyticus), group B streptococcus, enterococcus, Corynebacterium urealyticum
Yeast
Candida, Torulopsis

Fifty-sixty percent of those individuals with complicated UTIs resulting from underlying GU tract abnormalities will suffer recurrent UTIs within 2 months after treatment unless the underlying abnormality is corrected.

In some women with symptoms of recurrent UTIs, traditional urine cultures may not be positive. Cultures for fastidious organism such as Ureaplasma urealyticum, Mycoplasma hominis and Chlamydia trachomatis should be obtained. Urethral syndrome, trigonitis, or interstitial cystitis must be considered. Women with interstitial cystitis commonly present with symptoms of UTI that include urinary urgency, frequency, hesitancy, and suprapubic or pelvic pain. These patients are often treated empirically with antimicrobial agents and symptoms may improve temporarily, but then return. In this clinical situation, urine cultures should be obtained. When the cultures come back negative, this should lead the clinician into considering interstitial cystitis as a diagnosis.

Asymptomatic bacteriuria: Defined as a significant bacteriuria (greater than 10(5) CFU/mL) in a patient without any clinical symptoms.

Asymptomatic bacteriuria is generally benign in the nonpregnant woman, and prevalence increases with aging. The prevalence is 1% to 2% in school-aged girls, 5% in young, sexually active women, 10% to 15% in postmenopausal, community-dwelling women, and up to 50% of women in long-term care institutions. The more common bacteria in this group are Enterococcus species and coagulase-negative staphylococci. Asymptomatic bacteriuria is not associated with renal failure of hypertension, but these patients are at risk for bacteremia or septic shock if there is trauma to the genitourinary tract mucosa. If instrumentation is planned (i.e., catheterization in preparation for a surgical procedure), then a course of antibiotics is appropriate.

Asymptomatic bacteriuria occurs in approximately 5% to 10% of pregnant women, and 10% to 30% of these women will develop pyelonephritis later on in pregnancy. Acute pyelonephritis is a risk for preterm labor and delivery. It is imperative to identify asymptomatic bacteriuria early in pregnancy, as early treatment may prevent 50% to 80% of pyelonephritis cases.

Asymptomatic urinary tract infection is more common in women with diabetes than in those without, but symptomatic UTI does not differ.

There is a 25% to 50% prevalence of asymptomatic bacteriuria in women in long-term care facilities. The prevalence is the highest in the most functionally impaired, but there is not evidence to suggest that it is harmful.[20] Mortality and urinary incontinence rates are no different in the elderly population with or without asymptomatic bacteriuria.

Microbiology

Ninety percent of uncomplicated urinary tract infections are caused by gram-negative, aerobic bacilli from the Enterobacteriaceae family. Escherichia coli is the single most common and important organism, accounting for approximately 85% of infections. Klebsiella, Enterobacter, Serratia, Proteus, Pseudomonas, Providencia, and Morganella species make up the rest of the gram-negative bacteria. Staphylococcus saprophyticus is the second most common cause of cystitis in sexually active women and accounts for 10% of UTIs in this group of women. In older women, E. coli remains the most common uropathogen, but Proteus mirabilis and Klebsiella pneumoniae account for one third of infections. Pseudomonas aeruginosa infection is usually associated with urinary tract instrumentation. Staphylococcus epidermidis is a nosocomial pathogen often identified in those with indwelling catheters. Staphylococcus aureus is less commonly isolated and is most often associated with hematogenous spread. Other gram-positive organisms such as enterococci and Streptococcus agalactiae cause 3% of lower UTI. Enterococcus faecalis causes 15% of nosocomial infections, and Streptococcus agalactiae is associated with patients with diabetes.

Anaerobic fecal floras rarely cause infection, likely because the oxygen content present in the urine prevents their growth.

Candida species, Torulopsis glabrata, and other fungal organisms can cause UTIs in immunosuppressed patients and those with diabetes or indwelling catheters. Viruses can also cause UTI and gross hematuria and are usually associated with viremia (polyoma or cytomegalovirus).

Clinical Presentation

In otherwise healthy women, symptoms of UTI are typically urinary urgency, frequency, dysuria, and suprapubic discomfort. Generally, fever is not present. Acute, uncomplicated cystitis may be associated with gross hematuria. Occasionally, new-onset urinary urge incontinence may be a symptom. Pyelonephritis is associated with more constitutional symptoms such as fever, chills, nausea, vomiting, and flank pain. Differential diagnosis of urinary tract infection includes urethritis, non-bacterial cystitis (interstitial cystitis) and vaginitis. An algorithm helpful in the evaluation of women with acute dysuria is presented in Figure 12.1.

A history of a sexually transmitted disease, vaginal discharge or odor, pruritus, a partner with urethral symptoms, and no increased urinary frequency suggests urethritis or vaginitis. Pyuria occurs in chlamydial infections. Hematuria is not associated with vaginitis or sexually transmitted diseases, so its presence is usually associated with a UTI. Postmenopausal atrophic vaginitis can present with irritative voiding symptoms. Elderly patients may not manifest the classic symptoms and are more likely to present with gastrointestinal complaints.

Physical examination should include palpation of the abdomen and flank, as well as a pelvic examination if urethritis or vaginitis is suspected.

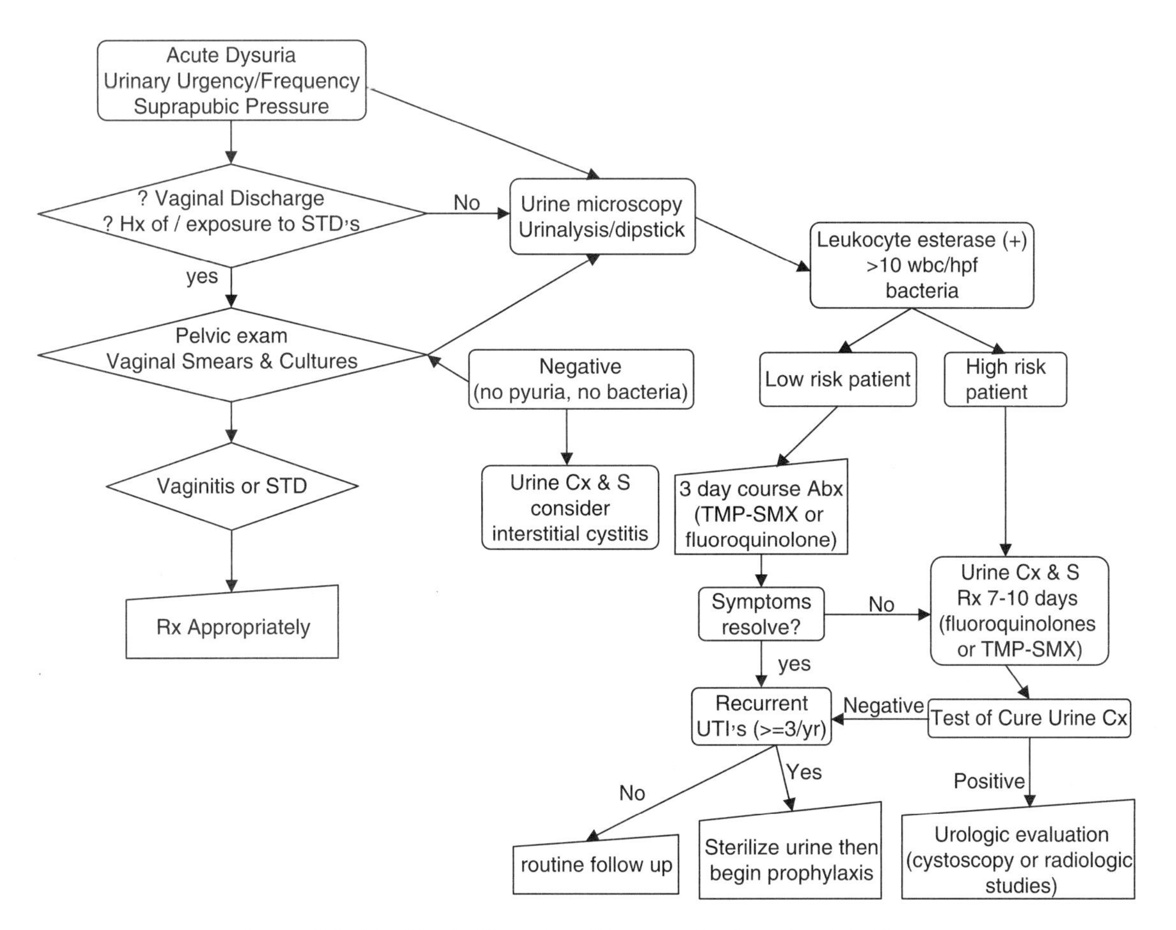

FIGURE 12.1. Algorithm for Diagnosis and Management of Acute Dysuria in Women.

Vaginal/cervical swabs and/or cultures for gonorrhea, chlamydia, trichomonas, and candida should be obtained as appropriate. Palpation of the urethra and anterior vaginal wall may reveal a mass or may result in urethral discharge, consistent with a urethral diverticulum. Costovertebral tenderness is often associated with pyelonephritis, whereas a flank mass may be associated with a perinephric abscess. Post-void residual volume measurement using a bladder scanner or straight catheterization should be obtained in those patients with diabetes, pelvic prolapse, or other neurological condition that may result in incomplete bladder emptying.

Diagnosis

A clean-catch, midstream urine sample should be obtained by instructing the patient to spread the labia and wipe the periurethral area from front to back with moistened towelettes. Obese women or those with physical disabilities may not be able to do this and urethral catheterization may be necessary.

Rapid Diagnostic Tests

Urinalyses by dipstick or microscopy are commonly used rapid screening tests to detect the presence of bacteria, pyuria, and hematuria. The nitrite test is a convenient and cost-effective test that detects the presence of bacteria that convert nitrates to nitrite. It has a sensitivity of 35% to 85% and a specificity of 92% to 100%. Enterococcus, staphylococcus, pseudomonas, and adenovirus, however, are not able to reduce nitrates.

Leukocyte esterase is an enzyme present in white blood cells and, when positive, indicates the presence of neutrophils. A positive test is equivalent to ≥4 WBC/high-power field (hpf). Ninety-six percent of UTIs have ≥10 WBC/hpf. The sensitivity of the leukocyte esterase test is 60% to 95%, with higher sensitivity in bacterial counts greater than 100,000 CFU/mL, and specificity is 94% to 98%. The positive predictive value is 50% and the negative predictive value is 92%.[21,22] Factors affecting the leukocyte count and nitrite test include hydration status (diuretic use). First morning urine collection is ideal.

Urine microscopy of an uncentrifuged urine sample can detect the presence of significant bacteria, leukocytes, and red blood cells. A hemocytometer is used to assess pyuria as defined as more than 10 white blood cells per milliliter of urine. In the absence of pyuria, UTI should be questioned. Gram-stained uncentrifuged urine can detect bacteriuria in over 90% of UTIs with colony counts greater than 100,000 CFU/mL. In cases where urine dipstick testing and microscopy are negative, and clinical suspicion is low urine cultures may be eliminated.

Urine Culture

No urine culture is required before treatment in otherwise healthy young women with typical symptoms of acute cystitis. Urine culture should be obtained in all pregnant and pediatric patients with positive urinalysis and/or high clinical suspicion for UTI. Patients with pyelonephritis and complicated UTI should also have a urine culture. Urine culture also helps to differentiate recurrent from persistent infection. Historically, urine cultures were considered positive when bacterial growth exceeded 100,000 CFU/mL. However, up to 40% of women with symptomatic UTI will have a lower colony count. This may be due to early stage of infection, recent use of antibiotics, time of day specimen is collected, and state of hydration. In symptomatic women, a colony count of 100 CFU/mL is acceptable for diagnosis of a urinary tract infection, with a sensitivity of 95% and specificity of 85%.[23]

Blood Cultures

Blood cultures are not usually indicated, as they have limited usefulness in the management of pyelonephritis in the adult or pregnant population. In high-risk groups, such as the immunosuppressed, pediatric population, or the elderly, blood cultures may be part of the sepsis evaluation.

Imaging Studies

Imaging studies for urinary tract infections have a low yield in otherwise healthy young women with acute or recurrent cystitis or pyelonephritis who respond to antimicrobial therapy. Ultrasound or contrast-enhanced CT scanning may be indicated if obstruction, renal masses, or renal infection is suspected or bacterial persistence occurs. Ultrasound is the preferred test to rule out obstructive disease, whereas CT scan is first choice for evaluating kidney integrity. Non-contrast spiral CT scan is ideal for evaluating nephrolithiasis. Intravenous pyelogram has no role in the evaluation of UTI in adults.

In children, the Technetium 99m labeled dimercaptosuccinic acid (99m Tc-DMSA) renal scan allows for accurate diagnosis of pyelonephritis in an acute febrile urinary tract infection and may reveal the extent of renal parenchymal damage. Voiding cystourethrogram and IVP are helpful in evaluating congenital abnormalities in children.

When a suburethral diverticulum is suspected, cystourethroscopy, double-balloon urethrogram, voiding cystourethrogram, or MRI studies are helpful.

Cystourethroscopy in young, otherwise healthy women does not impact management plans unless a urethral diverticulum is suspected. Cystourethroscopy in older women with recurrent cystitis or hemorrhagic cystitis eliminates the possibility of a bladder/urethral tumor as a cause. In women with a prior history of anti-incontinence surgery, permanent sutures or mesh eroding into the bladder or urethra must be considered as a nidus for recurrent urinary tract infections and may be visualized at the time of cystoscopy.

Urinary Tract Infections in the Elderly Female

Bacteriuria and urinary tract infections are more common in women older than 65 years of age. In the elderly living in nursing homes or long-term care facilities who have indwelling catheters, bacteremia is a significant risk. Risk factors for UTI in the elderly include estrogen deficiency, underlying medical and functional conditions that may cause urinary retention, poor perineal hygiene, and fecal soiling. Table 12.3 lists these risk factors. The most common uropathogen causing UTI in the elderly is E. coli, but is often polymicrobial.

TABLE 12.3. Risk Factors for Urinary Tract Infections in the Elderly

Increased vaginal pH due to decreased vaginal glycogen
Increased periurethral colonization with gram-negative bacteria
Fecal soiling, poor perineal hygiene
Incomplete bladder emptying due to
detrusor hypotonicity
pelvic prolapse
neurogenic bladder (diabetes, Parkinson's disease)
Increased episodes of urinary instrumentation due to increased hospitalizations
Alterations in cellular and immune response to infection
Increased prevalence of confounding medical conditions
diabetes, dementia, CVAs
Presence of indwelling catheters

Asymptomatic bacteriuria occurs in 20% of ambulatory women older than 65 years of age and 50% in those older than 80 years of age.[24] Asymptomatic bacteriuria is not an independent risk factor for increased morbidity or mortality and does not require treatment unless manipulation of the lower urinary tract is planned.[25]

Diagnosing UTI in the elderly is challenging, since many of the typical signs, symptoms, and laboratory data differ in this population. Urinary urgency, frequency, and dysuria may not be present or may be difficult to assess in the cognitively impaired. Malodorous or cloudy urine is not an accurate predictor of UTI. Altered mental state in a patient who is not cognitively impaired at baseline may be an indication of an infection.

The presence of a fever may be delayed, or hypothermia may be present, in those with infection. Studies conflict with respect to fever as a marker for UTI. Alessi et. al. concluded that fever is a sign of infection and antibiotics are warranted.[26] Warren, however, found that some fevers resolve spontaneously without treatment and that administering antibiotics without a clear indication of infection did not improve outcomes in the elderly.[27]

Urosepsis with a change in vital signs, respiratory or gastrointestinal symptoms, and abdominal pain in the presence of bacteriuria is an indication for antibiotic treatment.

Urinary incontinence is prevalent in 50% to 75% of the elderly in long-term care institutions. While new-onset incontinence may be caused by a UTI, chronic incontinence is not altered by sterilizing urine.[28,29]

Treatment of Urinary Tract Infection

Behavioral regimens such as increasing fluid intake and improving hydration may help relieve dysuria symptoms but have never been conclusively studied. Urinary analgesics such as phenazopyridine hydrochloride help relieve burning with urination and may be prescribed at 200 mg PO, tid, for 3 days. Discoloration of the urine occurs that then negates the use of dipstick urinalysis testing.

Antimicrobial therapy selection depends on the expected pathogen in the clinical scenario. Factors that influence choice of antimicrobial agents include efficacy, adverse effects, cost, and dosing interval. Therapy should target uropathogenic bacteria from the urinary tract without affecting the vaginal and fecal flora in order to reduce risk of developing resistant strains or causing yeast vaginitis. The Infectious Disease Society of America (IDSA) developed guidelines for use of antimicrobials in treating UTIs in women.[32] The guidelines for antimicrobial treatment are shown in Table 12.4.

Enterobacter such as E. coli, Proteus mirabilis, Staph saprophyticus, and Klebsiella make up more than 95% of all uropathogens causing UTIs. In a study of over 4000 urine isolates obtained from women with cystitis, nearly all isolates were sensitive to ciprofloxacin and nitrofurantoin. Eighteen percent were resistant to trimethoprim-sulfamethoxazole (TMP-SMX), and 25% were resistant to beta-lactams.[33] The prevalence of TMP-SMX resistant organisms rose from 9% in 1992 to 18% in 1996. Resistance to nitrofurantoin and ciprofloxacin did not change. Resistance of E. coli to TMP-SMX is likely due to its liberal use in treating and prophylaxis of UTIs. Travel to an area where TMP-SMX resistant strains exist may also be a problem. Therefore, the prevalence of resistant organisms in the community as reported by the local health departments must be considered.

Studies reviewed by the IDSA showed that single-dose trimethoprim was less effective than multi-day dosing in eradicating bacteria. Meta-analysis revealed that 3-day therapy vs. 7- to 10-day therapy had similar eradication rates, although a higher recurrence rate with the 3-day course. However, more adverse effects were seen in the 7- to 10-day course.[32]

Beta-lactams are not effective for single-dose therapy. Studies have shown that a 3-day course of amoxicillin had lower eradication rates and higher recurrence rates as compared to a 3-day course of TMP-SMX.[34] Beta-lactams are rapidly excreted, and the time in which they are concentrated in the urine is short. Beta-lactams, in general, are less effective in clearing gram-negative rods from the vaginal and colonic flora, predisposing to recurrence. Beta-lactams, especially amoxicillin, are the drugs of choice for treating Enterococcus faecalis, which is often resistant to TMP-SMX.

Nitrofurantoin is ineffective in the 3-day dosing regimen and must be used for 7 days. Eradication rates are approximately 80% and are lower than with other antimicrobials.[35]

Patients with uncomplicated UTIs who present with typical symptoms of urinary urgency, frequency, dysuria, and suprapubic pain may be treated without a urine culture and sensitivity. The IDSA recommends a 3-day course of TMP-SMX (or TMP) as long as the prevalence of resistant organisms in the community is less than 20%. Otherwise, a 3-day course of a fluoroquinolone (ciprofloxacin 250 mg bid or levofloxacin 250 mg qd) or a 7-day course of nitrofurantoin (100 mg bid) should be first-line. Nitrofurantoin spares the gut flora, thus possibly reducing the risk of developing resistant pathogens. Fluoroquinolones, while effective, are the most expensive and

Table 12.4. Antimicrobial Therapy For Uncomplicated Urinary Tract Infection

1st line therapy	TMP 100–200 mg BID or TMP-SMX double strength BID for 3 days (assuming E. coli resistance <20%)
2nd line therapy	Fluoroquinolones for 3 day course: Ciprofloxacin 250 mg BID Levofloxacin 250 mg qd Norfloxacin 400 mg BID
3rd line therapy	Nitrofurantoin macrocrystals 100 mg BID for 7 days
Other antimicrobials	Aminopenicillins (ampicillin or amoxicillin 250 mg TID for 7 days) (may be used 1st line for Enterococcus if no allergy) Cephalosporins (cephalexin 250–500 mg TID, cefuroxime 250 mg BID)

should not be used as first-line therapy unless there is a high rate of resistance to TMP-SMX.

In the older population, especially in those with high-risk conditions, E. coli remains the most common uropathogen, but Proteus mirabilis and Klebsiella pneumoniae account for one-third of infections. Eradication rates are lower in the elderly. In an uncomplicated UTI in the elderly, a 7- to 10-day course of antimicrobial therapy is indicated. First-line therapy in this group includes fluoroquinolones or TMP-SMX. Adverse effects are lower with fluoroquinolones. Nitrofurantoin requires a creatinine clearance of 40 mL/min.

In the younger population, Staphylococcus saprophyticus is a commonly identified uropathogen. This tends to be eradicated less frequently with a 3-day regimen than with longer therapy, especially with fluoroquinolones. Therefore, a 7-day course of fluoroquinolones should be used in this clinical scenario. Additionally, Proteus mirabilis is often resistant to nitrofurantoin.

Catheter-Related Urinary Tract Infection

Catheter-related UTI accounts for up to 40% of nosocomial infection. Within 5 days, 10% to 25% of catheterized patients become bacteriuric and 4% become bacteremic.[36] Bacteriuria is caused by migration of bacteria into the bladder after colonization by uropathogens along the surface of the catheter. The catheter itself impairs elimination of infected urine. Other complications of long-term catheterization include stone formation, periurethral abscess, bladder fibrosis, fistula formation, and a possible increased risk of bladder cancer.

Preventing infection in those with indwelling catheters requires maintaining a closed system and minimizing duration of catheterization. Breaking the seal to irrigate increases infection risk. Scheduled catheter changes every 2 to 4 weeks may be effective, but is expensive. Suprapubic and intermittent self-catheterization has not been evaluated in controlled trials. Use of disposable collection bags impregnated with an antibacterial polymer does reduce infection.[37] Silver impregnated catheters reduce infection for the first few days of catheterization but have no long-term benefit.[38]

Prophylactic antibiotics are not indicated for catheter use less than 3 days. If use is limited to 2 weeks, TMP-SMX or nitrofurantoin is effective. If catheter usage exceeds 2 weeks, resistant organisms will emerge such that continued antimicrobial therapy is less effective and treatment should be instituted when bacteriuria becomes symptomatic.

Catheter associated UTIs carry significant risk of multi-drug resistant bacteria, especially gram-negative rods. Catheter related UTI requires a 7- to 10-day course of TMP-SMX or fluoroquinolone. If urine culture shows gram-positive organism, amoxicillin/clavulanate is appropriate. Cure rates are lower with nitrofurantoin and beta-lactams.[39]

Methenamine mandelate, vitamin C, long-term antimicrobial suppression, topical urethral antisepsis, disinfection of the collection bag, bladder lavage with acetic acid, and one-way valve-equipped catheters are all ineffective in preventing catheter-associated UTI.

Complicated UTIs increase risk for recurrent, persistent, or resistant infections. Management of these patients includes treatment with a broad-spectrum antibiotic (fluoroquinolone) for 10 to 14 days, based on the results of a urine culture and sensitivity.

Pregnancy

Urinary tract infection is a common problem in pregnancy, leading to increased risk of pyelonephritis and premature labor and delivery. Risk factors for UTI in pregnancy include an antenatal history of UTI, presence of sickle-cell hemoglobin, lower socioeconomic status, sexual activity, anatomic anomalies, and diabetes mellitus.

Antimicrobial therapy in pregnancy includes beta-lactams (amoxicillin, cephalexin, amoxicillin/clavulanate) and nitrofurantoin. The latter should be avoided after the 36th week of pregnancy due to potential hemolysis in the fetus that is G6PD deficient. Trimethoprim sulfamethoxazole (TMP-SMX) is second-line since sulfonamides cross the placenta and can displace bilirubin from plasma-binding sites in the newborn, causing kernicterus. Therefore, use of sulfonamides in the third trimester should be avoided. Pregnant women with UTI should receive a full 7- to 10-day course of antibiotics. Fluoroquinolones are associated with cartilage degeneration and are contraindicated in pregnancy.

Recurrent UTI and Suppressive Antibiotics

Twenty-five percent of women who experience UTIs will develop 3 or more in a year. Recurrent UTI is defined as ≥3 culture-documented infections in a 1-year period, or 2 within 6 months. The pattern of culture-documented recurrences is important in determining subsequent treatment options and who may require further urologic evaluation.

For recurrent UTIs, correct the underlying cause (i.e., surgical relief of an obstruction, estrogenizing atrophic vaginal tissue, or eliminating diaphragm or spermicide use for contraception), if possible.

Prophylactic antibiotic suppression may be used. Once the urine has been sterilized (obtain a "test-of-cure" urine culture 2 weeks after completion of therapy), daily suppression with single-strength TMP-SMX, nitrofurantoin 50 to-100 mg, or ciprofloxacin 250 mg at bedtime for 6 months is an option. Breakthrough infections may still occur and should be treated with a full course of antimicrobial therapy. Once prophylaxis is stopped, 30% to 40% of patients will remain free of infection for the next 6 months.

Post-coital prophylaxis with single-strength TMP/SMX, nitrofurantoin 100 mg, or a fluoroquinolone may be offered to those women whose infections are coitally related.

In selected patients, self-administered standard 3-day therapy is also an option. If the symptoms do not improve within 5 days, a urine culture should be obtained.

Pyelonephritis

Pyelonephritis may present as fever, flank pain, or rigor, in the presence of a positive urinalysis (bacteriuria and pyuria) and culture.

Acute pyelonephritis in otherwise healthy women can be treated with a fluoroquinolone or TMP-SMX (if susceptible) for 10 to 14 days in an outpatient setting. If gram-positive cocci are present on gram stain, coverage for enterococcus (amoxicillin or amoxicillin/clavulanate) should be added.

In pregnant women or those with high-risk factors, hospitalization may be indicated. Intravenous fluoroquinolone should be first-line, or an aminoglycoside with ampicillin added, if enterococcus is present.

Key Summary Points

- In otherwise healthy women, symptoms of UTI are typically urinary urgency, frequency, dysuria, and suprapubic discomfort. Generally, fever is not present. Acute, uncomplicated cystitis may be associated with gross hematuria.
- The nitrite test (on a urine dipstick) detects the presence of bacteria that convert nitrates to nitrite. It has a sensitivity of 35% to 85% and a specificity of 92% to 100%. Enterococcus, staphylococcus, pseudomonas and adenovirus, however, are not able to reduce nitrates.
- Recurrent UTIs increase in frequency with sexual intercourse and advancing age.
- Except in neonates, the prevalence and incidence of UTIs is greater in females by a ratio of 30:1. In neonates and infants, UTI is more common in males and is usually associated with congenital anomalies.
- The periurethral area in women is colonized with intestinal flora.
- Behavioral factors such as direction of wiping after voiding, use of baths, frequency of voiding, type of menstrual protection, douching practices, and type of undergarments worn are not risk factors for developing UTI.
- *Persistent* UTI patterns (in contrast to *recurrent* patterns) generally require more definitive diagnostic testing, to rule out anatomic lesions preventing bacterial clearance. Referral for more formal urogynecologic evaluation should be considered.
- Women with a history of recurrent urinary tract infection *symptoms* who do not improve clinically with antimicrobial therapy should also have urine cultures obtained, as interstitial cystitis may be the underlying condition when cultures reveal no growth.

- If imaging studies are considered, ultrasound is the preferred test to rule out obstructive disease whereas CT scan is first choice for evaluating kidney integrity. Non-contrast spiral CT scan is ideal for evaluating nephrolithiasis. Intravenous pyelogram has no role in the evaluation of UTI in adults.

References

1. Hooton TM, Stamm WE. Diagnosis and treatment of uncomplicated urinary tract infection. *Infect Dis Clin North Am.* 1997:11:551–581.
2. Powers JD. New directions in the diagnosis and therapy of urinary tract infections. *Am J Obstet Gynecol.* 1991:164:1387–1389.
3. Patton JP, Nash DB, Abrutyn E. Urinary tract infection: Economic considerations. *Med Clin North Am.* 1991;75:495–513.
4. Johnson JR, Stamm WE. Urinary tract infection in women: diagnosis and treatment. *Ann Intern Med.* 1989;111:906–917.
5. Barnett BJ, Stephens DS. Urinary tract infection: An overview. *Am J Med Sci.* 1997;314:245–249.
6. Stamm WE, Hooton TM. Management of urinary tract infection in adults. *N Engl J Med.* 1993; 329:1328–1334.
7. Hooton TM, Scholes D, Hughes JP et al. A prospective study of risk factors for symptomatic urinary tract infection in young women. *N Engl J Med.* 1996; 335:468–474.
8. Gillenwater JY, Harrison RB, Kunin CM. Natural history of bacteriuria in schoolgirls: A long-term case-control study. *N Engl J Med.* 1979;301:369–371.
9. Ellis AK, Verma S. Quality of Life in women with urinary tract infections: is benign disease a misnomer? *J Am Board Fam Pract.* 2000;13(6):392–397.
10. Maranchie JK, Capelouto CC, Loughlin KR. urinary tract infection during pregnancy. *Infect Urol.* 1997; 10:152–157.
11. Connolly A, Thorp JM Jr. Urinary tract infection in pregnancy. *Urol Clin North Am.* 1999;26:779–787.
12. Klutke JJ, Bergman A. Hormonal influence on the urinary tract. *Urol Clin North Am.* 1995;22:629–639.
13. Hooton TM, Stapleton AE, Roberts PL, et al. Perineal anatomy and urine-voiding characteristics of young women with and without recurrent urinary tract infections. *Clin Infect Dis.* 1999;29:1600–1601.
14. Schaeffer AJ, Jones JM, Dunn JK. Association of vitro Escherichia coli adherence to vaginal and buccal epithelial cells with susceptibility of women to recurrent urinary-tract infections. *N Engl J Med.* 1981;304:1062–1066.
15. Sheinfeld J, Schaeffer AJ, Cordon-Cardo C, Rogatko A, Fair WR. Association of the Lewis blood-group phenotype with recurrent urinary tract infections in women. *N Engl J Med.* 1989;320:773–777.
16. Foxman B. Recurring urinary tract infection: incidence and risk factors. *Am J Public Health.* 1990;80:331–333.
17. Gupta K, Hillier SL, Hooton TM, Roberts PL, Stamm WE. Effects of contraceptive method on the vaginal microbial flora: a prospective evaluation. *J Infec Dis.* 2000;181:595–601.
18. Scholes D, Hooton TM, Roberts PL, Stapleton AE, Gupta K, Stamm WE. Risk factors for recurrent urinary tract infections in young women. *J Infec Dis.* 2000;182:1177–1182.
19. Warren JW. Catheter-associated urinary tract infections. *Infect Dis Clin North Am.* 1997;11:609–622.
20. Nicolle LE. Asymptomatic bacteriuria in the elderly. *Infect Dis Clin North Am.* 1997;11:647–662.
21. Pollock HM. Laboratory rechniques for detection of urinary tract infection and assessment of value. *Am J Med.* 1983;75:79–84.
22. Kusumi RK, Grover PG, Kumin LM. Rapid detection of pyuria by leukocyte esterase activity. *JAMA.* 1981;245:1653–1655.
23. Stamm WE, Counts GW, Running KR, Fihn S, Turck M, Holmes KK. Diagnosis of coliform infection in acutely dysuric women. *N Engl J Med.* 1982;307:463–468.
24. Baldassare JS, Kaye D. Special problems of urinary tract infection in the elderly. *Med Clin North Am.* 1991;75:375–390.
25. Abrutyn E, Mossey J, Berlin JA et al. Does asymptomatic bacteriuria predict mortality and does antimicrobial treatment reduce mortality in elderly ambulatory women? *Annals Intern Med.* 1994;120: 827–833.
26. Alessi CA, Harker JO. A prospective study of acute illness in the nursing home. *Aging (Milano).* 1998;10:479–489.
27. Warren JW, Palumbo FB, Fitterman L, Speedie SM. Incidence and characteristics of antibiotic use in aged nursing home residents. *J of Am Geriat Soc.* 1991;39:963–969.
28. Ouslander JG, Shapira M, Schnelle JF, Fingold S. Pyuria among chronically incontinent but otherwise asymptomatic nursing home residents. *J of Am Geriat Soc.* 1996;44:420–423.

29. Ouslander JG, Shapira M, Schnelle JG et al. Does eradicating bacteriuria affect the severity of chronic urinary incontiennce in nursing home residents? *Ann Intern Med.* 1995;122:749–754.
30. Strom BL, Collins M, West SL, Kreisberg J, Weller S. Sexual activity, contraceptive use, and other risk factors for asymptomatic and symptomatic bacteriuria. A case-control study. *Ann Intern Med.* 1987;107:816–823.
31. Avorn J, Monane M, Gurwitz JH, Glynn RJ, Choodnovskiy I, Lipsitz LA. Reduction of bacteriuria and pyuria after ingestion of cranberry juice. *JAMA.* 1994;271:751–754.
32. Warren JW, Abrutyn E, Hebel JR, Johnson JR, Schaeffer AJ, Stamm WE. Guidelines for antimicrobial treatment of uncomplicated acute bacterial cystitis and pyelonephritis in women. *Clin Infec Dis.* 1999;29:745–758.
33. Gupta K, Scholes D, Stamm WE. Increasing prevalence of antimicrobial resistance among uropathogens causing acute uncomplicated cystitis in women. *JAMA.* 1999;281:736–738.
34. Hooton TM, Winter C, Tiu F, Stamm WE. Randomized comparative trial and cost analysis of 3-day antimicrobial regimens for treatment of acute cystitis in women. *JAMA.* 1995;273:41–45.
35. Spencer RC, Moseley DJ, Greensmith MJ. Nitrofurantoin modified release versus trimethoprim or co-trimoxazole in the treatment of uncomplicated urinary tract infection in general practice. *J Antimicrob Chemother.* 1994;33:121.
36. Stamm WE. Catheter-associated urinary tract infections: epidemiology, pathogenesis, and prevention. *Am J Med.* 1991;91:65S–71S.
37. Hardyck C, Petrinovich L. Reducing urinary tract infections in catheterized patients. *Ostomy Wound Manage.* 1998;44:36–43.
38. Verleyen P, De Ridder D, Van Poppel H, Baert L. Clinical application of the Bardex IC Foley catheter. *Eur Urol.* 1999;36:240–246.
39. Brumfitt W, Hamilton-Miller JM. Efficacy and safety profile of long-term nitrofurantoin in urinary infections: 18 years' experience. *J Antimicrob Chemother.* 1998;42:363–371.
40. Wing DA, Hendershutt CM, Debuque L, Millar LK. A randomized trial of three antibiotic regimens for the treatment of pyelonephritis in pregnancy. *Obstet Gynecol.* 1998;92:249–253.

13
Interstitial Cystitis and Pelvic Pain: Understanding and Treating at the Primary Care Level

Deborah L. Myers

Introduction

Chronic pelvic pain is defined as pain in the pelvis of greater than six months' duration. It is estimated that 3.8% of women aged 15–73 have chronic pelvic pain which is more common than asthma or migraines.[1] Chronic pelvic pain directly costs society $880 million dollars per year.[2] It has been reported that approximately 10% of visits to the gynecologist, 20% to 40% of gynecologic diagnostic laparoscopies, and 12% to 20% of hysterectomies performed are for complaints of chronic pelvic pain.[3] Primary care providers will often be presented with these complaints from their female patients and can play a vital role in recognizing and treating this important women's health condition.

The diagnosis of chronic pelvic pain can be challenging, as the differential diagnosis encompasses more than one organ system and many symptoms overlap from one system to the other. As one views the female pelvis, it is evident that the pelvis is comprised of the bones and joints, muscles and ligaments, and contains three organ systems—the urologic, the gynecologic and the gastrointestinal systems. The anatomic juxtaposition of all these structures—musculoskeletal, urinary, reproductive and gastrointestinal systems—reminds the practitioner that any disease process that causes pain of one system can refer symptoms to another. Beyond the pelvis, neurotransmitters and neuromodulating substances of the brain and nervous system implicated in pain perception also account for the psychological factors that so often accompany patients with chronic pelvic pain.

The pelvic floor is innervated from sacral nerve roots S2, S3, and S4. These nerve roots include motor/efferent pathways and sensory/afferent pathways of both the somatic and visceral systems. This common innervation of the pelvis accounts for many of the overlapping symptoms. In the somatic system, the motor/efferent pathway of the somatic system innervates the pelvic floor and the perineal muscles, and the sensory/afferent pathways transmit mechanical, thermal, and chemical stimuli from the perineum, pelvic floor, and pelvic peritoneum.[4] In the visceral system, the motor/efferent pathways include both parasympathetic and sympathetic nerves of the organs, and the sensory/afferent pathways transmit information of noxious stimuli of the organs through the sympathetic system. Thus, it is not surprising that when one of the organs or muscles of the pelvis becomes diseased, the other pelvic organ/muscle systems are stimulated; diseases of the pelvic organs tend to have symptoms that mimic each other.

There are common embryologic origins of the pelvic organ systems that also contribute to the overlap of symptoms found in women with chronic pelvic pain. The urinary system and the reproductive system both develop from the intermediate mesoderm of the embryo called the urogenital ridge. The intermediate mesoderm that ultimately forms the bladder trigone is the same epithelium that forms the lower one-third of the vagina and vestibule.[5] Consequently, conditions that affect the bladder may produce vaginal/vulvar symptoms and vice versa.

It is also known that hormones affect both the gynecological and urinary tracts. Estrogen receptors have been found in the bladder trigone,[6] as have LH and HCG receptors.[7] There is also clinical evidence that chronic medical conditions such as migraine, epilepsy, asthma, and irritable bowel syndrome are exacerbated during the menstrual cycle. Estrogen and progesterone receptors are also known to affect bowel physiology.[8]

There are also known associations between chronic pelvic pain and history of psychosexual trauma and psychiatric disorders. Neuromodulators can affect the release and metabolism of neurotransmitters, thus affecting the perception of pain. Substance P, glutamate, and vasoactive intestinal peptide are excitatory substances. Endogenous opioid peptides, norepinephrine, serotonin (5-HT), and GABA (gamma amino butyric acid) are inhibitory. Current research in the neurobiology suggests that depression may be due to a deficit of GABA in association with depression.[9] Thus it is not surprising that perception of pain may be different in those who are depressed.

Goals of Diagnosis and Treatment

Often the clinician is faced with the challenge of determining whether or not the patient's pain is due to a physical or psychological disorder. It is important to recognize that both causes may coexist. However, all causes affecting the patient's pain need to be addressed; thus, whether or not psychological causes are primary or secondary becomes a non-issue. It is also important for the primary physician taking care of the patient to set realistic expectations of diagnosis and treatment for the patient. The primary care physician should explain to the patient that the cause of her pain may or may not be determined and that her pain most likely will not be "cured" but rather, "managed". The goals of treatment should be (1) relieving severe pain; (2) restoring the patient to daily living; (3) improving her family and spousal relationships and quality of life; (4) preventing relapse to severe pain with the patient's commitment to treatment regiments, be they physical or psychological; and (5) explaining to the patient that the process will be ongoing and long-term.

Differential Diagnosis and Treatment

A comprehensive list of the causes of chronic pelvic pain is presented in Table 13.1. This discussion, however, will be limited to the more common diagnoses encountered in the primary care setting. Conditions of the musculoskeletal systems (levator ani myalgia, abdominal wall trigger points, postural problems), gastrointestinal system (irritable bowel disease), the reproductive system (endometriosis, pelvic inflammatory disease, pelvic adhesions, vulvodynia and pudendal neuralgia), and the genitourinary system (interstitial cystitis) will be discussed. The influence of psychological factors is also addressed.

Pain of Musculoskeletal Origin

Abdominal Wall

Referred pain from the abdominal wall can cause pelvic pain. Cyriax, in 1919, first described that

TABLE 13.1. Differential Diagnosis of Chronic Pelvic Pain

Musculoskeletal
Abdominal wall Levator ani myalgia
Gastrointestinal
Diverticulitis Irritable bowel syndrome Malignancy
Adhesive disease Gynecologic
Endometriosis Pelvic inflammatory disease Pelvic adhesions Vulvodynia Pudendal neuralgia
Psychological Urologic
Interstitial cystitis Bladder stones Malignancy Radiation therapy to bladder

abdominal wall pain can originate from structures other than the abdominal viscera.[10] Carnett, in 1926, described a diagnostic maneuver (the Carnett test) that involves palpating the abdomen while the person tenses the abdominal wall by raising either the legs or head while supine.[11] If, while palpating the painful area, the pain is increased, then the pain is likely to be from the abdominal wall and not the viscera. Conditions such as nerve entrapment, inflammation of an intercostal nerve root or anterior cutaneous nerve, rib tip syndrome, myofascial pain, trigger points, and hernias may be among the sources. One can further confirm the pain is from the abdominal wall by injecting the area with a local anesthetic, such as 2 ml to 3 ml of 2.5% bupivacaine. If the pain is abolished, then the pain is most likely due to neuralgia. In women who have had prior pelvic surgery, entrapment of the ilioinguinal (L1), genitofemoral (L1, L2) or iliohypogastric (T12, L1) nerves in the lower abdominal scar can occur. Entrapment of these nerves will cause pain in the lower abdomen and the inner thighs.[12] Hernias in various sites—inguinal, femoral, umbilical, incisional, Spigelian line (lateral border of the rectus muscle), sciatic, obturator canal or perineum—may also cause chronic pain. Ultrasound or MRI may aid in the diagnosis, and muscle strengthening and/or surgical treatment is indicated.

Levator Ani Myalgia

Levator ani myalgia is a condition that can represent a cause of chronic pelvic pain or result from chronic pain originating from another source. The levator ani muscle is comprised of three muscle groups—puborectalis, pubococcygeus, and iliococcygeus. Patients who have chronic disease processes of the gastrointestinal, reproductive, or urinary systems can develop spasm of the levator ani and other pelvic floor muscles as a secondary problem. The low back (Iliopsoas, quadratus lumborum), sacroiliac region, external muscles of the pelvic girdle (piriformis muscle), and internal muscles of the pelvis (obturator internus muscle) can be involved. Women with chronic pelvic pain will often develop faulty posture typically characterized by persistent lumbar lordosis and a forward pelvic tilt.[13] The muscles of the back can be assessed externally and the muscles of the pelvis assessed internally by intravaginal palpation. These muscles should be assessed bilaterally, as unilateral abnormalities can be detected. The bulk of the muscle, defects in the muscle, and trigger points can be determined. Pelvic examination of the internal muscles will reveal a tight pelvic floor; yet most women will, surprisingly, demonstrate a weak pelvic muscle contraction or Kegel squeeze, as the pelvic muscles are already contracted and thus cannot be contracted any further. Women with difficulty relaxing their pelvic muscles may also have dysfunctional voiding, urinary urgency and frequency, or constipation and defecatory dysfunction. Women with levator myalgia will often have a history of frequent prolonged periods of unilateral standing or sitting, inactive lifestyles, and sleeping on the side or stomach.[13] Referral to a physical therapist who has special training in treatment of pelvic floor disorders is ideal. Treatment will often include a series of exercises, myofascial release, and biofeedback/electrical stimulation to rehabilitate the pelvic floor muscles.

Pain of Gastrointestinal Origin

Benign or/malignant colorectal tumors, colitis, diverticular disease, and irritable bowel syndrome can all cause abdominal/pelvic pain. Irritable bowel syndrome is a poorly understood condition of the gastrointestinal tract characterized by abdominal pain, bloating, and alternating constipation and diarrhea. It is a functional disorder that predominates in women more than men, often beginning in the late teen years.[14] Its etiology is unknown. Women will often complain of a flare-up of symptoms premenstrually, which may be related to the abrupt decrease of progesterone.[15] Women with irritable bowel syndrome may also complain of painful intercourse. The common term "spastic colitis" is not accurate, as irritable bowel syndrome is not characterized by inflammation. Patients with irritable bowel syndrome can be categorized into three groups: (1) abdominal pain, gas and bloating, (2) diarrhea dominant and (3) constipation dominant. The Rome II criteria in diagnosis of irritable bowel include 2 of the 3 features present for 12 weeks within the past year. The three features are (1) pain relieved following defecation, (2) onset of pain associated with change in stool frequency, and (3) onset of change associated with change in stool appearance. These criteria are supported by abnormal stool form, abnormal stool passage, passage of mucus, and bloating.[16] Diagnosis is made by history, physical exam, and diagnostic testing, depending upon the level of suspicion, to rule out other gastrointestinal conditions. Thus, diagnosis may require food diaries, lactose intolerance tests, sigmoidoscopy, barium enema, or abdominal ultrasound and/or CT scan. Referral to a gastroenterologist or surgeon for colonoscopy may be necessary. Treatment encompasses dietary changes that may include elimination or restriction of lactose, sorbitol, carbonated beverages, fructose, and caffeine. Medications include bulking agents (psyllium), osmotic laxatives (polyethylene glycol), antispasmodics (dicyclomine, hyoscyamine), antidiarrheal agents (loperamide, atropine/diphenoxylate), and tricyclic antidepressants. Newer medications Paroxetine, an SSRI, Tegaserod, a serotonin 5-HT4 agonist (for constipation dominant), and Alosetron, a serotonin 5-HT3 antagonist that requires a special license to prescribe (for diarrhea dominant) also show promise. Interestingly, preliminary research has shown an improvement of symptoms when these patients are treated with GnRH agonists.[17]

Pain of Gynecologic Origin

Pain in the pelvis can be due a variety of gynecological disorders. One must consider benign or malignant tumors, endometriosis, pelvic adhesions in women with prior pelvic surgery or infection, and chronic pelvic inflammatory diseases. Careful pelvic examination, pelvic ultrasound/CT scan and laparoscopy/pelviscopy will help to delineate these conditions. Pelvic masses will need to be evaluated for malignancy.

Endometriosis

Endometriosis is a condition of the female reproductive tract in which functioning endometrial tissue is outside the uterine cavity. The symptoms of endometriosis are typically those of chronic cyclic pelvic pain, occurring before and during the menses, but pain can also occur on a daily basis. Women can also have associated complaints of urinary frequency. Dyspareunia and infertility are often presenting complaints. Endometriosis occurs in 5% to 15% of women of reproductive age and can be a cause of infertility at a rate of 38%.[18] Endometrial implants are most frequently found along the posterior cul-de-sac and uterosacral ligaments at a rate of 69% which can lead to complaints of dyspareunia.[19] Implants can also be found on the appendix, bowel, and in the bladder.

There are findings on pelvic examination that suggest endometriosis. Nodular implants can be palpated on the uterosacral ligaments rectovaginally. The uterus may be scarred and fixed to the posterior cul-de-sac or lateral pelvic walls. Ultrasound may be helpful in suggesting the diagnosis by showing the presence of ovarian endometrioma. The definitive diagnosis of endometriosis is made by pelviscopy with biopsy of peritoneal lesions; thus, referral to a gynecologist may be necessary. There are reports that advocate the empiric use of Lupron (Tap Pharmaceutical Inc., Lake Forest, IL) therapy in patients with pelvic pain to aid in the diagnosis of endometriosis. If relief of symptoms occurs after administration of Lupron, then the diagnosis of endometriosis may be inferred. Contraindications for empiric therapy include undiagnosed uterine bleeding, pelvic masses, and suspicion of pregnancy.

The treatment of endometriosis is directed at suppressing the hormonal implants and promoting shrinkage of existing ones. Oral contraceptives, used either in cyclic or continuous fashion, and nonsteroidal anti-inflammatory medications have proven effective in reducing symptoms.[17] Lupron can be also be used for short-term treatment. In the 1980s, an androgenic agent, Danazol, was popular in treatment of endometriosis, but is no longer commonly used since the introduction of the GnRH agonists. Surgical treatment of endometriosis will depend on the woman's desire for pregnancy. If a woman plans future childbearing, then conservative therapy such as cauterization, laser vaporization, or excision of implants can be performed.[20] This is often followed by hormonal therapy with either a GnRH agonist or oral contraceptive pills to further suppress development of endometrial implants. Definitive therapy for endometriosis is hysterectomy with bilateral salpingo-oophorectomy. This radical surgical intervention would be performed if a woman has completed childbearing or has failed prior conservative surgical/medical treatment. However, it has been found that even after adequate treatment of endometriosis, problems of pelvic pain persist or recur, despite the resolution of the endometriosis. For the relief of pelvic pain, overall success rates resulting from medical treatment are roughly the same as after surgical treatment. Therefore, the decision to proceed with surgery should be highly individualized, and patients should be carefully counseled with respect to goals and expectations.[21]

Pelvic Inflammatory Disease

Women with acute pelvic inflammatory disease will have more obvious clinical signs of infection, such as cervical motion tenderness, fever, elevated white count; and an elevated sedimentation rate. Wet preparation of the vagina reveals white cells. Treatment for pelvic inflammatory disease is directed at the use of appropriate antibiotics, whether prescribed for inpatient or outpatient therapy.

Women with chronic ("subacute") pelvic inflammatory disease, on the other hand, may have only complaints of chronic pain unassociated with systemic signs of illness. To aid in diagnosis, DNA probes/cultures can be done to detect Gonorrhea and Chlamydia. An endometrial biopsy to look for plasma cells and confirm endometritis, or a diagnostic pelviscopy to look for pelvic adhesive disease or inflammatory changes of the pelvis, may be needed.[22] Chronic pelvic inflammatory disease may require long-term antibiotics (doxycycline, clindamycin, ceftriaxone) or, ultimately, hysterectomy.

Pelvic Adhesions

Pelvic adhesive disease is a potential cause of pelvic pain and may result from pelvic inflammatory disease, endometriosis, ruptured appendicitis, and diverticulitis. Thus, in a patient who complains of chronic pelvic pain, obtaining prior surgical reports to review for presence of adhesions can be useful. Treatment of adhesions by lysis is problematic since adhesions can simply reoccur. Howard et al. performed laparoscopic pain mapping under conscious sedation to determine whether adhesions were the cause of patients' pain.[23] Adhesions were the source of pain in approximately 50% of patients who were successfully mapped. After lysis of adhesions, immediate relief can be obtained; but within 4 months, it is common for symptoms to recur. Patients with dense intestinal adhesions, however, may experience significant reduction of pain for a longer period of time after adhesiolysis.

Vulvodynia

Vulvodynia is defined as a condition of chronic vulvar discomfort with symptoms of burning, stinging, irritation, and rawness whose symptoms are usually confined to the vulva, but can be perceived by the patient as pelvic pain. It predominates in white women (97%) as well as nulliparous women (62%). The mean age of patients is 32 years with a range of 11–75 years.[24] Vulvodynia can be grouped into five syndromes: cyclic vulvitis, vulvar dermatoses, vulvar papillomatosis, vulvar vestibulitis, and essential "dysesthetic" syndrome. All of these conditions can cause painful intercourse—a common complaint in women with chronic pelvic pain—but essential dysesthetic vulvodynia is the subtype that is characterized by chronic pain. Patients with essential vulvodynia describe a constant or intermittent superficial burning pain as well as urethral and/or rectal discomfort; these symptoms occur even without intercourse or contact with the vulva. Patients have symptoms similar to those seen in neuralgia. Patients can have pain with light touch (allodynia), paroxysmal stabbing pains, and hyperesthesias. Causes of neuralgia in the vulva or pelvis include prior pelvic or back surgery, back pain, cycling or horseback riding injuries, muscle spasm, or multiple sclerosis.

Essential dysesthetic vulvodynia is characterized by the lack of physical findings seen in the other subtypes. A careful examination of the vestibule to Hart's line is essential in diagnosing these subtypes. Hart's line is defined as the point where the edge of the outer vestibule meets the squamous epithelium of the vulvar skin

(Figure 13.1). Using a moistened cotton swab, the vestibule is carefully examined out to Hart's line, looking for pinpoint painful areas and red irritated vestibular glands of the hymenal ring. In vestibulitis, the Skene's glands, posterior fourchette, minor vestibular glands and the Bartholin's glands are often tender. If needed, a dilute solution of acidic acid can be applied with a 4 × 4 gauze to the perineum to highlight abnormal areas. Colposcopy of the vulva and vestibule may be helpful in diagnosing these conditions; referral to a gynecologist will be needed. Abnormal areas should be biopsied to rule out vulvar intraepithelial neoplasia. Often these patients have already seen many other physicians and are applying various creams and using other local measures. The provider may need to have the patient stop all treatment regimens, allow the patient a "drug holiday" with a return to baseline symptoms, and then repeat the assessment and physical examination. In essential vulvodynia, there will be pain over the entire vulva and allodynia. Careful neurologic examination of the low back, lower extremities, spinal X-rays, and MRI may all be necessary.

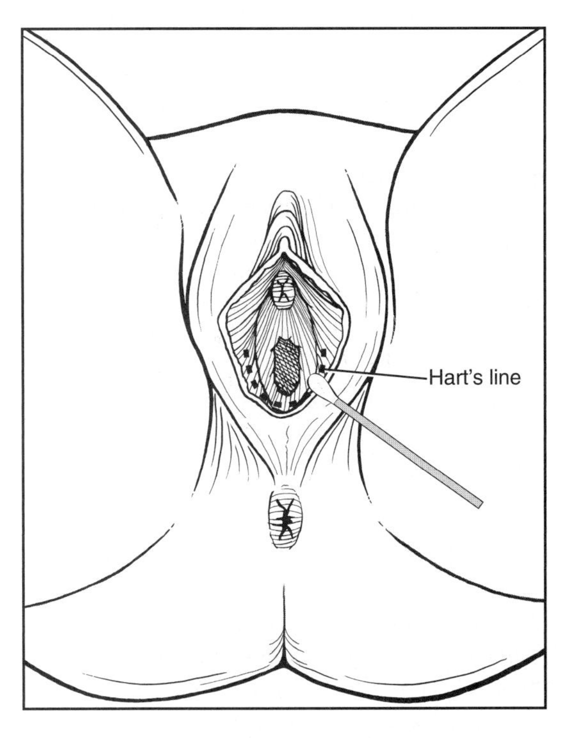

Figure 13.1. Vestibule examination using a cotton swab.

Treatment will be directed at the underlying cause if found. Self-help measures can be instituted for these patients. Recommendations for women are to wear loose clothing, void while cool water is poured over the perineum, use mild soaps for bathing, double rinse their laundry to thoroughly remove any detergent, and avoid self-applied black hair coloring dyes in the shower, as the dye rinses over the perineal skin. A hair blow dryer on a cool setting is recommended to remove moisture from the vulvar region. Dietary changes have been recommended that involve a low calcium oxalate diet and supplementation with calcium citrate.[25]

Topical anesthetics such as Xylocaine jelly can be applied to the perineum for reduction of pain. Medications used for neuropathic pain such as Nortriptyline, Amitriptyline (25 mg to 75 mg QHS), Gabapentin, or Carbamazepine can reduce pain.[26] These medications change the pain threshold, thereby reducing symptoms of burning.[27] Surgical procedures should be limited in these patients. Referral to a pain clinic may be needed for challenging patients.

Pudendal Neuralgia

Another cause of chronic pelvic pain is neuralgia of the pudendal nerve caused by herpes virus. Diagnosis will be based upon a history of herpes type-II infections. Acute herpetic lesions and outbreaks are characteristically found on the vulva and appear as a painful blister; diagnosis is made by culture. The initial infection is often the most severe and can be associated with fever, lymphadenopathy, urinary burning, and difficulty voiding. Recurrent outbreaks are usually less acute and are common just prior to menses. Recurrent outbreaks often have a prodromal syndrome, with paresthesias resulting from the virus harboring in the dorsal nerve root ganglion. If the herpes virus should invade the pudendal nerve, pudendal neuralgia can develop. For patients with recurrent outbreaks or pudendal neuralgia, antiviral agents such as acyclovir, valacyclovir, and famciclovir can be used in suppression therapy. The time course of the outbreak may be shortened by using a variety of anti-viral agents.[28]

Pain of Psychological Origin

Chronic pelvic pain can be of psychological origin, but whether or not the patient has a psychological disorder, the clinician is obligated to rule out physical causes of chronic pelvic pain. Several studies have looked at the psychological profiles of patients with complaints of chronic pelvic pain and have demonstrated an increased incidence of psychiatric disorders and history of abuse and sexual assault.[3] Conversely—and not surprisingly—chronic debilitating pain can lead to depression, anxiety, and domestic and marital discord. It has also been shown that neurotransmitters of depression, anxiety, and psychological states affect the neurotransmitters of pain syndromes. Medications (tricyclics, GABA-ergic and serotonin reuptake inhibitors) that increase the inhibitory neuromodulators are useful for treatment. It is reported that 50% of chronic pelvic pain patients have depression.[3] Diagnosis and treatment of depression should not be overlooked; if ignored, the management of the underlying disorder of the pain will not be as successful. Untreated depression may promote the patient to obtain secondary gain from the office visit and the provider; pain will persist even after the pain stimulus has resolved.[29]

Pain of Urologic Origin

Interstitial Cystitis

Painful bladder syndrome can result from a number of etiologies including interstitial cystitis, tuberculosis, stones, malignancy, previous chemotherapy of the bladder, and pelvic irradiation. Interstitial cystitis is a chronic condition of urinary urgency, frequency, and suprapubic pain in the absence of bacteruria. It often represents a diagnosis of exclusion when no known cause of painful bladder can be identified.

Interstitial cystitis is a great impersonator of gynecologic conditions and can easily be misdiagnosed. Within gynecological practices it is estimated that approximately 38% to 85% of women with chronic pelvic pain may actually have interstitial cystitis.[30,31] It affects more women than men, in a ratio of 9:1. The average age for a woman to be diagnosed is 40–46 years, with an age range of 30–50 years.[32,33] Currently, two integrated theories—(1) "leaky glycosaminoglycan layer-epithelium" and (2) "neurogenic up-regulation", involving mast cell release of vasoactive substances (histamines and substance P)—are proposed to explain the pathogenesis of interstitial cystitis.

Patients with interstitial cystitis complain of urinary frequency (>8 voids during the day), nocturia (>2 voids during sleep) and either cyclic or constant pelvic pain.[29] Patients, during flare-ups, may complain of voiding every 30 minutes. Patients can complain of difficulty voiding and post-void fullness. Symptoms are often increased with intercourse and near the menses.[34] Some patients may report exacerbation of symptoms with certain foods and beverages such as coffee, alcohol, citrus fruits, tomatoes, and chocolate (see Table 13.2). Questionnaires have been developed to improve screening of patients with symptoms of urinary frequency, urgency, and pain. O'Leary et al. in 1997 developed two validated self-administered questionnaires to monitor symptoms[35] (Figure 13.2). Parsons et al. developed the PUF (pelvic pain and urgency/frequency) questionnaire as another tool to detect interstitial cystitis[36] (Figure 13.3).

Table 13.2. Dietary Irritants to Avoid

All alcoholic beverages
Apples
Apple juice
Cantaloupes
Carbonated drinks
Chili,
Spicy foods
Citrus fruits (lemons, limes, oranges, etc.)
Coffee
Cranberries
Grapes
Guava
Lemon juice
Peaches
Pineapple
Plums
Strawberries
Tea
Tomatoes
Vinegar

Adapted from Gillespie L. *You don't have to live with cystitis.* New York: Avon, 1988:241–258.

Interstitial Cystitis Symptom Index	Interstitial Cystitis Problem Index During the past month, how much has each of the following been a problem for you?
Q1.During the past month, how often have you felt the strong need to urinate with little or no warning? 0.___not at all 1.___less than 1 time in 5 2.___less than half the time 3.___about half the time 4.___more than half the time 5.___almost always	Q1. Frequent urination during the day? 0.___no problem 1.___very small problem 2.___small problem 3.___medium problem 4.___big problem
Q2. During the past month, have you had to urinate less than 2 hours after you finished urinating? 0.___not at all 1.___less than 1 time in 5 2.___less than half the time 3.___about half the time 4.___more than half the time 5.___almost always	Q2. Getting up at night? 0.___no problem 1.___very small problem 2.___small problem 3.___medium problem 4.___big problem
Q3. During the past month, how often did you most typically get up at night to urinate? 0.___none 1.___once 2.___2 times 3.___3 times 4.___4 times 5.___5 or more times	Q3. Need to urinate with little warning? 0.___no problem 1.___very small problem 2.___small problem 3.___medium problem 4.___big problem
Q4. During the past month, have you experienced pain or burning in your bladder? 0.___not at all 2.___a few times 3.___almost always 4.___fairly often 5.___usually	Q4. Burning pain, discomfort, or pressure in your bladder? 0.___no problem 1.___very small problem 2.___small problem 3.___medium problem 4.___big problem
Add the numerical values of the checked entries; total score:__________	Add the numerical values of the checked entries; total score:__________

O'Leary MP, Sant GR, Fowler FJ, Whitmore KE et al. The interstitial cystitis symptom and problem index Urology;49(suppl 5A), May 1997

FIGURE 13.2. The O'Leary validated, self-administered IC questionnaires to monitor symptoms.

Physical examination in a patient with interstitial cystitis often reveals few specific findings. The suprapubic tubercle or sacroiliac joints may be tender. Pelvic examination may reveal tenderness of the bladder or urethra or tender "trigger points" along the levator muscles. Pelvic examination will serve primarily to evaluate and rule out other causes of urinary urgency, frequency, and pelvic pain such as urethral diverticula, bladder stones, malignancy, and recurrent urinary tract infection.

Office Testing

Urinalysis and urine culture are required laboratory studies. A culture for acid-fast bacilli or yeast may be done depending upon index of suspicion. Assessment of post-void residual urine volume should be performed, either by bladder ultrasound or by catheterization. Urine cytology would be obtained in patients who have risk factors for bladder cancer, such as smoking, occupational exposure to organic dyes, hematuria, or age over 50.

Identifying Patients Is Important
A New Screening Questionnaire for
Pelvic Pain and Urgency/Frequency (PUF)

Circle the answer that best describes how you feel for each question.

		0	1	2	3	4	Symptom Score	Bother Score
1	How many times do you void during waking hours?	3-6	7-10	11-14	15-19	20+		
2	a. How many times do you void at night?	0	1	2	3	4+		
	b. If you get up at night to void, to what extent does it usually bother you?	None	Mild	Moderate	Severe			
3	Are you currently sexually active? YES _____ NO_____							
4	a. If you are sexually active, do you now have or have you ever had pain or urgency to urinate during or after sexual intercourse?	Never	Occasionally	Usually	Always			
	b. Has pain or urgency ever made you avoid sexual intercourse?	Never	Occasionally	Usually	Always			
5	Do you have pain associated with your bladder or in your pelvis, vagina, lower abdomen, urethra, perineum, testes, or scrotum?	Never	Occasionally	Usually	Always			
6	Do you still have urgency shortly after urinating?	Never	Occasionally	Usually	Always			
7	a. When you have pain, is it usually—?		Mild	Moderate	Severe			
	b. How often does your pain bother you?	Never	Occasionally	Usually	Always			
8	a. When you have urgency, is it usually—?		Mild	Moderate	Severe			
	b. How often does your urgency bother you?	Never	Occasionally	Usually	Always			

SYMPTOM SCORE (1, 2a, 4a, 5, 6, 7a, 8a)

BOTHER SCORE (2b, 4b, 7b, 8b)

TOTAL SCORE (Symptom Score + Bother Score) =

Patients with IC are likely to have higher scores (>15)

FIGURE 13.3. Parson's PUFF scale for IC evaluation.

On a voiding diary, patients with interstitial cystitis demonstrate abnormally low bladder capacity, with average voided volumes of 75 cc-to 100 cc, and maximum volumes around 250 cc. The voiding diary also allows the clinician to assess whether specific fluids represent potential bladder irritants.

The potassium chloride sensitivity test (KCL test) can be performed as a quick, low-cost means to detect interstitial cystitis in the primary care setting. Potassium chloride, when instilled into the bladder of a patient with interstitial cystitis, should trigger symptoms of urinary urgency, frequency, and pain. Symptoms are generally not triggered by KCL in a non-inflammatory bladder. An active or recent urinary tract infection needs to be ruled out before performing the test. The KCL test is performed as follows: 30 cc to 50 cc of room temperature solution #1(sterile water) is instilled into the bladder through a catheter, held for 2 to 4 minutes, and symptoms assessed. Solution #1 is drained, and then 30 cc to 50 cc of room temperature solution #2 (40meq KCl/100cc H_2O) is instilled, held for 2 to 4 minutes, and symptoms assessed again. An increase of 2 or more on the symptom scale with solution #2 indicates a likely diagnosis of interstitial cystitis. The potassium sensitivity test can be significantly painful to some patients. A rescue solution composed of 10,000 units of Heparin and 30 cc of 1% Xylocaine can be instilled to relieve the provoked symptoms. Although Parson's study demonstrated that 30% of women with interstitial cystitis were not KCL sensitive, it is still a useful, simple office diagnostic test.[36,37]

Treatment

Behavorial and Dietary. The chronic nature of IC, including the possibility of relapses, should be explained to the patient. Physicians should encourage their patients to read self-help books, obtain information from the National Kidney and Urologic Diseases Information Clearinghouse (3 Information Way, Bethesda, MD 20892-3580. Phone: 1-800-891-5390) and the Interstitial Cystitis Association (110 North Washington Street, Suite 340, Rockville, MD, 20850. Phone: 301-610-5300, 1-800-HELPICA). The Interstitial Cystitis Association (ICA) provides patients with support group information, conferences, and medical information. Suggested web site addresses are www.ichelp.org and www.ic-network.com.

Clinicians have found that avoidance of certain food and beverage groups improves symptoms (Table 13.2) Increasing water intake is recommended; dilute urine is less irritating to a sensitive bladder. Urine acidity can also be reduced by using a teaspoon of baking soda in a glass of water QD to BID, using the OTC product calcium glycerophosphate (Prelief, AK Pharma Inc., Pleasantville, NJ) sprinkled directly onto the food, or by prescribing Potassium Citrate (Urocit-K, Mission Pharmacal Co. San Antonio, TX) 5–10 meq po TID. Anecdotally, chondroitin sulfate (often found in combination with glucosamine), 1000 mg daily, has been reported to relieve bladder symptoms.[35] The amino acid supplement L-arginine taken 500 mg PO TID for 6 months can provide relief of symptoms.(37). Other herbal alternatives (Algonot Plus and Cysto Protek, Algonot LLC, Sarasota FL; and Cysta-Q, Farr Laboratories, Westwood, CA) are found at various web sites on the Internet. However, patients should understand that the majority have not undergone rigorous scientific testing to establish their risk profile or efficacy.

Bladder retraining to increase bladder capacity and extend voiding intervals can be introduced if symptoms are mild or after symptoms are controlled. Generally, it is reasonable to try to increase the voiding interval by 15 minutes each month until a 3- to 4-hour voiding interval is attained. Monthly physician visits assist with maintaining compliance, providing motivation, and monitoring of patient progress.

Stress reduction techniques including self-visualization, self-hypnosis, baths, deep breathing, and meditation can be utilized.[38] Development of coping mechanisms, problem solving, and also sex therapy, with the help of a psychologist, may be a valuable element of care, particularly for IC patients with unremitting pain.

Pharmacologic Therapy. Pentosan polysulfate (Elmiron, Ortho-McNeil, Raritan, NJ) is the only FDA approved oral medication for the treatment of interstitial cystitis. Elmiron is prescribed 100 mg PO tid. Possible side effects include gastrointestinal distress, headache, and reversible hair loss, and it should be used with caution in women with bleeding ulcers or bleeding diasthesis. Only 60% of patients will experience relief of symptoms, and relief may not be seen until 4 to 6 months of use. Therefore, other treatment options may be needed during this hiatus.[39]

Tricyclic anti-depressants such as amitriptyline and nortriptyline are frequently prescribed "off- label" for interstitial cystitis. Tricyclics can give prompt relief of symptoms in most patients. Tricyclic anti-depressants have been shown to (1) reduce bladder urgency by their anticholinergic properties, (2) raise the pain threshold, (3) improve sleep by sedation, and (4) elevate mood. When prescribing in a younger population, one can start out at 25 mg QHS and increase to 50 mg to 75 mg QHS; but these medications should be used with caution in the elderly, as they can cause confusion and electrocardiogram changes.

The antihistamine Hydroxyzine (Atarax, Vistaril, Pfizer, New York, NY) is used off-label and may be especially useful in a patient with a history of allergies. Possible mechanisms of action include stabilization of mast cells, anticholinergic properties, and a sedative effect. The recommended starting dose is 25 mg at bedtime, which can be titrated up to 50 mg after one to two weeks. The allergy/asthma medication montelukast (Singulair, Merck & Co., West Point, PA), a leukotriene inhibitor, may prove to be effective.

Phenazopyridine (Pyridium, Warner Chilcott, Rockaway, NJ) is a bladder analgesic that can relieve symptoms on a PRN basis for symptom flares. Urised (Poly Medica Pharm, Woburn, MA) or Urimax (Integrity Pharm Corp, Fishers, IN) can be used in a similar manner. The antispasmodic medications used to treat overactive bladder may improve symptoms. However, based upon our current understanding of the pathophysiology of interstitial cystitis, this group of medications does not affect the cascade pathway and is, therefore, unlikely to be effective if used alone.

Specialized Diagnosis and Management

If initial diagnostic maneuvers are not conclusive and/or initial treatments have not proven to be effective, referral to these specialty providers is indicated: urogynecology, urology, physical therapy, psychology, psychiatry, or pain clinics for further diagnostic steps and/or treatment.

Specialized diagnostic techniques that may be performed include urodynamic testing and cystoscopy under anesthesia with hydrodistention. Cystoscopic findings of interstitial cystitis are petechial hemorrhages (glomerulations) and Hunner's ulcers.

Therapy may include intravesical installations. Medications used for installations include dimethylsulfoxide (DMSO), FDA approved in 1978; heparin; hyaluronic acid (Cystistat, Bioniche, Ontario, Canada—available only in Canada) BCG (Bacillus Calmette Guerin), anesthetic agents such as Xylocaine and Marcaine, and cocktails of different combinations of Xylocaine, corticosteroid, heparin, antibiotics, and sodium bicarbonate. Depending upon the medication used, the frequency of installations will vary.

Hydrodistention of the bladder or cystoscopic destruction of glomerulations/ulcerations with either electrocautery or the neodymium (Nd): YAG laser may be employed. End-stage patients may require radical surgical procedures such as enterocystoplasty, cytolysis, urinary diversion, or urinary diversion into a continent pouch combined with cystectomy.[40] These extirpative procedures, however, have not shown to be beneficial, as patients continue to suffer from phantom sensory urgency and pain.[41]

Physical therapists who specialize in treatment of pelvic floor dysfunction may utilize biofeedback and/or electrical stimulation of the pelvis. Sacral neuromodulation (InterStim, Medtronic Corp., Minneapolis, MN) has been used to treat the symptoms of urinary frequency and urgency associated with IC.

Optimal management of IC should involve close collaboration between the primary care physician and the specialist. The primary care physician should stay involved in the management of these patients as part of a multidisciplinary team to provide the best overall care for the patient.

Patient Evaluation

History

In evaluating a patient with chronic pelvic pain, detailed history taking and physical examination are the most important components to diagnosis.

A history addressing all of the above possible causes (musculoskeletal, gastrointestinal, gynecological, urinary, psychological) needs to be queried and can be lengthy. To assist the provider in doing so, a questionnaire developed by The International Pelvic Pain Society (www.pelvicpain.org) is available free of charge from their web site. This questionnaire will assist the provider in screening the differential diagnosis of chronic pelvic pain and in directing the history taking into specific areas. It also helps to determine if there was an event (e.g., an accident, previous surgery, psychological trauma, severe urinary tract infection, episode of severe abdominal pain, menarche, or pregnancy) related to when the patient's pain started. It is important to obtain detailed information about the pain—location, severity, quality (sharp, dull, burning), and cyclic or constant nature. Patients can complete a pain map[12] and rate the severity of their pain using either a visual analogue scale, or a rating scale of 0 to 10, with 10 indicating the worst possible pain.

The clinician should ascertain what makes the pain worsen or improve; whether the pain interferes with daily activities; and whether the pain is associated with urination, bowel movements, intercourse, physical activity, or the menstrual cycle. Though by no means diagnostic, there are certain areas of described pain that correlate to an organ system or systems (Table 13.3).

Physical Examination

Physical examination will be directed by the history but can be performed, in general, according to the following guidelines. As the patient stands, walks, or bends, one can notice gait problems, limping, asymmetry, and posture that may indicate musculoskeletal dysfunction. Tenderness or pain elicited upon palpation of joints, ligaments, and/or bony structures may indicate musculoskeletal problems. An assessment of the strength and reflexes of the lower extremities should be performed with the patient sitting. While the patient is supine, a careful examination of the abdominal wall should evaluate for trigger points, painful scars, hyperesthesia, and hernias and perform general screen for abdominal or pelvic pathology. Assessment of spinal disc problems with straight leg raising can be carried out. The examination is then continued in the lithotomy position. Careful examination of the perineum and vestibule is performed. On speculum exam, the vaginal walls and cervix should be inspected. When starting the internal exam, it is best to gently insert a single digit, evaluating the pelvic muscles (levator ani and obturator internus) for spasm and strength, the uterosacral ligaments for nodularity, and the bladder and urethra for tenderness. Routine bimanual examination of the pelvic organs is then completed. Rectal examination should include a check for masses and tenderness of the piriformis muscle and coccyx and Hemoccult testing.

TABLE 13.3. Pain Location and Associated Organ System

Location of pain	Involved organ/organ system
lateral pelvic pain	adnexa or sigmoid/colonic
midline infraumbilical pain	uterus/cervix
pubic bone/groin pain	bladder/vagina
lower sacral pain	uterosacral ligaments/posterior cul de sac,
low back pain alone	musculoskeletal
both ventral and dorsal pain	intrapelvic pathology
pain that relieves with rest	musculoskeletal or adnexal

Adapted from Howard FM, El-Minawi AM, Sanchez RA. Conscious pain mapping by laparoscopy in women with chronic pelvic pain. *Obstet Gynecol.* 2000;96:934–939.

Laboratory, Radiological, and Specialized Tests

Basic laboratory studies such as CBC, UA, C&S, and ESR are indicated; but beyond these, other blood work ordered should be based upon history-taking and physical findings. Routine radiological tests (ultrasound, CT, and MRI scans) can be costly and are often of low yield. Simple tools such as a pain diary, menstrual diary, food diary, and voiding diary are more cost-effective and also more likely to reveal a diagnosis. Other diagnostic studies such as laparoscopy, colonoscopy, and cystoscopy will require referral to the appropriate specialist.

Treatment and Follow-up

Psychological support of the patient with chronic pelvic pain is often needed to sustain the patient for long-term relief and recovery, even if a discrete physical etiology is identified. With respect to analgesics, the regular use of non-steroidal anti-inflammatory medications is the usual first-line regimen. The use of medications on a PRN basis may in some cases be counterproductive, as it places the patient in the position of policing and monitoring for pain episodes. Policing encourages the patient to focus more on her pain and pain episodes. Thus, each episode becomes an emergency, the pain may be perceived as more severe, and the patient is not free to focus on her daily living activities. It is also recommended that regular follow-up visits be scheduled with an adequate amount of time allotted, as opposed to a "*call me when you have pain*" plan, to minimize disruption to the office schedule with add on visits, as well as emergency room visits.

If narcotics are needed to control the pain, a firm policy should be established between the patient and provider. Such a pain contract is available on line from the International Pelvic Pain Society web site. The contract needs to address the strength of the medication and number prescribed, the type of pain for which the medication is prescribed, and the need for regular follow-up visits. If such an understanding cannot be maintained, then narcotics should not be prescribed and the patient referred to a pain clinic.

Neuroleptic pain medications such as gabapentin (Neurontin, Parke Davis, Morris Plains, NJ) and carbamazepine (Tegretol, Novartis Consumer Health Inc., Parsippany, NJ) used for neuropathies are used off-label for chronic pain. These medications down-regulate the hyperesthesia seen in these patients. Nonsurgical management of pain relaxation therapy and transcutaneous electrical nerve stimulation (TENS) units have been used to raise the pain threshold for patients with interstitial cystitis. Additionally, patients may seek out alternative non-Western treatments such as acupuncture. Surgical treatment of pain, or neurolytic procedures, include the transection of nerves, injection of chemicals (alcohol, phenol, and hypertonic saline) to destroy the nerves, nerve blocks, and denervation procedures. These secondary-line treatments would be provided through a pain specialist or multi-disciplinary pain clinic.

Conclusion

The diagnosis and management of chronic pelvic pain is a challenge, as there are musculoskeletal, psychological, gynecological, gastrointestinal, and urological causes. The primary care provider is in an ideal position, seeing the patient as a whole, to screen and diagnose for the different causes and institute therapeutic management. When necessary, the primary care provider can make the appropriate referrals for more specialized diagnostics and treatments. The provider is in the position to oversee the patient's care plan, thus providing a focused, but comprehensive, approach to the patient's overall health.

Key Points

- Chronic pelvic pain is defined as pain in the pelvis of greater than six months' duration.
- The diagnosis of chronic pelvic pain can be challenging, as the differential diagnosis encompasses more than one organ system, and many symptoms overlap from one system to the other.
- Often, the pain will not be "cured", but rather, "managed."
- Patients who have chronic disease processes of the gastrointestinal, reproductive, or urinary systems can develop spasm of the levator ani and other pelvic floor muscles as a secondary problem.
- Gynecologic conditions that can produce chronic pain include benign or malignant tumors, endometriosis, pelvic adhesions in women with prior pelvic surgery or infection, and chronic pelvic inflammatory diseases.
- Among pelvic pain sufferers with known adhesions, those adhesions are the source of the pain only about 50% of the time.
- IC often represents a diagnosis of exclusion when no other cause of painful bladder can be identified.

References

1. Zondervan KT, Yudkin PL, Vessey MP, Dawes MG, Barlow DH, Kennedy SH. Prevalence and incidence

of chronic pelvic pain in primary care: evidence from a national general practice database. *Br J Obstet Gynaecol.* 1999;106:1149–1155.
2. Mathias SD, Kuppermann M, Liberman RF, Lipschutz RC, Steege JF. Chronic pelvic pain: prevalence, health-related quality of life, and economic correlates. *Obstet Gynecol.* 1996;87:321–327.
3. Reiter RC, Gambone JC. Demographic and historic variables in women with idiopathic chronic pelvic pain. *Obstet Gynecol.* 1990;75:428–432.
4. Rogers RM. Basic pelvic neuroanatomy. In Steege JF, Metzger DA, Levy BS, eds. Chronic Pelvic Pain: An Integrated Approach. Philadelphia: W.B. Saunders Co., 1998:31–58.
5. Moore K. The Developing Human: Clinically Oriented Embryology. 4th ed. Philadelphia, W.B. Saunders Co., 1988.
6. Bussolati G, Tizzani A, Casetta G et al. Detection of estrogen receptors in the trigonum and urinary bladder with an immunohistochemical technique. *Gynecol Endocrinol.* 1990;4:205–213.
7. Tao YX, Heit M, Lei ZM, Rao CV. The urinary bladder of a woman is a novel site of luteinizing hormone-human chorionic gonadotropin receptor gene expression. *Am J Obstet Gynecol.* 1998;179:1026–1031.
8. Xiao ZL, Pricolo V, Biancani P, Behar J. Role of progesterone signaling in the regulation of G-protein levels in female chronic constipation. *Gastroenterology.* 2005 Mar;128(3):667–675.
9. Shiah IS, Yatham LN. GABA function in mood disorders: an update and critical review. *Life Sci.* 1998;63(15):1289–1303.
10. Cyriax EF. On various conditions that may stimulate the referred pains of visceral disease, and a consideration of these from the point of view of cause and effect. *Practitioner.* 1919;102:314–322.
11. Carnett JB. Intercostal neuralgia as a cause of abdominal pain and tenderness. *Surg Gynecol Obstet.* 1926;42:625–632.
12. Carter JE. Surgical treatment for chronic pelvic pain. *JSLS.* 1998;2:129–139.
13. Howard FM. Chronic pelvic pain. *Obstet Gynecol.* 2003 Mar;101:594–611.
14. Ringel Y, Sperber AD, Drossman DA. Irritable Bowel Syndrome. *Annu Rev Med.* 2001;52:319–338.
15. Case AM, Reid RL. Menstrual cycle effects on common medical conditions. *Compr Ther.* 2001;27:65–71.
16. Vanner SJ, Depew WT, Paterson WG et al. Predictive value of the Rome criteria for diagnosing the irritable bowel syndrome. *Am J Gastroenterol.* 1999 Oct;94:2912–2917.
17. Eliakim R, Abulafia O, Sherer DM. Estrogen, progesterone and the gastrointestinal tract. *J Reprod Med.* 2000;45:781–788.
18. Speroff L, Glass RH, Kase NG. Clinical Gynecologic Endocrinology and Infertility. 5th ed. Baltimore, MD: William and Wilkins, 1994.
19. Koninckx PR, Meuleman C, Demeyere S, Lesaffre E, Cornillie FJ. Suggestive evidence that pelvic endometriosis is a progressive disease whereas deeply infiltrating endometriosis is associated with pelvic pain. *Fertil Steril.* 1991;55:759–765.
20. Marcoux S, Maheux R, Berube S. Laparascopic Surgery in Infertile Women with Minimal or Mild Endometriosis. Canadian Collaborative Group on Endometriosis. *N Engl J Med.* 1997;337:217–222.
21. Howard FM. An evidence-based medicine approach to the treatment of endometriosis-associated chronic pelvic pain: placebo-controlled studies. *J Am Assoc Gynecol Laparosc.* 2000 Nov;7:477–488.
22. Hemsell DL. ACOG educational bulletin: Antibiotics and gynecologic infections. In: American College of Obstetrics/Gynecology 2001 Compendium. Washington, DC: ACOG; 2001;237:302–309.
23. Howard FM, El-Minawi AM, Sanchez RA. Conscious pain mapping by laparoscopy in women with chronic pelvic pain. *Obstet Gynecol.* 2000;96:934–939.
24. Baggish MS, Miklos JR. Vulvar Pain Syndrome: A Review. *Obstet Gynecol Surv.* 1995;50:618–627.
25. Metts JF. Vulvodynia and vulvar vestibulitis: challenges in diagnosis and management. *Am Fam Physician.* 1999;59:1547–1556.
26. Byth JL. Understanding vulvodynia. *Australas J Dermatol.* 1998;39:139–148.
27. Bergeron S, Binik TM, Khalife S, Pagidas K. Vulvar vestibulitis syndrome: a critical review. *Clin J Pain.* 1997;13(1):27–42.
28. Harger JH. Genital herpes simplex infections. *Contem OB/Gyn.* 1997;April:21–41.
29. Walling MK, Reiter RC, O'Hara MW, Milburn AK, Lilly G, Vincent SD. Abuse history and chronic pain in women: I. Prevalences of sexual abuse and physical abuse. *Obstet Gynecol.* 1994 Aug;84(2):193–199.
30. Clemons JL, Arya LA, Myers DL. Diagnosing interstitial cystitis in women with chronic pelvic pain. *Obstet Gynecol.* 2002 Aug;100:337–341.
31. Parsons CL, Dell J, Stanford EJ et al. Increased prevalence of interstitial cystitis: previously unrecognized urologic and gynecologic cases identified

using a new symptom questionnaire and intravesical potassium sensitivity. *Urology*. 2002 Oct;60(4): 573–578.
32. Oravisto KJ. Epidemiology of interstitial cystitis. *Ann Chir Gynaecol Fenn*. 1975;64:75–77.
33. Parsons CL. Interstitial cystitis: clinical manifestations and diagnostic criteria in over 200 cases. *Neurourol Urodyn*. 1990;9:241–250.
34. Simon LJ, Landis JR, Erickson DR, Nyberg LM. The Interstitial Cystitis Database Study: concepts and preliminary baseline descriptive statistics. *Urol*. 1997;49(5A):64–75.
35. O'Leary MP, Sant GR, Fowler FJ Jr., Whitmore KE, Spolarich-Kroll J. The interstitial cystitis symptom and problem index. *Urol*. 1997 May;49(5A Suppl): 58–63.
36. Parsons CL, Stein PC, Bidair M, Lebow D. Abnormal sensitivity to intravesical potassium in interstitial cystitis and radiation cystitis. *Neurourol Urodyn*. 1994;9:515–520.
37. Parsons CL, Greenberger M, Gabal L, Bidair M, Barme G. The role of urinary potassium in the pathogenesis and diagnosis of interstitial cystitis. *J Urol*. 1998;159:1862–1866.
38. Ripoll E, Mahowald D. Hatha Yoga therapy management of urologic disorders. *World J Urol*. 2002 Nov;20:306–309.
39. Parson CL, Mulholland SG. Successful therapy of interstitial cystitis with pentosanpolysulfate. *J Urol*. 1987;138:513–516.
40. van Ophoven A, Oberpenning F, Hertle L. Long-term results of trigone-preserving orthotopic substitution enterocystoplasty for interstitial cystitis. *J Urol*. 2002 Feb;167:603–607.
41. Nielsen KK, Kromann-Andersen B, Steven K, Hald T. Failure of combined supratrigonal cystectomy and Mainz ileocecocystoplasty in intractable interstitial cystitis: is histology and mast cell count a reliable predictor for the outcome of surgery? *J Urol*. 1990;144:255–259.

14
Getting Your Urogynecology Visits "Up and Running": Key Questionnaires, Forms and Coding Tips

Vincent R. Lucente and Marie C. Shaw

Introduction

In today's competitive and ever-changing marketplace, no medical practice has an unlimited budget; more often, there is barely enough cash flow to meet current needs and obligations. Resources such as money, time, and space seem to be literally shrinking. Unfortunately, when the ink on the bottom line turns red, many physician leaders forced to cut costs often do so by laying off valuable staff. This downsizing often serves to further strain the productivity of the practice. An alternative to such downsizing can usually be found by adding nontraditional services or products, expanding existing products, or creating new service offerings.

In a recent survey, the Medical Group Management Association (MGMA), a professional organization for medical group practice managers, surveyed physicians as to recently added services within existing practices. The most common answers included in-practice laboratory, radiology, or other procedure-based services; ambulatory surgery centers; and the use of alternative medicine providers.[1] Opportunities exist within the field of Urogynecology to add each of these types of services to an existing primary care practice.

Michael Porter, noted business strategist and frequent author for *The Harvard Business Review*, defines strategy as "the positioning of a business to maximize the value of the capabilities that distinguish it from its competitors." He believes that the central focus of strategy is achieving a sustainable competitive advantage.[2]

Product differentiation is a positioning strategy used to distinguish products or services from the competition. These distinctions can be either real or perceived. The key to a solid differentiation strategy is creating a unique advantage that can be sustained over time. Differentiation can be obtained through such features as convenience, unconditional service guarantees, better hours, more nursing care, quick follow-up, better technology, or specialized diagnostic equipment.[2] But remember, if the office across town can easily copycat your differentiation strategy, your competitive edge will not last very long.

One interesting differentiation strategy worth noting is house calls. Reminiscent of an old Marcus Welby, MD rerun, doctors are incorporating in-home medical treatments into their practices. Not only is it the ultimate service differentiator, a doctor who makes a house call can be paid as much as 45% higher than for a typical office visit. Many pelvic floor disorders such as urinary and fecal incontinence lend themselves to evaluation via house calls (possibly in a nursing home environment), because their initial workups are largely based on patient histories.

Differentiation can also be obtained by carving out niche services for your patients based on their wants and needs. Think about your market. It is not homogeneous, and it can be broken down into several layers. You can create specialized services or niches within your overall practice to meet the needs of each of these smaller groups. Abandoning the "one-size-fits-all" approach to reaching female patients in favor of creating different messaging points, customizing services and communication vehicles used to reach each of these groups can prove to be a very successful service differentiator. Offering comprehensive screening for pelvic floor disorders can attract the very desirable niche market of women 35 years of age and older. But before you start, there a few questions you need to ask yourself.

In their book, *Health Care Market Strategy*, authors Hillestad and Berkowitz[2] propose four key questions to ask when exploring a new service or niche market.

Who are the possible customers?
Where do they get care now?
What are their needs?
How do they make decisions?

Let's explore these four questions for developing a niche service offering of primary care for female urinary incontinence. The first question is perhaps the easiest to answer: *Who are the possible customers*? They include your *current* patients. A recent survey, conducted by the National Association For Continence, revealed that women ranked their PCP only second to their OB-GYN physician as the provider they wanted to see for incontinence care.[3]

Where do they get care now? Sixty-four percent of women who seek treatment for stress urinary incontinence generally talk to their family/primary care doctor. As the prevalence of female urinary incontinence continues to rise, the number of women receiving treatment has not risen proportionately. Obviously, this mismatch represents an opportunity. Embarrassment and the lack of awareness regarding treatment keep women from seeking help, even within an educated consumer market segment. A poll of incontinent women found that 62% wait a year or longer before discussing their condition with a physician, and 17% wait five or more years. While postponing treatment, women tend to give up many of their favorite physical or recreational activities.[3] In an even more disturbing statistic, nine out of ten patients who discussed their bladder symptoms with their physician had to bring it up themselves.[4] Primary care providers are not in the habit of asking patients about pelvic floor symptoms. Urinary incontinence is the number one reason listed when families are asked for the reason they institutionalized a loved one into a nursing facility.[5] Simply starting a conversation with your patients can open up a market growth opportunity. It is also good medical practice.

What are their needs? Perimenopausal women want alternative/complementary options, in conjunction with traditional medical care—usually with an emphasis on wellness and prevention. They want their services to be coordinated and convenient. To the extent that your office can provide pelvic floor treatment options, without requiring referrals, you will improve the convenience to the patients. Women will demand knowledgeable and expert providers who share decision-making and discuss alternatives. The most up-to-the minute information and technology will become the standard.

As is the case with any medical condition, women suffering from incontinence want to be properly evaluated and effectively treated. One characteristic that sets urinary incontinence apart from other chronic medical conditions, however, is the negative impact on quality of life. While hypertension or diabetes may pose greater threats to overall health, your patients' day-to-day quality of life is impacted more by their incontinence. In fact, one study found that the negative impact on one's quality of life from urinary incontinence, when compared to other common chronic illnesses, to be second only to major depression. Incontinence often affects a women's self-esteem, which can actually worsen her underlying anxiety and depression. Incontinence also negatively impacts work productivity, sexual satisfaction, sleep patterns, and even interactions with children, as physical play becomes more difficult. There are also economic issues surrounding the expenses associated with purchasing absorption protection items and the increase in laundering.

The caregiver's level of awareness regarding treatment options directly impacts patient care. Women, frustrated by inappropriate or inadequate treatments, may abandon intervention altogether when, in fact, their condition could have been cured through proper evaluation and medical treatment. Efficient, quality incontinence care management is good for your practice. As a primary care provider, you have a unique opportunity to effectively evaluate and manage this condition and, in doing so, significantly increase the quality of your patients' lives.

How do they make decisions? It is widely know that women tend to direct the healthcare decisions within the household. Word-of-mouth referral and provider reputation consistently rank high as influencers. Recent market research by Solucient, a company that specializes in health care business intelligence, indicates that women select hospitals on three principle factors: their family health insurance, the quality of the medical staff, and a strong reputation.

Public ratings are also gaining popularity among female consumers. While nearly two-thirds of women surveyed reported that they would be either very likely or somewhat likely to research public ratings when selecting a hospital, they did express skepticism about trusting the sources of the ratings. Interestingly, more women indicated a strong level of trust regarding internet-based rankings of physicians than those of hospitals (57 to 16%).

Incorporating the Management of Female Incontinence into Your Practice

Getting Started

Perhaps the best place to start when considering incorporating evaluation and treatment of female urinary incontinence into your practice is the education of your staff. This should begin with stating the precise reasons for offering this service line to your patients, especially if you have never done so in the past. It is important for the staff to understand the importance of providing this service, as well as their role in its execution. Take the appropriate time to educate your staff on the basic pathophysiology of urinary incontinence, as well as the various medical, behavioral, and dietary therapies you are planning to offer. It is also important that they understand when a referral may be necessary.

It is helpful to utilize good basic review articles, as well as chapters from easy-to- read textbooks and selections from various nursing publications. To further energize their interest in this service expansion, it may be prudent to send some members of your staff to a local or regional course on female pelvic floor disorders.

Lastly, it could be extremely helpful to have your staff shadow a nurse or a physician extender who currently works in a subspecialist's office. Doing so will help them learn not only clinical information, but also the patient flow and operational aspects of incontinence care.

Your Staff's Attitudes Toward Bladder Function

Health professionals typically pride themselves on being able to discuss difficult or embarrassing subjects with their patients. However, some of your staff may harbor negative attitudes regarding pelvic floor dysfunction. Many of us grew up with negative attitudes—or at least inhibitions—about bowel and bladder function. As a young child, you might have felt shame and guilt if you had a bowel or bladder accident. These unhealthy social attitudes can influence feelings about urinary incontinence and the ways in which your staff interact with patients with this condition. Communication and education may help you break down these barriers.

Your patients may also subscribe to certain negative attitudes about bladder function. Be aware that these attitudes can affect how patients talk about their problem. Your patients with urinary incontinence may not be able to approach this subject if your professional relationship is not perceived as supportive. If they bring themselves to mention their problem at all, they may do it in such a veiled, roundabout way that you may not even initially understand.

Some patients may use vernacular terms to describe their condition or joke about the problem as though it were of no concern to them. Be prepared to listen and observe closely—not only to what patients say, but to their body language as well. Listen and watch for their unspoken anxiety, and do your best to encourage them to talk about their condition.

The Patient Flow Process

Once the staff has a solid working understanding of what it takes to develop this service line, it is important to incorporate their input as you develop the patient flow process. This process starts from the moment a patient calls your office complaining of urinary incontinence or checks the "yes" box on your screening questionnaire. Each step of the patient flow must be carefully orchestrated to avoid fragmentation and inefficiency. It is extremely helpful to have the patients complete a dedicated incontinence questionnaire and a 24- to 48-hour urinary diary. These documents will provide helpful insight into establishing the underlying diagnosis. In fact, these documents often make the diagnosis for you. One excellent validated questionnaire is the 20-question Pelvic Floor Dysfunction Inventory (PFDI), available at www.augs.org. Patients completing this survey often report feeling "understood" or "listened to."

The next step in getting started is to develop your documentation process. By spending some time up front thinking about key questions, symptoms, pertinent related medical conditions, and medications you can save valuable time in the office. There is no better way to accomplish this than by incorporating streamlined, easy-to-use physician evaluation forms. This is especially true when it comes to performing and documenting the comprehensive physical examination. One such form was developed by The American Urogynecologic Society and is available at www.augs.org.

Lastly, you should collect and organize patient education materials. Be sure to read these materials yourself before making them available. Remember, pamphlets that use easy-to-read, straightforward language (preferably in larger type) are best. Resources for these educational materials are included in the resource list at the end of the chapter.

Patient Evaluation

It is not practical to try to treat urinary incontinence on the tail end of a visit for a blood-pressure check or a routine annual exam. During those visits, it is more effective to simply inquire about your patient's possible pelvic floor dysfunction via a few open-ended questions. Any affirmative answers should prompt you to encourage thoughtful completion of the above-mentioned questionnaires and the bladder diary, to be reviewed during a future *problem-focused* visit. The key here is to emphasize to the patient your recognition of how much they are suffering from this medical condition and that it is NOT a normal part of aging. Let your patient know that the best way you can help them is through another visit dedicated strictly to their specific pelvic floor problem.

The patient should present to that dedicated visit with a full bladder. This allows the nurse to perform a standing stress test (to capture the sign of stress urinary incontinence). Your nurse can also measure the patient's voided volume and her catheterized post-void residual. It is even possible to calculate the patient's average flow rate by asking her to measure her complete voiding time via a stopwatch. While the nurse is accomplishing these tasks, you can familiarize yourself with the patient's specific complaints by reading her symptom questionnaire.

After you have completed your evaluation and discussed treatment, it is valuable to have your nurse reinforce any and all of your instructions to the patient. Over time, as your nursing staff becomes more experienced, time-intensive instructions, such as bladder retraining, can easily be communicated to the patient after you have left the room.

Once the appropriate treatment plan has been established, it may be cost-effective for a nurse practitioner or other such physician extender to see the patient for her next appointments as the "fine tuning" of the plan takes place.

After the Visit: The Reimbursement Process

Why Coding is Important

It is a fact of life in healthcare today that physicians must assign codes and document the care given patients in order to assure appropriate reimbursement. Understanding the basics of coding is essential to that process. It is highly recommended that every physician take coding courses on a frequent basis, because the rules change constantly. Attending a coding course is probably the best way to learn the rules and guidelines surrounding proper coding. This section cannot replace that experience or convey the information in a coding book, but it contains the basics of what you need to know to get started.

So many physicians we work with say, *"I have someone in my billing department to take care of that,"* and they have no idea of what they are or are NOT receiving reimbursement for. Don't let this important practice responsibility rest solely on the shoulders of the billing people. We are not saying that you should be actually doing the billing, but you should have a very comprehensive and clear understanding of the process.

Codes condense a lot of information. Medical procedures, diagnoses, and supplies are identified by codes. The same codes are used by healthcare providers, managed care groups, insurance companies, government agencies, and research organizations. When everyone uses the same codes, it streamlines the cycle from treatment to payment and makes it easier to monitor health care treatments and outcomes.

Just as physicians look at serial lab studies to find a pattern, payers look at the codes that are submitted to discover a pattern. Examining submitted codes this way, a profile can be developed of the way each physician conducts his or her practice. Questionable coding patterns or profiles trigger inquiries from insurers. The federal government, intent on eliminating fraud and abuse, has increased the attention paid to coding profiles. Other payers also profile providers and practices to determine the need for further review of records and claims. Understanding coding can help keep your practice from being audited and, if you should have to go through one, good coding practices will assure you pass with flying colors.

Coding Basics

The basic rules of the road of medical reimbursement are really not that difficult to comprehend. In general, third-party payers are obligated to pay for services provided by physicians if they fulfill the following criteria:

- Service must be covered within the patient's insurance policy or healthcare contract.
- Given the patient's condition, this service provided must be a medically appropriate treatment.
- The service is medically necessary and in accordance with the appropriate standards of care consistent with the medical diagnosis. Also, more so than ever before, the service must also be determined to be the most appropriate level of care in the most appropriate setting (i.e., office, ambulatory care surgery unit, or hospital).
- Lastly—perhaps equally important—the service is also coded correctly. Physicians must realize that although payers are under an obligation or contract to pay for services that meet these criteria, they are never really eager to pay. Actually, they are often reluctant to pay; so, in order to collect the allowable reimbursement for your services, it is important that you have an in-depth familiarity of what is covered by the major payers in your patient population. Unfortunately, almost all payers reserve the right to pass judgment on what is necessary and appropriate as deemed by their internal review process. This often is the underlying reason for denials as insurance companies seek an opportunity to avoid payment. What you can control is the coding process; therefore, it is in your best interest to learn how to code correctly.

There are three main coding systems: (1) ICD-9, which describes why you are performing the service, (2) CPT, and (3) HCPCS, which describes what service you provided.

Current procedural terminology (CPT) is copyrighted in 2004 and updated yearly by the American Medical Association. No fee schedules, basic units, relative values, or related listings are included in the CPT. You are probably well familiar with the codes listed in the CPT regarding evaluation and management services; however, providing urodynamic testing (or even simply inserting a catheter) is considered a surgical service and is also listed in the CPT manual. Perhaps more practical is to ensure that your master office encounter form or billing sheet includes the ICD-9 diagnostic codes for common urinary tract conditions. Some of the more common conditions are listed in Table 14.1.

Coding should be thought of simply as a vehicle for communicating information regarding what medical service you provided and the reason you did so. Procedural codes enable the physician to

TABLE 14.1. Common Pelvic Floor Conditions and ICD-9 Codes

Bladder Codes
Overactive bladder (596.59)
Stress incontinence (625.6)
Mixed incontinence (788.33)
Intrinsic sphincter deficiency (599.82)
Incomplete bladder emptying (788.21)
Urge incontinence (788.31)
Urinary frequency (788.41)
Slowing of the urinary stream (788.62)
Acute cystitis (595.0)
Interstitial cystitis (595.10)
Other chronic cystitis (595.20)
Prolapse Codes
Uterine prolapse (618.2 or 618.3)
Vaginal vault prolase after hysterectomy (618.5)
Cystocele (618.01)
Rectocele (618.04)
Other
Fecal Incontinence (787.60)
Constipation (564.00)

communicate exactly what was done; and the diagnostic codes communicate the nature of the disease, illness, condition, or symptom of the patient that established the medical necessity for the service or procedure. Unfortunately, simple coding errors by either the physician or the office staff can be interpreted as fraudulent acts by insurance carriers. It is, therefore, extremely important that you and your staff understand the ground rules of coding in order to avoid common errors. If you, yourself, have not taken a coding course recently, it should be on the top of your to-do list.

Are You Ready to Market?

Contrary to common belief, most companies, organizations or products DO NOT build awareness or recognition with big advertising budgets. To build this valuable equity, an organization must start with a solid strategy and involve everyone in the organization to reinforce the "promise" behind the service. Your practice is no different. Practices build strong brands by consistently delivering quality services, nurturing customer relationships, and delivering consistent, meaningful messages.

It is extremely important to lay the foundation of the first two bullet points prior to advertising or communicating about the service. So many people make the mistake of thinking that *marketing* is the advertisement or brochure. Those documents are only the communication tools. They are supported by having all employees engaged in the service promise, identifying the right target audience, and researching how to effectively reach that audience.

To see if your practice is ready to move forward to creating communications tools in the marketing process, take the quick self-assessment quiz (Table 14.2) at the end of this chapter. If you check "no" to any of the boxes, work on that area before you proceed.

Getting The Word Out

Once you have decided to implement this service line into your practice and the groundwork is in place, educating women about incontinence—along with the message that help is readily available—is key to having the service grow.

It is important to recognize that many patients are still reluctant to seek treatment for urinary incontinence. Just because they are afflicted by this condition, it is not a guarantee that they will automatically seek treatment. According to various surveys, certain conditions must be met before a patient will seek treatment for a medical problem. Keeping these points in mind will help guide the "what" you say about your service.

1. The patient needs to be aware of the medical problem and experience a desire or need to change it.
2. The patient needs to be aware that a treatment modality for the condition exists.
3. The patient needs to be aware that the treatment modality or modalities that are available are efficacious.
4. The patient needs to believe that the benefits of treatment are worth the effort, not only monetarily, but regarding time as well.
5. The patient must know where to go for treatment, and the treatment must be relatively accessible.

TABLE 14.2. Self-assessment Quiz

If your process is not in place for offering evaluation and management of female urinary incontinence, then you are not ready to proceed to the communication phase of marketing. Take this self-assessment quiz to see where your practice is.

Female Urinary Incontinence Service Evaluation	YES	NO
I (physician) have been to recent postgraduate education courses or seminars and am up-to-date on the latest advances.		
In my practice all front office staff have written guidelines and procedures on how to schedule patients with incontinence.		
In my practice all clinical staff have written guidelines and procedures on how to deal with patient with incontinence.		
I (physician) am conscious of how my staff and I speak to patients about these conditions.		
The office had adequate forms and patient education materials available.		
All staff has a clear understanding of the clinical evaluation, procedures and services we offer and the appropriate staff understands how to correctly code and bill for those services.		
We have an established relationship with a subspecialist(s) for necessary referrals.		

As can be seen in the daily life of most Americans, the use of the Internet is significant across all age groups. In a poll released in December 2004 by Harris Interactive, 73% of all adults in the U.S. reported using the Internet, up from 49 % who did in December 2000. Topping the list of online activities are e-mail (66%), research for work or school (46%), checking news and weather (43%) and getting information about hobbies or special interests (40%). Researching information about health or diseases ranked at 21% and was in close ranking with making travel plans and looking up local events and activities.

If your practice does not have a web site—get one NOW! There are many online resources and professional medical organizations that can guide you through a simple turnkey operation, or you can contact a local web designer or a local college; many have students who can assist you in this process. Web design and hosting have become very inexpensive, and the investment is well worth the effort. At a minimum, your site should include the following section on an easy to navigate tool bar:

- Home—Welcome & Introduction
- About Us—Practice overview (add in here your service line in female incontinence) and bios of staff with photos
- Contact Us Information
- Privacy & Disclaimer and Disclosures
- Patient Education—Resources for patients
- Office logistics—Appointment information, directions and financial policies
- Patient Forms—Available to download (include the incontinence questionnaire and 48-hour voiding diary)
- Links—Internet links to informative sites (some provided at the end of the chapter)

The elements of the web site described above have one main purpose—disseminating information. Many physician and hospital sites are becoming interactive where patients can make their own appointments, fill prescriptions, view test results, and e-mail providers. For many, these uses of the Internet and e-mail have raised concerns about ethics, appropriateness and liability. To assist you in evaluating this for your practice, the American Medical Association publishes extensive Internet guidelines at www.ama-assn.org/ama/pub/category/2386.html.

We advocate a very grassroots approach to creating public awareness. Ask the question: *Where do the women (over 50 years of age) you want to reach live, work and play?* While the answer will vary from community to community, some that we have found to be consistent include diners, health clubs, churches, and beauty/nail salons. Advertising in these places is a very targeted approach and can be cost effective. Local newspapers can also offer competitive advertising rates if you place more than one ad, and many publish special pullout health sections. People tend to keep these special sections longer than the daily or Sunday paper. As with all advertising, repetition is key; one ad placed one time in any of these vehicles will not produce results.

The best place to start is in your office, with patient information booklets, posters, and tabletop displays. Many of these educational tools are supplied by pharmaceutical and medical device companies and are informative and professionally produced. Patient information and questionnaires are also ideal for your web site—you do have one, don't you? Be sure to include links to credible national sources (included in the back of the chapter).

Always remember that the best marketing is still simply word of mouth. Every woman you care for is a potential champion for your practice. Although reluctant to tell anyone about their incontinence, women love to share their success stories of how they no longer have "that problem" and have regained their life back. That advertisement is priceless.

Conclusion

As a primary care provider, you have a unique opportunity to develop the evaluation and management of female pelvic floor disorders as a successful service line for your practice. Hopefully, the information in this chapter was practical in terms of how to get started or refine what you already are doing. We can assure you that you will find it not only extremely gratifying from a clinical point of view, but also from a CEO's view of the bottom line.

Key Points

- Many primary care providers are reluctant to ask about pelvic floor dysfunction, because their time with each patient is limited.
- When patients require evaluation of pelvic floor disorders, scheduling a problem-oriented visit focusing on those issues alone is the most cost-effective approach.
- Establishing an efficient approach to the evaluation and treatment of pelvic floor dysfunction will benefit primary care providers both emotionally and financially.

How to get started

- Educate Staff
- Develop patient flow process
- Streamline documentation
- Use pre-printed exam sheets
- Collect and organize patient educational materials

Initial Patient Counseling

- Validate urinary incontinence as an important problem, not a normal part of aging
- Provide educational pamphlets
- Request patient complete a symptom questionnaire, voiding diary, and perform a urinalysis
- Schedule follow-up, dedicated office visit.
- Ensure patient presents with a "full" bladder

Patient Examination

- Collect patient history
- Physical/pelvic examination

  Assess for concurrent prolapse

- Focused neurologic examination
- Perform standing stress test (SST)
- Measure patient voided volume and post-void residual

References

1. Pulse Survey, www.mgma.org. April 1, 2003.
2. Hillestad S, Berkowitz E. *Health Care Market Strategy: From planning to action.* Boston, MA: Jones and Bartlett Publishers. 2004.
3. NAFC, Affiliates Bulletin, Volume 8, Number 2–2003.
4. Wyman JF, Harkins SW, Choi SC, Taylor JR, Fantl JA. *Obstet Gynecol.* 1987;70:378–381.
5. Ekelund P, Rundgren A. Urinary incontinence in the elderly with implications for hospital care consumption and social disability. *Arch Geront Geriatrol.* 1987;6:11–18.

Resources

The following is a list of web-site resources for your patient education booklets and additional materials. Several of these sites are also appropriate for links on your web site.

National Association for Continence
www.nafc.org
American Academy of Home Care Physicians
www.aahcp.org
Medical Group Management Association
www.mgma.org
American Foundation for Urologic Disease
www.afud.org
National Institute for Diabetes & Digestive & Kidney Disease
www.niddk.nih.org
American College of Obstetrics and Gynecology
www.acog.org
Simon Foundation
www.simonfoundation.org

Index

Printed in the United States of America.